D1630122

OXFORD MEDICAL PUBLICATIONS

Health economics research
in developing countries

Health Economics Research in Developing Countries

Edited by

Anne Mills

Department of Public Health and Policy,
London School of Hygiene and Tropical Medicine;
Department of Social Science and Administration,
London School of Economics and Political Science

and

Kenneth Lee

Centre for Health Planning and Management,
Keele University

Oxford   New York   Tokyo
OXFORD UNIVERSITY PRESS
1993

Oxford University Press, Walton Street, Oxford OX2 6DP
Oxford New York Toronto
Delhi Bombay Calcutta Madras Karachi
Kuala Lumpur Singapore Hong Kong Tokyo
Nairobi Dar es Salaam Cape Town
Melbourne Auckland Madrid
and associated companies in
Berlin Ibadan

Oxford is a trade mark of Oxford University Press

Published in the United States
by Oxford University Press Inc., New York

A catalogue record for this book is available from the British Library

Library of Congress Cataloging in Publication Data
Health economics research in developing countries / edited by Anne Mills
and Kenneth Lee.
(Oxford medical publications.)
Includes index.
1. Medical economics — Developing countries. I. Mills, Anne. II. Lee,
Kenneth, 1944–. III. Series.
[DNLM: 1. Delivery of Health Care — economics. 2. Developing Countries.
3. Economics, Medical. W 74 H4357]
RA410.55.D48H4 1993 338.4'73621'091724 — dc20 92–49379

ISBN 0–19–261620–X (h/b)

Typeset by The Electronic Book Factory Ltd, Fife, Scotland
Printed and bound in Great Britain by
Dotesios Ltd, Trowbridge, Wilts

Preface

In 1983 we published *The economics of health in developing countries*. Its aim was to illuminate the ways in which economic concepts and techniques can be (and are) applied to health and health services. Each chapter reviewed 'the state of the art' in a particular area, together with some theoretical developments and a limited selection of research findings.

Since 1983, there has been a rapidly growing interest in the economics of health in developing countries. One striking feature has been considerably increased research effort, providing the basis for a publication which concentrates on reporting research methodologies and empirical findings.

The purpose of this book, therefore, is to present a number of in-depth studies involving the application of economic concepts and techniques to health and health services. It illustrates the application of the theories and concepts reviewed in the first volume. Its aim is both to clarify the ways in which health economics can be used in practice and to report research results that are of general importance to policy-makers.

We invited those economists most active in researching the health sector in developing countries to contribute chapters. The resulting collection of studies thus reflects current research emphases: particularly on the evaluation of the desirability of alternative means of financing health care; and on measures to improve health sector efficiency. All the contributors have had direct experience of working in developing countries, whether for governments, educational institutions, or international agencies.

It is intended that this book should be of use to all those interested (as policy-makers, managers, or academics) in economic issues concerning the health sector and in the application of health economics to improve the efficiency and equity of resource use. We expect that the work will be of interest to fellow health economists, but our aim throughout has been to keep professional as well as academic needs in mind.

We are most grateful to all the contributors who share with us the desire to make the fruits of their research efforts more widely available.

London and Keele   A.M.
November 1992   K.L.

Contents

Contributors

John S. Akin is a Professor of Economics at the University of North Carolina, Chapel Hill, where he teaches public sector economics and health economics. He was previously senior economist in the Office of Population, Health, and Nutrition Research at the World Bank, where he co-authored the Bank's official policy paper on health finance, *Financing health services in developing countries: an agenda for reform*. Before joining the World Bank, Dr Akin worked extensively on the topics of contraceptive choice, infant and maternal health, and the economics of government transfer programmes, and numerous others in applied microeconomics. He co-authored the book *The demand for primary health care in the Third World*. Dr Akin received his Ph.D. in economics from the University of Michigan, and has furthered his professional experience through affiliations at the Institute for Research on Poverty and the Department of Economics at the University of Wisconsin, Madison; the Brookings Institution; the US Departments of Health, Education and Welfare, and of Agriculture; and the Centre for the Economics of Education of the London School of Economics.

Peter Berman is a Lecturer in International Health Economics at the Harvard School of Public Health in Boston, USA. He has a Ph.D. in Agricultural Economics from Cornell University, and was Assistant Professor at Johns Hopkins University School of Hygiene and Public Health. He has held several long-term international postings, including two periods in Indonesia. Most recently, he completed almost four years as a Programme Officer with the Ford Foundation in New Delhi, India, where he was involved in developing a new programme in health economics and financing.

Ricardo Bitran-Dicowsky is a senior economist with Abt Associates Inc., of Cambridge, Massachusetts. He has twelve years of experience in health economics and corporate finance in developing countries and the United States. His work in health economics focuses on the determinants of health-care demand and provider costs, and on the interactions between the demand for and the supply of health services. He teaches at the Boston University School of Public Health and at Tufts University. He holds an MS in Industrial Engineering from the University of Chile, and an MBA in Finance and a Ph.D. in Economics from Boston University.

Guy Carrin is Professor of Economics at the University of Antwerp, Belgium, and Adjunct Professor of Public Health at Boston University, USA. At present he is seconded to the World Health Organization, Geneva, where he holds the position of health economist in the Director-General's Office. He has acted as a consultant to the Belgian Ministry of Public Health, the European Development Fund, Medicus Mundi Belgium, Médecins sans Frontières, USAID, and the World Bank. During the academic year 1985–6 he was Takemi Fellow in International Health at the Harvard School of Public Health. He is the author of *Economic evaluation of health care in developing countries* and *Strategies for health care finance in developing countries – with a focus on community-financing in sub-Saharan Africa*.

Avi Dor received a Ph.D. in Economics from the City University of New York – Graduate School in 1986. While in graduate school he was also adjunct lecturer at Lehman College and Baruch College, where he taught various courses in microeconomics. In December 1984 he began work as a consultant at the World Bank's Development Research Department, where he wrote his dissertation. His dissertation and other World Bank research activities focused on household demand for health services in developing countries, with special emphasis on the role of user fees and alternative financing schemes. In 1987 Dr Dor joined the Urban Institute's Health Policy Centre as a Research Associate, where he pursued a variety of research topics related to the US health-care system, including the impact of alternative reimbursement mechanisms on Medicare, and multi-service costs of institutional providers such as nursing homes and renal dialysis facilities. In 1990 Dr Dor joined the newly formed Agency for Health Care Policy and Research as Research Fellow. His current work focuses on the market for hospital care in the US, with emphasis on anti-trust issues and the impact of third-party-payers on hospital performance. Dr Dor has published widely in the health economics, law, and medical literature.

David W. Dunlop is Professor of Health Economics in the

Department of Family and Community Medicine at Dartmouth Medical School in Hanover, New Hampshire, where he has had various academic appointments since 1979. Concurrently he has also held academic appointments at Boston University and the University of North Carolina at Chapel Hill. For the last three years, he has held a long-term consulting assignment in the Economic Development Institute (EDI) of the World Bank to assist in the development of an educational programme in health economics and financing in developing countries. Previously, he initiated the health economics focus of *Social Science and Medicine* as one of its editors. In the early 1980s he worked for the United States Agency for International Development, and was instrumental in launching that organization's work in health economics and financing. He has also served as a consultant for the World Bank, WHO, PAHO, the Inter-American Development Bank (IDB), and many countries in Africa and US-based agencies and organizations. He received his Ph.D. at Michigan State University.

Susan Foster is a Lecturer in Health Economics in the Department of Public Health and Policy of the London School of Hygiene and Tropical Medicine. Previously she was an economist in the Action Programme on Essential Drugs and Vaccines of the World Health Organization in Geneva, writing and researching on the economics of the production, distribution, and use of pharmaceuticals. She has travelled widely in developing countries, assisting a number of countries to develop and implement rational drugs policies. Prior to joining WHO, she worked as a project officer in the Population, Health, and Nutrition Department of the World Bank. Her current research interests include the economic impact of HIV disease and AIDS in developing countries, especially the costs of treatment and of preventive programmes, and the impact of the HIV epidemic on food production; and also the distribution and use of antimalarial drugs.

Jacques van der Gaag has written extensively on the economics of health, the equity of health-care systems, and the provision of health care in developing countries. The subject matter of his books and articles include the efficiency of labour markets, the economic returns to education, and the development of comprehensive health-care indices. He recently published *The willingness to pay for medical care* (with Paul Gertler), and

Including the poor (with Michael Lipton). He is a staff member of the World Bank.

Charles Griffin is an Associate Professor of Economics at the University of Oregon. He is currently on leave and working at The Urban Institute, where he is a Senior Research Associate and Senior Health Economist on the AID-funded Health Financing and Sustainability Project. Charles Griffin earned his Ph.D. in economics from the University of North Carolina in 1983, specializing in economic development and public finance. He also holds an MA in policy analysis from Duke University, and was a postdoctoral fellow in economic demography at Yale University. His research has been on social sector financing in developing countries, emphasizing health and population programmes. He has co-authored a book on the demand for primary health services, and is the author of another on health-sector financing in Asia. He has written numerous papers and articles on health financing.

Geoffrey Hoare is a Senior Research Fellow in the Centre for Health Planning and Management at Keele University, UK. After a first degree in Economics from City University, he completed a Master's degree in health economics and health planning at the Nuffield Institute, University of Leeds, staying on to undertake postgraduate studies into the links between strategic planning and the planning of human resources in the British National Health Service. Since then, his interests and activities have focused primarily on the developing world. Current interests encompass health economics and its application to improve performance and outcomes, and include health financing; financial planning and resource allocation; cost analysis and economic evaluation; microcomputer applications in planning and evaluation; and the development and use of health information systems. He has undertaken numerous research, consultancy, and training activities on behalf of international agencies such as ODA, WHO, the World Bank, FINNIDA, and the International Health Policy Program. These have included work in Botswana, Malawi, Namibia, Pakistan, Uganda, Zambia, and the British Caribbean Dependent Territories.

Abdulai Issaka-Tinorgah graduated from the University of Ghana Medical School in 1979, and worked in various clinical posts until 1983. He then joined the Technical Unit of the Northern Region

Rural Integrated Programme (NORRIP), where he stayed until 1991. In 1985 he completed the Master's degree in Community Health at the Liverpool School of Tropical Medicine. In 1991 Dr Tinorgah rejoined the Ministry of Health in Ghana.

Kenneth Lee is Director of the Centre for Health Planning and Management at Keele University, UK, and Director of its international MBA (Health, Population, and Nutrition) Programme. A graduate in Economics and in Business Studies from the Universities of Hull and Keele, Professor Lee joined the staff of the School of Economic Studies and Nuffield Centre for Health Services Studies, University of Leeds, in 1971. Before establishing the Centre at Keele in 1986 he was Senior Lecturer in Health Economics at Leeds, and Director of its Master's Programme in Health Services Studies. Professor Lee's main teaching and research have been in the fields of health economics and health-care management, planning, and evaluation. He has written over a hundred texts in health economics, strategic management, health-care financing, community health care, care of the elderly, health promotion, emergency medical services, and human-resource management, including *Economics and health planning* (1979), *Policy making and planning in the health sector* (1982, with Anne Mills), and *The economics of health in developing countries* (1983, co-edited with Anne Mills). He is a regular consultant and adviser to the World Bank, the Overseas Development Administration, the World Health Organization, the United Nations Development Programme, and the Commission of the European Communities, involving work in Africa, South-East Asia, the Western Pacific, the Caribbean, and Europe. He is founder and Editor-in-Chief of the *International Journal of Health Planning and Management* and serves on the editorial board of *Socio-Economic Planning Sciences*.

Maureen Lewis, currently with the Latin America Region of the World Bank, was Senior Research Associate at The Urban Institute in Washington, DC between 1985 and 1990, where she established a research programme in health policy and demographic studies in developing countries. Before that she was Senior Human Resource Economist at USAID. For the last decade and a half she has been engaged in research and policy advisory activities in Asia, Africa, and Latin America. Dr Lewis received her doctorate in Population Economics from the Johns Hopkins University. Her research has focused on the financing of health services and family planning in developing countries, and she has published in the areas of human-resource economics, health economics, and development economics.

Anne Mills is a health economist and Reader in the Department of Public Health and Policy, London School of Hygiene and Tropical Medicine, and the Department of Social Science and Administration, London School of Economics and Political Science. She is also Head of the Health Economics and Financing Programme at the London School of Hygiene and Tropical Medicine. She graduated from the University of Oxford and then worked in Malawi as Overseas Development Institute Fellow and economist in the Ministry of Health. Since 1979, when she joined the London School of Hygiene and Tropical Medicine, she has worked extensively abroad in the field of health economics and health financing for agencies such as ODA, WHO, and the World Bank, in countries such as Malawi, The Gambia, Nepal, Thailand, Jordan, and the Caribbean. Her particular research interests have been generally in the application of health economics to health policy and planning issues, and more specifically in the application of economic evaluation methodologies and the evaluation of financing policies. Particular research projects have included a cost-effectiveness analysis of malaria control in Nepal (for which she gained her Ph.D.), an assessment of the impact of malaria control in Nepal on the historical development of the Terai and currently on households, and an analysis of hospital costs and resource-allocation patterns in Malawi. She is the author of numerous books and articles on issues in health economics and health planning, including *The economics of health in developing countries* (co-edited with K. Lee).

Prosper Nyandagazi was Director of Finance and Administration at the Ministère de la Santé Publique et des Affaires Sociales of the Republic of Rwanda. At present he is a staff member of UNICEF.

Vincente B. Paqueo is an economist at the World Bank, currently working in the population and human-resources sector operating division of the Asia Country Department V. Prior to his current assignment, he worked with the Policy, Planning, and Research complex of the World Bank. He joined the World Bank in 1985 as a Consultant, and then worked as an economist in the Population, Health, and Nutrition Department (Policy and Research Division). Before 1985 he was a professor at the University of the Philippines

School of Economics, and executive director of the Council for Asian Manpower Studies. He holds a Ph.D., and has published various articles on health, education, labour, and demographic economics.

Margaret Phillips is a health economist currently working in Mexico. She graduated from the Australian National University in Science (1976) and Economics (1979), and spent five years working in Australia's government aid agency. After completing an M.Sc. in Community Health in Developing Countries at the London School of Hygiene and Tropical Medicine in 1984 she continued at the School, and was involved in empirical research on a number of topics, including the cost-effectiveness of interventions to control diarrhoeal diseases, the preparation of manuals and guidelines on cost-effectiveness analysis, and, on behalf of WHO, UNICEF, ODA, and the EEC, in evaluation and cost studies of immunization and diarrhoeal disease-control programmes in a number of countries, including Nigeria, Mozambique, Nepal, and Mexico. Most recently she has been working on the economic dimensions of adult ill health for The World Bank, and on the economic aspects of diabetes in Mexico for the Health Economics and Financing Programme, LSHTM. She is the author of a number of articles reporting empirical research, and co-editor of *The health of adults in the developing world.*

Barry M. Popkin, a human-resource economist, is Professor of Public Health Nutrition and a Fellow of the Carolina Population Centre, University of North Carolina at Chapel Hill. He has been actively involved in research in low-income countries related to the demand for health care for a number of years. This has included co-authoring with Dr Akin a number of studies on the demand for health care, including the book *The demand for primary health care in the Third World.* Dr Popkin's survey research experience in the Philippines began in the early 1970s, and included a two-year period of helping to set up a health economics curriculum at the University of the Philippines School of Economics. He was overall director of the longitudinal survey research project which provided the data for the study reported in this book. Dr Popkin received his Ph.D. in agricultural economics from Cornell University and his Master's degree in economics from the University of Wisconsin, and has additional professional research experience at the Institute for Research on Poverty at the University of Wisconsin, Madison;

the Rockefeller Foundation; the Office of Economic Opportunity; and several national and international agencies.

Nicholas Prescott is an economist on the staff of the World Bank. He has published a number of articles on health economics in developing countries. His publications for the World Bank include *China: the health sector; Indonesia: health planning and budgeting*; and *World development report 1984*.

Suomi Sakai is a physician with a Dr P.H. from Johns Hopkins University School of Hygiene and Public Health. Her doctoral research involved modelling alternative pricing strategies for public health-centre services, based on data from a national health-centre cost study. She is currently a Project Officer in Health with UNICEF in Beijing, People's Republic of China.

Donald S. Shepard is engaged in teaching, research, and project management in health economics. He is Research Professor at the Florence Heller School of Social Welfare, Brandeis University and a member of the faculty of the Harvard School of Public Health, and has been a Research Associate at the Harvard Institute for International Development. He is involved in economic analysis of health-care programmes in developing countries and in the United States. His publications and reports include projections of costs and financing for hospital and primary health-care services in Honduras, Rwanda, and Zaire, and studies of user fees and health insurance in Rwanda, Zaire, and Lesotho. He has evaluated the cost-effectiveness of immunizations and oral rehydration therapy in Indonesia, the Ivory Coast, Honduras, The Gambia, Ecuador, and Zaire for the US Agency for International Development, the World Bank, and the World Health Organization. His studies in the United States developed methods to incorporate cost-effectiveness analysis into clinical trials and mathematical models in the health sector. Dr Shepard holds an MPP and a Ph.D. in Public Policy from the Kennedy School of Government at Harvard University.

J. Brad Schwartz, a public finance economist, received his Ph.D. in economics from the University of North Carolina at Chapel Hill. He taught at the University of South Florida before returning to the University of North Carolina as Lecturer in the Department of Economics and Research Associate at the Carolina Population Center. He is currently Senior Economist, Center for International

Development at the Research Triangle Institute. Dr Schwartz has conducted studies on the financing of health, education, and welfare programmes in both developed and developing countries. In addition to the demand for modern infant delivery, his health economics research includes studies on neonatal mortality, the pricing of contraceptives, the demand for adult and child outpatient care, the determinants of breast feeding, and the financing of public- and private-sector health services. The study of infant delivery in the Philippines was conducted while he was affiliated with the Carolina Population Center.

Catriona Waddington has a Master's degree in health economics from York University. Since 1984 she has been a lecturer in health economics at The Liverpool School of Tropical Medicine. She has written several general articles and has published original data on resource allocation in Fiji, primary health-care costs in Guinea Bissau, and cost-sharing in Ghana. From 1989–91 she was seconded to The Ministry of Health in Ghana as Regional Health Economist in Volta Region.

Dieter Zschock, who received his Ph.D. from the Fletcher School of Law and Diplomacy of Tufts University, is professor of economics at the State University of New York at Stony Brook, where he specializes in economic development with an emphasis on human resources and social policy. He has worked for the Ford Foundation in Latin America, held visiting research appointments at Princeton University, and participated in a number of social-sector assessments under the auspices of the World Bank and the US Agency for International Development. More recently, he has directed large-scale research projects funded, through his university, by USAID and the Pew Charitable Trusts. Among his publications are *Health care financing in Latin America and the Caribbean, Health care in Peru: resources and policy*; and 'Medical care under social insurance in Latin America'.

1

Health economics research in developing countries: an overview

Kenneth Lee, Anne Mills, and Geoffrey Hoare

Introduction

Those responsible for the planning, delivery, and evaluation of health and health-related services increasingly recognize that systematic approaches are necessary, in the face of limited and often shrinking resources for health, to make the inevitable difficult choices. In the developing world, this recognition has been longer established than elsewhere, and sharpened by recent and continuing economic difficulties. Economics, which is concerned with issues of choice related to production, exchange, and consumption, provides a ready vehicle for the consideration of how best to use scarce resources for the production of health. Certainly, the potential contribution that techniques of economic analysis can bring to the improvement of health is being given much attention, and rightly so.

Economists have applied many of their traditional analytical techniques, methods of analysis, and ways of approaching problems to the study of the health sector: sometimes with difficulty, often with considerable modification; and sometimes with questionable success. As the established body of mainstream economic theory is both applied to, and refined for, the study of the health sector, a clearer understanding is emerging of the ways in which the health-production process might be improved.

This book illustrates the range of analytical methods and tools of economics; demonstrates how they can, and do, contribute towards the objective of improving health; identifies the difficulties involved in applying them to the study of the health sector; and outlines the ways in which traditional theory has been modified or adapted for application to health. This is done through chapters which each present a particular piece of research. Throughout the book, the emphasis is on the methods used and on the relevance of the results to the formulation of health policy and to the improvement of the efficiency, effectiveness, and equity of the health sector.

Interest in the economics of health has been greatly stimulated by the gravity of the global economic crisis and its impact upon the economies of the Third World and their people. The 1980s saw a slowing down and in many cases a reversal of earlier progress in economic growth in developing countries. A significant proportion of the world's population experienced a fall in its standards of existence (Abel-Smith 1986). Real social expenditure per capita (on health care and education) fell in one half of all developing countries in the 1980s (Edel 1991). All the countries in Africa with a per capita Gross National Product of less than $300 had declining real per capita expenditures on health care.

The immediate external causes of the economic problems faced by many developing countries are twofold: rising debt repayments – the total debt repayments of the developing world now exceed the value of all new aid and loans received each year, and amount to 25 per cent of their export revenues; and falling commodity prices, which have exacerbated the debt-repayment problems by reducing exports' earning capacity. The last decade has seen commodity prices for the principal commodities of many developing countries fall substantially in real terms.

Responses to these economic problems have typically involved Structural Adjustment Policies, aimed at resolving balance of payment crises and meeting debt obligations while maintaining essential imports and encouraging economic growth. In most instances, this has involved attempts to reduce domestic demand and boost exports. The need for such adjustment policies is generally accepted, although many have questioned the means adopted (Cornia *et al.* 1987). Adjustment programmes have typically involved significant cuts in government expenditure and subsidies on foodstuffs and primary products; currency devaluation; and drastic demand-management policies. In many countries, health expenditures have fallen faster than government expenditures overall (Edel 1991). In countries with strict adjustment programmes, real health expenditure per capita fell by nearly 20 per cent (Kakwani *et al.* 1989).

The effects on the health sector, particularly in Africa, have been dramatic. Immediate victims of the spending cuts have been those items most easily varied in the short run, such as drugs, transport, and fuel (Edel 1991). Ability to purchase items bought on international markets has been severely limited by the effects on prices of devaluation. Resulting shortages have severely impeded both the effectiveness of health services and the confidence of the public in them. While it has not been possible to reduce significantly the numbers of those employed, expenditure control has been executed through reductions in real salaries (Lindauer *et al.* 1988). Perversely, while salaries and wages as a proportion of recurrent expenditure have increased rapidly as a result of the reduction in other expenditures, the efficiency of manpower has declined as a result of low salaries and lack of complementary resources. Essential repairs and maintenance have suffered, while infrastructure developments, including both upgrading and new construction projects, have had to be postponed.

Economic issues in the health sector

Faced with this backcloth and other continuing concerns, what are the key problem areas in health policy and health services, and to what extent can economics, and more especially health economics, assist in addressing and overcoming them? Problems are considered below under two main headings: macro resource-allocation issues; and strategic and operational efficiency.

Macro resource-allocation issues

In most developing countries, public expenditure grew rapidly during the 1960s and 1970s. However, the economic climate of the 1980s led to lower levels of growth in public expenditure, with some countries experiencing a reduction either in total or in per capita public expenditure. Health expenditures, as mentioned above, generally fared less well than other items of expenditure.

Even were resources in the health sector used to maximum effect, it is unlikely that they would be sufficient to meet basic health needs. Current economic circumstances (and also current ideologies) in general preclude increased public expenditures, whether financed through debt or through increased taxation; while political realities make reallocations from other areas to health (however justifiable on economic or social criteria) unlikely.

Consequently, many developing countries have been looking at alternative and additional ways of generating the additional resources required. The challenge is to find ways of raising resources which distribute the burden according to ability to pay; which encourage the provision of appropriate services; and which make those services available in accordance with need rather than solely in accordance with willingness to pay.

At the same time, low per capita expenditures on health are frequently exacerbated by the use of health-sector resources on interventions of limited effectiveness and/or efficiency. As much as 70 per cent of government health expenditures may be spent on high-cost, high-technology hospital services (Mills 1990) provided by relatively highly trained medical professionals; and focused on the provision of episodic curative care for individuals most of whom reside in urban areas. These services are often little related to the major determinants, dimensions, or distribution of health status in developing countries. Put bluntly, if some of the resources used for hospital services were transferred to primary health-care (PHC) services, many conditions could be treated earlier, at a less severe stage, or even prevented altogether. Where inefficiencies exist, such a shift need not be at the expense of the volume of hospital services provided.

Health services should be appropriate to both the needs and the means of developing countries. It follows that they should be both technically appropriate (i.e. they should effectively address the determinants and dimensions of the major health problems) and economically appropriate (i.e. they should take account of the volume, composition, and alternative uses of the resources likely to be available for health purposes). Clearly, many health sectors (including those in developed countries) fail in these respects.

Strategic and operational efficiency

Poor macro resource-allocation decisions are compounded by strategic and operational inefficiencies; the reasons are many.

Accessibility and utilization. Utilization of health facilities has been shown to be highly correlated with distance to the nearest facility. Poor transport and communication systems (especially in rural areas) effectively limit the coverage radius of health facilities for outpatient services to walking distance; which, for maternal and child health services, may be very short. Consequently, present patterns of service-provision effectively limit coverage to a small proportion of the population. To improve coverage, greater consideration needs to be given to the relationship between the population to be served and the location, type, and number of the facilities from which they are served.

Inefficient, low-quality, and unreliable public services. It is unrealistic to expect consumers to travel any distance (or indeed pay money) to health facilities for treatment unless they can be confident that they will receive the quality and quantity of services appropriate to their needs. However, poor financial and service planning often means that the supply of essential resources to health facilities is at best erratic. Recurrent expenditures on items such as drugs, fuel, and essential maintenance are often under-funded. Support services such as procurement, storage, distribution, and transportation are often beset with logistical and management problems. These factors and others effectively limit the capability of (sometimes expensively trained) health workers to work effectively; limit their capacity to provide outreach services to those outside the immediate catchment areas; and discourage those within these areas from attending. Often, these problems are most acute for isolated rural facilities. As a result, these low-level facilities are often under-used, whilst higher-level facilities and staff are overworked, distorting still further who gets what, and who is denied.

Poorly functioning referral systems. Highly specialized medical care is neither necessary nor desirable for the majority of conditions found in developing countries. The organizational structure aspired to is a hierarchical referral system whereby patients are treated in the community, and only when a particular level of care cannot cope are patients referred to higher levels. In practice, however, referral systems rarely operate as intended.

Isolation of PHC workers. Attempts to extend health-service coverage have led to the increased use of minimally trained health workers working in often remote rural locations. However, for such workers to function effectively, they must not be isolated from the rest of the health-care system. Peripheral health workers require management and professional support and supervision from the higher levels of care. Conversely, effective planning and resource-allocation require a flow of information to the centre relating to health problems and needs, activity levels, and operational efficiency (for instance, performance levels and costs). Information systems are often poorly designed, so that much of the information that is transmitted to the centre is inappropriate for planning and management purposes.

Inefficiencies in the drug-supply systems. A considerable proportion of recurrent budgets is devoted to drugs, dressings, and vaccines. However, considerable inefficiencies often result from inefficient procurement and selection procedures; poor storage and stock-control arrangements; and inadequate transportation and distribution systems, particularly to rural areas.

Poor systems of financial planning and management. Health sectors have generally performed poorly in the areas of planning and financial management. Seldom do actual patterns of resource-use correspond with statements of national priorities or objectives. Indeed, poor accounting systems often make it difficult to obtain timely and reliable information on actual expenditures, as opposed to budgetary allocations. Costly investments in physical infrastructure and specialist human capital have often been made without reference to the additional recurrent costs that they generate (Waddington and Thomas 1988). Inevitably, health-sector investments require complementary expenditures on items such as drugs, dressings, transport, fuel, and essential maintenance; and, in many instances, on administrative and professional support. Not uncommonly, the pressure on recurrent budgets has been exacerbated by donor support for highly visible investments in physical infrastructure.

The nature of economics and health economics

Economics as a topic is concerned with the study of economic activities as a subject in its own right (i.e. production, consumption, and trading relationships between people; the characteristics of market and non-market frameworks for these activities; and the relationships between them) (Williams 1987). Economics as a discipline, however, is concerned with the use of economic techniques of analysis, and conceptually distinct modes of thought, in the study of a whole range of topics. This distinct mode of thought is primarily concerned with the exercise of choice in recognition of the scarcity of resources relative to the desire for them. The discipline of economics may therefore be applied to the study of a whole range of human activities (including, of course, the health sector).

Central to economics are a number of deceptively simple concepts and techniques. However, the terminology employed may make it difficult for non-economists to understand them. These key concepts and techniques include: scarcity; opportunity cost; costs; production functions; supply; demand; elasticity; the margin; shadow pricing; externalities; equity; and techniques of economic evaluation (Lee and Mills 1978).

Health economics, in its broadest sense, attempts to apply the theories, concepts, and techniques of economics to the institutions, actors, and activities that affect health. Historically, the focus of health economics was on how to calculate the value of health to the economy (Lee and Mills 1983). Now, increasingly, attention is being given to the study of how to achieve a socially optimal allocation of resources (i.e. economic analysis of how to allocate resources between alternative health activities). In the recent past (and to a considerable extent still in developed countries), health economics has been focused rather narrowly on health services (and in particular on medical services). However, a greater understanding of the determinants of states of health in populations is bringing with it a willingness to address wider areas of health-related activities.

In the sphere of health, the application of principles and techniques of economic analysis is complicated by the unusual characteristics of the commodities health and health care. For instance, it is difficult to specify precisely the nature of the health-production process; that is, the process by which resource inputs are transformed into health improvements. Clearly, health is not produced in the same way as a manufactured consumer item such as a car. Health as an output is difficult to define, measure, and value. Definitions vary according to who is responsible for definition, and the purposes to which definitions are put. The health-care professions often favour an approach which emphasizes the presence or absence of pathological factors. Other definitions measure health in terms of its impact on the capacity of individuals to perform their normal daily functions or activities; the amount of distress associated with conditions; or some combination of both. This particular issue exemplifies the complexities in applying economics to the health sector; equally, the challenges and opportunities for empirical study are many.

Health economics research: topics and methods

The range of topics now embraced by health economics is illustrated by the chapters of this book. It should be noted, however, that the selection here is by no means comprehensive: it reflects the topics that economists are currently working on, and the gaps in coverage are perhaps as interesting as the topics covered, since they indicate where more attention is required.

The subject of the relationship between health and economic development is a perennial one (Cumper 1983): the attention it receives seems to wax and wane, perhaps depending on the relative affluence (or poverty) of the health sector and the degree to which it feels bound to justify its activities by reference to their positive impact on economic development. The chapter by Mills critically examines the claims that malaria control (in this case in Nepal) promoted economic development by permitting the exploitation of previously uncultivated land. It illustrates the analytical methods that can be used to explore the relationship between health and economic development. It concludes that malaria control certainly contributed to land exploitation, though perhaps not to the extent that has been claimed, and that its cost was minor compared to that of the other investments required to render the land productive and in relation to the returns from the cultivated land.

Because of the financing crisis facing the health sector in many countries, many health economists have in recent years focused their attention on financing issues. Obtaining information on financing and expenditure patterns is a necessary first step to making policy decisions on changes (Griffiths and Mills 1983). Zschock in Chapter 3 summarizes some of the major findings of the Health Sector Analysis of Peru, which was designed to test the premiss – shared by Peruvian health-sector authorities and foreign aid officials – that current patterns of resource-allocation in the country's health sector were inappropriate for the implementation of the Peruvian government's major health-sector policy goal: to make primary health care and essential hospital services geographically and financially accessible to all Peruvians. Extensive data-gathering efforts were undertaken in order to be able to analyse the expenditure, resources, and coverage of the three main components of the health sector: the Ministry of Health, the Peruvian Institute of Social Security, and private health institutions. Serious imbalances were found in the distribution of health services, with a third of the population with no access to modern health care. Recommendations were made to improve this situation.

In discussions of alternative options for the financing and provision of health care, the role of the private sector is receiving increasing attention. The chapter by Griffin and Paqueo is concerned – as is the chapter by Zschock – with illustrating the types of data that can be collected, and what they reveal about the health system. However the former authors' focus is particularly on the relative growth and distribution of private-sector services. Their data come from the Philippines. On the basis of these data, the authors challenge the common assumption that the private sector serves only the urban rich: they show that the private sector played a much larger role than did the public sector in the expansion and geographical equalization of services that took place in the 1970s.

Perhaps the most hotly debated of the various financing options facing developing countries is the use of user fees in the public sector. Not surprisingly, economists have been foremost in that debate, and it has stimulated a great increase in work on the revenue consequences of fees and their impact on users. This work is reflected in the book in the chapters by Lewis; Shepard, Carrin, and Nyandagazi; Schwartz, Akin, and Popkin; and Dor and van der Gaag.

Lewis in Chapter 5 looks at the desirability of fees largely from the providers' perspective. She reports a study in the Dominican Republic of user fees in public hospitals, which investigated the background and context to fees, the different systems operated, the resources generated and how they were used, and the means devised to exempt patients unable to pay. She concludes that the revenue raised was of considerable value to hospitals (even if in absolute amounts it was not very much), and draws lessons on the design of user-fee policies.

Shepard, Carrin, and Nyandagazi also look at revenue raised

by fees, but use the means of a household survey to provide supplementary data on utilization, expenditure on health services, and willingness to pay. They looked at the health centre level, surveying a government and a mission facility in each of two areas of Rwanda. They concluded that their methods were of considerable use for rapidly assessing the potential for user fees and advising policy-makers.

A crucial issue in the discussion of the desirability of user fees has been the effect of fees on utilization: to what extent will fees deter use? This question can be examined using classic economic techniques of demand analysis (albeit with adaptations to allow for the specific features of demand for health care). This has become an area of considerable controversy, mainly centring on the specification of the demand function and the measurement of the necessary variables included in the model. Two chapters present economic demand models and their results. Schwartz, Akin, and Popkin investigate the economic determinants of demand for modern infant delivery in the Philippines. They examine a number of different delivery options, and explore the extent to which their use is influenced by factors such as cash price, time-price of travelling, perceived quality, and various household characteristics. They conclude that the choice of delivery type was relatively insensitive to changes in money price, and suggest policy options to improve the coverage and quality of delivery services.

Dor and van der Gaag investigate demand in a situation where health care is free of charge. They argue that travel time acts in a similar way to price, and develop models to identify the impact of travel time and other economic variables on health-care utilization by adults in rural Côte d'Ivoire. They conclude that even free services do not guarantee equitable use because of travel costs, and suggest that imposing user fees could improve equity if fee income is used to improve the geographical distribution of services.

From chapter 9 onwards the authors turn their attention to issues of health-sector efficiency, and demonstrate the usefulness to policy-makers of particular approaches to assessing efficiency. Two chapters, Chapter 9 by Phillips and Chapter 11 by Prescott, use techniques of economic evaluation to identify approaches to delivering particular interventions that are likely to be efficient. The chapter by Phillips represents a slightly unusual use of economic evaluation techniques: to advise an international agency (in this case WHO) on which strategies it should be promoting for the control of diarrhoeal disease. Unlike the preceding chapters, it does not draw its data from a particular country study, but rather relies on published literature from a number of countries. After describing how the data were obtained and analysing and presenting the cost-effectiveness results, the chapter discusses factors that influence cost-effectiveness ratios, and the limitations of this analytical approach.

Prescott presents another variant of the cost-effectiveness technique: the use of modelling to identify the most cost-effective option. He examines alternative chemotherapy regimes for schistosomiasis, involving choices of whether or not to screen for infection prior to treatment, and if screening is not done, whether to treat everyone, or only high-risk groups. Through a resource-allocation model he is able to determine the sensitivity of the optimal choice of chemotherapy regime to behavioural and economic parameters, which will vary both between countries and within countries. He calls for more attention to be paid to compliance rates and costs of treatment.

Study of the costs of health institutions is vital to improve efficiency. Until recently, most studies have used an accounting approach which provides useful data but cannot allow for the variety of factors which influence facility costs. Chapter 10 presents one of the very few developing country examples of an econometric analysis of hospital costs, which attempts to specify a cost function and to assess whether larger facilities are more efficient (economies of scale), and whether it is more efficient to deliver services together rather than separately (economies of scope). A model is developed and is used to analyse data on hospital costs from Ethiopia. Despite data problems, preliminary conclusions on economies of scale and scope could be drawn, and the approach is considered promising.

The next chapter by Foster takes pharmaceuticals as its subject, and reviews the range of ways in which economists and economics can improve the efficiency and equity of drug supply and use. She considers drug selection and cost-effectiveness considerations, local production, drug prices and procurement, distribution and logistics, prescription and compliance, and financing (particularly fees for drugs). She concludes that much remains to be done to rationalize the production, purchase, and use of drugs, and that good economic research is needed to help decision-makers select from the options for rationalization and improve efficiency without sacrificing equity.

Chapter 13 by Berman and Sakai illustrates yet another approach to investigating efficiency: the detailed study of costs and resource-use at facility level. They identify measures of operating efficiency in the use of manpower and expendable supplies for rural health services in Java, Indonesia, and present their results. They argue we should not write off the public sector as hopelessly inefficient: much can be done by administrative and management improvements involving the collection and analysis of data on performance and the development of incentives to encourage facility managers to improve efficiency.

This theme, of improving public-sector performance, is continued in the final chapter, by Issaka-Tinorgah and Waddington. They review past attempts to use budgetary reform to improve efficiency, and point out the reasons why such attempts have failed though a case study of the introduction of programme budgeting into the Ministry of Health in Ghana. They go on to suggest that more modest budgetary reform measures are required, for example functional analysis and functional budgeting, and describe a pilot study from The Gambia.

These chapters exemplify not only the range of topics studied by health economists, but also the range of methods used. Some are highly accessible to non-specialists; others less so. One of the features of the development of health economics research in the last ten years has been the increased use of mathematical techniques of analysis, as exemplified here in the chapters on demand and cost functions. Such techniques, widely used in developed country studies, have been little employed until recently in developing countries. Their data requirements are usually greater than can be met by routine information systems, and special expensive surveys may be needed; none the less they complement the smaller, more applied and pragmatic studies that have until recently been the norm.

Future prospects and directions for health economics research

The various chapters in this book have sought to demonstrate the practical value of health economics as an aid to improved decision-making and resource use, and the areas to which health economics has usefully been directed. Attention in this chapter finally turns to questions of how to increase the supply of health economics expertise, and who should conduct health economics studies.

Relative to the developed world, the number of economists working within and/or on the health sectors of developing countries is small (Phillips 1988). Most of them are located in universities in developed countries, or in international agencies such as the World Bank. It appears that, in relation to other employment opportunities in the private sector and other Ministries, the health sector remains a comparatively unattractive option for trained economists (Drummond and Mills 1989). Where economists are found in the health sector, they are often poorly utilized, or unable to influence decision-making.

If the application of economics to the health sectors of developing countries is to be extended, a number of developments are necessary. It is vital that there should be an increased supply of indigenous health economists: fortunately a number of agencies wish to fund local researchers, and in time and with the necessary back-up an expansion of supply should occur. In addition better use should be made of available skills and resources. Too many health economists from developed countries work in developing countries for short periods only, and on consultancy assignments rather than on research. More medium- to long-term projects, involving collaboration between developed and developing country institutions as equal partners, are required.

However, if economic approaches to decision-making in the health sector are to have greater impact, they cannot remain the sole preserve of health economists. Given some training in the basic concepts and techniques of economic analysis, it is possible for health planners or health-service providers to assess the value and methodological rigour of studies, and to undertake useful studies on their own behalf. From the centre to the periphery of the health-care system, there is an urgent need, and widespread scope, for improvements in approaches to resource-allocation choices and financial planning and budgeting.

Until comparatively recently, the dissemination of the economist's approach was effectively limited by a paucity of relevant teaching materials and opportunities for training. Recently, a number of international agencies have been involved in attempts to provide training in health economics for health-sector managers, planners, and service-providers. Activities have encompassed seminars and the production of training materials for decision-makers. Key initiatives have attempted to promote closer ties between senior staff in ministries of health, finance, and economic planning and development. Discussions have attempted to promote the use of economic evaluation techniques and a deeper understanding of the politics and mechanics of budgetary processes.

These and other attempts to broadcast the philosophy of health economics should bring forth new recruits from existing areas of economics and from related fields. Induction courses in epidemiology, health policy, and planning would allow new entrants to health research to contribute to the development of the relevant disciplines.

In developing countries, where resources are especially scarce, the potential benefits to be derived from the application of economics to decision-making should be clear. Seldom are policies the outcome of a systematic evaluation of the costs and benefits of alternative options. Indeed, it is rare for health objectives to be formally articulated, still less to be quantified and have their implementation monitored. Consequently, few developing countries are maximizing the impact they could have upon health status, given the resources available to them. In the present austere environment, even greater attention needs to be given to the role that economics can play in improving health standards. A number of broad areas can be identified:

- exploring the relationships between inputs and outputs, with the objective of increasing productivity;

- identifying the costs of the resources used in interventions in relation to the value of the benefits they produce;

- re-ordering priorities using the information derived from the above;

- exploring the options for new or increased sources of funding, and their implications; and

- identifying the efficiency and equity consequences of alternative pricing, revenue-generating, and organizational strategies.

Encouragingly, recent developments have seen a growing willingness to employ both economists and economic techniques in the systematic analysis of the ways in which resources are used within the health sector. It is unlikely that this trend will reverse in the foreseeable future. Considerable progress has been made in the development, adaptation, and refinement of theory, and in empirical investigation. This book is a reflection of that growth and influence over the last decade, and a timely reminder of both what is possible and what remains to be done. The agenda is forbidding but crucial: we hope that this text demonstrates that health economics research, though daunting, is rewarding. If the reader imbibes even a little of the enthusiasm of the contributors for progress on this research agenda, then the text will have served its purpose well.

References

Abel-Smith, B. (1986). The world economic crisis. Part 1: repercussions on health. *Health Policy and Planning*, 1(3), 202–13.

Cornia, G. A., Jolly, R., and Stewart, F. (ed.) (1987). *Adjustment with a human face*. Vol. 1. *Protecting the vulnerable and promoting growth*. Oxford University Press.

Cumper, G. (1983). Economic development, health services, and health. In *The economics of health in developing countries* (ed. K. Lee and A. Mills), pp. 23–42. Oxford University Press.

Drummond, M. and Mills, A. (1989). Developing economics expertise for the evaluation of primary health care. *Public Administration and Development*, 9, 83–96.

Edel, B. (1991). *Patterns of government expenditure in developing countries during the 1980s: the impact on social services*, Innocenti Occasional Papers Economic Policy Series No 18. International Child Development Centre, Florence.

Griffiths, A. and Mills, M. (1983). Health sector financing and expenditure surveys. In *The economics of health in developing countries* (ed. K. Lee and A. Mills), pp. 43–63. Oxford University Press.

Kakwani, N., Makonnen, E., and van der Gaag, J. (1989). Structural adjustment and living conditions in developing countries. Population and Human Resources Department, World Bank, Washington DC. [Draft].

Lee, K. and Mills, A. (1978). The role of economists and economics in health service planning. In *Economics and health planning* (ed. K. Lee), pp. 156–79. Croom Helm, London.

Lee, K. and Mills, A. (1983). Developing countries, health, and health economics. In *The economics of health in developing countries* (ed. K. Lee and A. Mills), pp. 1–22. Oxford University Press.

Lindauer, D. L., Meesok, O. A., and Suebsang, P. (1988). Government wage policy in Africa: some findings and policy issues. *The World Bank Research Observer*, **3**(1), 1–25.

Mills, A. (1990). The economics of hospitals in developing countries. Part 1: expenditure patterns. *Health Policy and Planning*, **5**(2), 107–17.

Phillips, M (1988). Health economics research – report of a meeting. *Health Policy and Planning*, **3**(4), 315–19.

Waddington, C. and Thomas, M (1988). Recurrent costs in the health sector of developing countries. *International Journal of Health Planning and Management* **3**(3), 151–66.

Williams, A. (1987). Health economics: the cheerful face of the dismal science? In *Health and economics* (ed. A. Williams), pp. 1–11. Macmillan, London.

2

The impact of malaria control on the economic development of Nepal

Anne Mills

Introduction

Travellers have noted for centuries the dangers of malaria in the Nepal Terai (the areas of the Terai are identified in Fig. 2.1). A detailed account was given by Landon in 1928, when he published a description of his visit to Nepal:

We are now in the twelve-mile-wide strip of raw forest, which has not unjustly earned for the Terai its famous reputation of being the unhealthiest region in all Asia. But there is nothing to betray its evil nature unless, perhaps, like the upas valley in Java, the extra luxuriance of its vegetation suggests a warm marshy soil and therewith, to a modern mind, mosquitos.

Throughout the hours of daylight the Terai is safe enough. It is the evening that man may not spend in this beautiful park. Sundown in the Terai has brought to an end more attempted raids into Nepal and has buried more political hopes than will ever be known. The English learnt their lesson early, for within forty years of Plassey a column – moving to the help of hard-beset Nepal – withered and retreated before the miasma of this paradise. The English had been told of its dangers, but they had to learn from experience what all India had known and feared for centuries . . . The tribe of the Tharus alone – an indigenous race of the Terai, fit only to act as carters – are immune . . . Perhaps after all this zone is only affected by an unusually virulent form of the fever, but of its mortal effect there is no question. The records of Nepal and of the Indian army are crowded with the names of its victims. This local pestilence is known far and wide as *awal*, a name which hums an undertone of death throughout the chronicles of Nepal. Between October and March its teeth are drawn. (Landon 1928, Chapter X).

There are earlier similar accounts also, by Father Giorgi, an Augustinian, in the mid-eighteenth century (reported by Landon

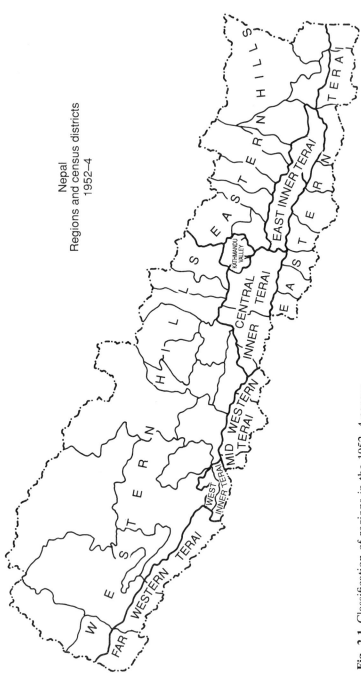

Nepal
Regions and census districts
1952–4

Fig. 2.1 Classification of regions in the 1952–4 census.

1928) and Colonel Kirkpatrick, in 1793 (Kirkpatrick 1811). Landon also comments on the importance of villages such as Hetaura, a town in the Chitwan Valley in the Central Inner Terai where malaria control was first started, as commercial centres and trading posts during the winter months.

From Lady Day (March 25th) to Michaelmas (September 29th) there is nothing in this fever-haunted district of Hetaura but a few houses, deserted by all except a handful of carters and a native traveller or two . . . But during the winter it is a well populated centre from which diverge four or five of the main routes of South Nepal. (Landon 1928, Chapter X).

In contrast to the malaria-ravaged towns of the Terai, Landon notes the decreasing prevalence of malaria as the Terai gives way to the foothills of the Himalayas. He comments of Butwal (in the foothills north of the Terai) that 'it is possible to live in Butwal all the year round, though the climate cannot be said to be healthy and epidemics of *awal* occasionally paralyse its industries', and at Palpa (Tansing, about 4000 feet in altitude) that 'the town is well drained and rarely suffers from epidemics' (Landon 1928, Chapter XI).

Many commentaries on Nepal have attributed the economic development of the Terai to the malaria control programme. Indeed, malaria control in the Nepalese Terai is one of the most often quoted examples of the economic benefits to be obtained when disease control permits fertile land to be cultivated. Taylor (1965), for example, stated:

One instance (of the benefits of disease control) I observed personally is the opening of the Rapti Valley in Nepal by a malaria control programme . . . For centuries the severe hyperendemic malaria of the Terai forests below the Himalayan foothills had made this area uninhabitable for any except local jungle tribes who had developed a high degree of resistance. A mass mosquito control programme with insecticide spraying has now opened up this fertile area for settlers from the grossly overpopulated hillsides of Nepal. Within five years, local immigration produced a tenfold increase in population with dramatic and spreading economic development.

The same argument has been applied to the whole of the Terai:

Prior to 1960 the Terai was relatively sparsely populated, largely as a result of the prevalence of malaria and other diseases; since that time, however, with effective malaria eradication and the dramatic reduction of cholera and smallpox, the Terai is being settled rapidly and often illegally (Blaikie *et al.* 1980).

Virtual eradication of malaria from the Terai after World War II . . . dramatically increased the marginal productivity of agricultural labour and, in large part in consequence of migration thereby induced, the population of the Terai grew at about 2.4% per annum between the 1952–4 and the 1961 censuses whereas that of the hills grew at only 1.2% (Jamison 1980).

The objective of the research reported here was to investigate the validity of the claims that have been made for malaria control and to explore and evaluate its contribution to the economic development of the Terai. The methodological framework is, in conceptual terms, straightforward. A convenient summary indicator of economic development is per capita national income. Malaria control affects per capita income through influencing, firstly, the population size and, secondly, the level of aggregate income (Prescott 1979). A change in the population size results from removing the effect of malaria on mortality and fertility. A change in the level of aggregate income results from the effect of malaria control on the supply and productivity of land, labour, and capital.

The effect on *land* is straightforward: land (or other natural resources) may be unexploited because malaria inhibits settlement and exploitation. The effect on *labour supply* is more complex: reduced mortality increases the current and future labour force; reduced disability and debility increases the supply and produc- tivity of the current labour force, and the productivity of the future labour force if malaria affected the school performance of children. The effect on the supply of *capital* stems from the potential influence of malaria control on rates of private and public saving and thus investment. A common assumption is that a larger *population* will lower the rate of private saving, because if incomes remain constant or increase at a rate lower than that of the population, a greater proportion of income will need to be spent on consumption. A larger population also demands a higher level of investment in social infrastructure (for example, health services), thus reducing the availability of public savings for what some would argue to be more productive physical capital.

The effect of malaria control on per capita income and, by implication, on economic development can thus be traced through its effect on population size and the supply of labour, capital, and land. However, applying this evaluative framework presents major theoretical difficulties, and demands extensive information. In order to develop the research methodology, past studies on the economic benefits of malaria control were reviewed (see Mills 1989) in order to see how they tackled these difficulties. A list of data requirements was then drawn up, to enable the research to trace over time (distinguishing as far as possible between areas of no malaria, little malaria, and much malaria) the changes in demographic variables, population distribution, land area cultivated, and crop production and yields. Of particular interest was the phasing of these variables over time compared with the phasing of the malaria control programme. The list also included the cost of malaria control and other resource costs of opening up new land. The results of this search for historical information are reported in Part 1 of this chapter. Part 2 then uses this information to identify, quantify, and value the gains and losses associated with malaria control.

A final introductory word is in order. The focus of this evaluation on *economic* development should not be taken as indicating that malaria control has no intrinsic value *per se*, or that improvements in indicators of economic development adequately capture all the private and social benefits of malaria control. Clearly, an improved standard of living (from the perspective of households) and increased levels of economic development (from the perspective of the government) are but elements of the overall benefit. Households and society value the extension of life and improvement in the quality of life as benefits in their own right, and not merely as means to improvement in economic circumstances. However, this research concentrated on changes in economic indicators for three main reasons. Firstly, malaria control in Nepal has frequently been justified by reference to its contribution to opening up the Terai. Secondly, there is no satisfactory or unambiguous way of valuing improvement in health *per se* (Mills 1985). Thirdly, in a poor, subsistence economy people do place a high priority on improving their economic circumstances.

Part 1: The historical evidence

The history of malaria and malaria control in Nepal

Pre-malaria control Nepal can be divided into four broad areas in terms of their malaria characteristics (see Fig. 2.2):

- The southern edge of the Outer Terai was flat, cultivated, and hypoendemic, with relatively limited malaria, though it was liable to more severe outbreaks from time to time;

- the northern forested edge of the Outer Terai, the Inner Terai, and the lower forested slopes of the hills (below 2000 feet) that enclosed it were hyperendemic and intensely malarious;

- the cultivated valleys situated further to the north between 2000 and 4000 feet were hypoendemic, with some transmission of malaria at a low level; and

- parts of the country above 4000 feet had little or no transmission of malaria.

Very limited information on parasite rates pre-control (NMEO 1970) gives the following picture:

hyperendemic areas: infant parasite rate 9 per cent to 85 per cent; child parasite rate 12 per cent to 70 per cent;

hypoendemic areas: infant parasite rate 0.0 per cent to 0.5 per cent; child parasite rate 0.2 per cent to 7.8 per cent.

No population base is available for these rates, and incidence cannot therefore be calculated. In the hyperendemic areas *Plasmodium falciparum* was found to be the most common parasite, and in hypoendemic areas, *P. vivax*.

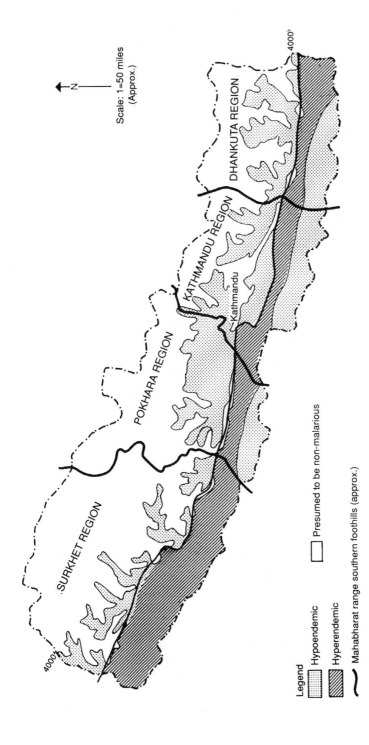

Fig. 2.2 Original endemicity of malaria in Nepal.

Legend

Hypoendemic

Hyperendemic

Mahabharat range southern foothills (approx.)

Presumed to be non-malarious

Scale: 1=50 miles
(Approx.)

N

SURKHET REGION

POKHARA REGION

KATHMANDU REGION

DHANKUTA REGION

Kathmandu

4000'

4000'

An earlier survey carried out in the Rapti Valley (Central Inner Terai) during 1956–7 found that the infant parasite rate was 63 per cent, the child parasite rate 57–77 per cent, and the child spleen rate 92 per cent (NMEO 1966). A much earlier survey of this area (Phillips 1925) found differing levels of morbidity and mortality amongst different ethnic groups, the indigenous race (the Tharus) being the least susceptible to malaria, and one of the groups of recent migrants (the Kumalaya) the most. One group of settlers he described as 'doomed to extinction'. In this particular part of the Inner Terai, malaria is likely to have had the characteristics of holoendemicity: high spleen rates in children, but low rates in adults for the indigenous population.

Unfortunately, this is the only evidence available on the morbidity and mortality in Nepal caused by malaria before control began in the 1950s. It is not known to what extent it is representative of the Inner Terai as a whole, nor is there similar information available for hypoendemic areas. It can only be hypothesized, therefore, that in the hyperendemic areas it is likely that immunity in adults gave some considerable degree of protection to indigenous farmers, though at the expense of relatively high infant and child mortality. New settlers, both adults and children, seem to have been at high risk of illness and death. In hypoendemic areas, the relatively low infant and child parasite rates and the predominant species (*P. vivax*) suggest that malaria prevalence in adults was relatively low, and symptoms were relatively mild. Repeated relapses may have caused severe debility in a small proportion of the population. Occasional epidemics, causing morbidity and mortality, are likely to have occurred.

Pilot projects in the late 1950s showed that residual spraying of DDT inside houses stopped the transmission of malaria, and suggested that malaria eradication was feasible. A nation-wide campaign was started, with spray coverage achieved in 1960–2 in the Central and West zones, in 1964 in the East, and in 1965–6 in the Far West. The campaign had rapid results. The combination of DDT spraying and clearing of the forest by settlers which destroyed breeding-places resulted in the virtual elimination of the most important vector *Anopheles minimus* (none have been found in recent years), and a dramatic reduction in transmission, though not complete cessation. By 1968 only a few thousand cases were being detected, and control was subsequently maintained, though at a rather higher level of cases (Mills 1989). When compared with countries like India and Sri Lanka, Nepal has been remarkably successful in maintaining control.

Three important points should be emphasized from this brief survey. Firstly, the whole of the Terai was not equally malarious before malaria control. Infant and child parasite rates varied considerably in hyperendemic areas, and were low in hypoendemic areas. Secondly, there is evidence that the Tharus, an indigenous tribe, had some inherited immunity to malaria, and that some settlers were able to develop sufficient immunity to establish themselves in the hyperendemic areas, though others failed to do so. Finally, the main vector *A. minimus* proved to be vulnerable to changes in its habitat. This raises the possibility, considered further later, that settlement itself might produce a degree of malaria control, even in the absence of an organized campaign.

Expenditure in malarious areas

Malaria control expenditure. The total cost to the public sector of malaria control between 1955 and 1985 was calculated by summing all expenditures by all agencies involved in malaria control, and converting expenditure to the base-year of 1980, giving Rs 1193.93 million (1980 prices). The total annual cost of control in 1980 prices varied surprisingly little between 1965/6, when total coverage was achieved, and the present. Expenditure declined to a low point in the early 1970s, but had to be rapidly increased to keep a resurgence of malaria in check. A similar pattern can be seen in the early to mid-1980s. Given the current mix of malaria control strategies, an annual cost (1980 prices) of around Rs 40 million seems to be the consequence. To this should ideally be added the amounts households spent on treatment and prevention. A survey in 1984 (Mills and Colbourne 1985) indicated that private expenditure on malaria was certainly not insignificant; but it would be dangerous to extrapolate from a single year's estimate to the whole of the period of malaria control.

The cost of malaria control is not likely to have been the same throughout the country: although the strategies of control were common, accessibility, location, and terrain influenced costs. No historical evidence is available on geographical cost differences. A recent analysis is available (Mills 1989), but reflects the current malaria control situation – particularly the persistence of malaria transmission in the Outer Terai and the resistance of one vector to DDT. Perhaps the best guide to the relative costs of control in different areas is likely to be current fixed costs per capita, which reflect the cost of maintaining a malaria control infrastructure in each district. They suggest that the malaria control infrastructure is cheapest in the Outer Terai, though becoming more expensive from East to West, and most expensive in the Hill (Mills 1989). Inner Terai districts vary, some being closer to the per capita fixed costs of the Hill, and others to the Outer Terai.

Other expenditure. No geographical breakdown of development expenditures is available, though several sources comment on the disproportionately high allocation (relative to population size) to the Kathmandu Valley and to a lesser extent the East and Inner Terai (IBRD 1975). Of all development projects in the first four plans (1956–1974/5), 29 per cent were in the Terai, 34 per cent in the Kathmandu Valley, 14 per cent in the Hills and Mountains, and 23 per cent were devoted to national development (Sainju and Ram, undated). Of total externally funded agricultural project costs between 1951 and 1970, just over 50 per cent were for projects located in the Terai (Sakiyama 1971). From somewhat scanty evidence on irrigation schemes, it appears that parts of the East Terai were irrigated prior to malaria control; malaria control coincided with or preceded a substantial expansion of government-funded irrigation in the East Terai; and malaria control was followed by the extension of government-funded irrigation to the West and Far West Terai (Reejal 1979; Dixon 1975). A considerable proportion of development-plan expenditure was devoted to roads, much of it in the Terai, on the East-West Highway. While this certainly contributed to opening up the Terai for development, its aims were also to unify Nepal, to facilitate communications, and to provide alternatives to routes that previously went through India.

A portion of the development-plan expenditure on agriculture was spent on formal settlement schemes in the Terai, which settled around 73000 families between 1965 and 1985 (Sainju and Ram, undated; CBS 1985). The cost of World Bank schemes was estimated to be $1400 per settler in the mid 1970s (Dixon 1975). However, official programmes played a minor role in the settlement of the Terai: the World Bank estimated that between 1965 and 1975 9000 hectares were settled under government programmes and 120000 hectares spontaneously.

Other costs of opening up the new areas included seeds, fertilizers, and animal or machine power. To what extent might improved inputs such as these have contributed to increased agricultural production? The answer appears to be very little. While the consumption of chemical fertilizers, high-yielding seeds, and plant-protection materials increased, they did so from a low level; and the quantity of improved seeds and chemical fertilizers used was small relative to the land area cultivated.

In summary: malaria control costs amounted to some Rs 1194 million over the first thirty years of the programme. At the same time, substantial government resources were spent on other forms of investment in the Terai, particularly irrigation, roads, and settlement schemes.

Demographic change in Nepal

There is no direct evidence in Nepal of the effect of malaria control on mortality, fertility, or population growth-rates; nor is there good evidence on the mortality due to malaria before control. Indeed, opinions of the severity of malaria in Nepal before control are somewhat contradictory. On the one hand, malaria is believed to have been severe, causing significant mortality. For example, White (1982) stated that population growth undoubtedly accelerated because of reduction in malaria mortality, and the World Bank (IBRD 1982) suggested that malaria control may have resulted in a slight rise in fertility. On the other hand, malaria is believed to have inhibited settlement, implying that the malarious areas were very sparsely populated, though clearly a certain level of population would have been necessary to maintain transmission. This population, especially the Tharus and possibly one or two other indigenous tribes, is believed to have had some genetically-based immunity to malaria. This fact, together with the scarcity of people, implies that large numbers of people cannot have been severely affected by malaria prior to the introduction of control measures.

A starting-point in exploring the probable demographic consequences of malaria control is to estimate the proportion of the population exposed to different levels of malaria. According to the 1952–4 census, 21 per cent of the Nepalese population lived in the East Outer Terai and 4 per cent in the mid-West Outer Terai, both classified as hypoendemic. In addition a proportion (unknown, but likely to be small) of the Hill population lived in hypoendemic areas. Approximately 9 per cent of the population lived in areas classified as hyperendemic. Of these, 32 per cent were Tharus (though Tharus made up 57 per cent and 64 per cent of the population in the West Inner Terai and Far West Terai respectively). Something over 25 per cent of the population was therefore exposed to hypoendemic malaria, and 9 per cent to hyperendemic malaria.

What evidence is there of changing demographic variables before and after malaria control? Table 2.1 shows population growth-rates from 1911 to 1981. The large rise in 1952–4 was thought to be mainly due to underestimates in the three previous censuses. Seddon (1984) reviewed this and other evidence on population growth. He concluded that the Nepalese population was growing, if slowly, from the early nineteenth century onwards, and particularly from the 1930s onwards. He attributed this to immigration, land-reclamation policies, a more unified state which reduced the severity of local famines, and developments in agriculture in the eighteenth and nineteenth centuries (particularly the introduction of new crops).

Table 2.1 shows that the growth-rate has been increasing since 1952–4. The crude death-rate markedly fell, from 27 in the period 1952/4–1961 to 21 in the intercensal period 1961–71, and to 13.5 in 1971–81 (CBS 1985). Infant mortality also fell markedly though

Table 2.1 *Population size and growth, 1911 to 1981*

Census year	Population	Population growth-rate Unadjusted	Adjusted*
1911	5638749		
1920	5573788	–0.13	
1930	5532574	–0.07	
1941	6283649	1.16	
1952–4	8256625	2.27	
1961	9412996	1.64	
1971	11555983	2.05	1.99
1981	15022839	2.62	2.63

Source: Central Bureau of Statistics (1985)

* For under-enumeration of children aged 0–4.

regional differences persisted, infant mortality being highest in the Mountain, lowest in the Hill, and in between in the Terai (Banister and Thapa 1981).

It is thus clear that mortality began falling *before* malaria control (the only continuing campaign in the 1950s was in the Rapti Valley, covering a very small proportion of the population). The population growth-rate accelerated in the 1960s and 1970s: yet, at most, only around 35 per cent of the population had been at risk of malaria, and the great majority of people lived in hypoendemic areas. Malaria control may, therefore, have been a direct stimulus to population growth, though clearly it was not the initial cause of the rising population, nor necessarily the main factor in the declining mortality rates.

Evidence of the reasons for Nepal's declining mortality rates is very limited. Cassen (1981) warns against attributing too great an importance to one cause alone: 'in general, in populations subject to high mortality and multiple risks of infection and disease, removal of a single source of risk may make little difference'. He suggested that improvements in nutrition and a variety of disease-control programmes may together provide part of the explanation. There have indeed been control activities against diseases other than malaria in Nepal, for example smallpox and cholera, and it may be that settlers in the Terai in the 1960s and 1970s improved their nutritional status through immigration. To the extent that malaria control facilitated this migration it may have indirectly affected nutritional status, and thus mortality rates.

Fertility has remained high, with no obvious change between 1952–4 and 1981. There has been some speculation that malaria control may have had a small effect on fertility because of higher than expected fertility in Terai women in the early 1960s (Banister and Thapa 1981). Even so, it seems that if malaria control did increase fertility, the effect was sufficiently small to have had only a slight influence on population growth.

The geographical distribution of population

There is little direct information on the movement of people into areas freed from malaria. Information, therefore, has to be pieced together from census data on population distribution, racial origin, and place of birth, and from specific surveys and studies.

Population distribution by geographical region. Although changes in census boundaries in 1961 and 1971 make direct comparison impossible (Kansakar 1977), the change in population distribution by broad geographical region over time can be described. Before 1952–4, allowing for the inaccuracies of the censuses, there was no clear tendency for population distribution between the regions to change. In 1952–4 and 1961 (which was before malaria control everywhere except in the Central Inner Terai) population density outside the Kathmandu Valley was highest in the East Terai and next highest in the West Terai (see Table 2.2). Despite the hyperendemic malaria, population density in the three Inner Terai regions was around or over 100 per square mile.

The growth-rates in Table 2.2 for the period 1952–4 to 1961 indicate that in the East, the population of the Outer Terai was increasing relative to that of the Inner Terai and the Hills. The Central Inner Terai had the highest growth rate, presumably reflecting the development project (including malaria control) in the late 1950s. In the West, the West Hills grew at around the national average, the West Inner Terai slightly more slowly, and the West and Far West Terai slightly faster. Their lower growth-rates suggest net migration from the East Hills, the East Inner Terai, the Western Hills, and the West Inner Terai: this is confirmed by

Table 2.2 *Change in population density 1952–4 to 1971*

| Region | Population per square mile | | | Average annual growth | | Adjusted* |
	1952–4	1961	1971	1952/4–61	1961–71	1952/4–61
Nepal	151	173	213	1.7%	2.1%	1.6%
E. Hills	169	186	201	1.2%	0.8%	1.1%
E. Inner Terai	103	106	142	0.4%	3.0%	0.3%
E. Terai	353	433	581	2.6%	3.0%	2.3%
Kathmandu Valley	1885	2110	2839	1.4%	3.0%	1.3%
Central Inner Terai	91	112	227	2.6%	7.3%	2.3%
W. Hills	157	175	206	1.4%	1.6%	1.6%
W. Inner Terai	125	138	235	1.2%	5.5%	1.4%
W. Terai	266	306	343	1.8%	1.1%	2.0%
Far W. Terai	83	96	150	1.8%	4.6%	2.1%

* For difference in enumeration years in 1952–4 census between East and West Nepal.

data on lifetime internal migration from the 1961 census. The main regions with a net gain in migrants were the Central Inner Terai and the East and Far West Terai (Seddon 1984).

The population of some Terai regions does appear, therefore, to have grown at a rate in excess of the natural rate of increase before malaria control was extended to these regions. However, the change in the regional population distribution accelerated markedly in the 1960s. In the East, the East Inner Terai joined the East Terai in experiencing considerable growth, and the growth-rate of the East Hills fell. The Central Inner Terai had the highest growth-rate of all regions (7.3 per cent p.a.), followed by the West Inner Terai (5.5 per cent). The Western Hills and the West Terai grew at less than the national average, but the Far West Terai showed rapid growth.

Table 2.3 shows the change in population density between 1971 and 1981 (note that the regions cannot be directly compared with those in Table 2.2, because of boundary changes). The highest growth-rate is now in the Far West Terai (called West Terai in the Table), and the West (Central) Terai and Western Inner Terai are also growing fast. The Western Mountain and Hill shows a surprisingly high growth-rate, apparently largely due to local development projects. Elsewhere, the growth-rates of the

Table 2.3 *Change in population density, 1971 to 1981*

Region	Population per sq. km.		Av. annual growth 1971–81
	1971	1981	
Nepal	79	103	2.7%
E. Mountain and Hill	78	87	1.1%
E. Inner Terai	55	73	2.9%
E. Terai	212	306	3.7%
Kathmandu Valley	566	714	2.4%
Central Mountain and Hill (previously called Western Hill)	74	88	1.7%
Central Inner Terai	74	105	3.6%
W. Mountain and Hill	27	43	4.8%
W. Inner Terai (includes Surkhet)	49	73	4.1%
Central Terai (previously called Western Terai)	159	241	4.2%
W. Terai (previously called Far-Western Terai)	55	105	6.7%

Source: Gurung (1982). 1971 figures adjusted to 1981 boundaries.

Hill and Mountain populations remain well behind the national average growth-rate. In the East, the growth-rate of the East Terai exceeds that of the East Inner Terai. The growth rate of the Central Inner Terai has slowed down, though is still well in excess of the national average. Again, this picture of changing regional population distribution is confirmed by information on lifetime migration from the 1971 census (Seddon 1984).

To what extent do other types and sources of data shed light on these population movements? One area of interest is population distribution and movement before control. It is clear from various accounts that there had been considerable movement of people into the Terai before malaria control. Kansakar (1979), for example, commented that 'by the time the Terai and Inner Terai had been opened up to the hill people after the eradication of malaria, large tracts of reclaimable Terai and the Inner Terai had been already cultivated, tilled and owned by people of Indian origin as well as the indigenous people like Tharus, Kumhal, Dhimal, Sattar etc who were immune from malaria'. He also commented that the most fertile areas had been cultivated, leaving areas for later settlement which were less appropriate for cultivation. Rana (1971) made similar points.

Blaikie *et al.* (1980) noted a marked growth in population in the Terai in the nineteenth and early twentieth centuries, particularly in the plains adjoining India. In the late nineteenth century there was also a considerable increase in the volume of trade with India, trading centres in the Terai owing their importance to their situation on the trade routes between Tibet, the Nepal Hills, and India, and to the availability of Terai products (grain, timber) for trade. Although this trade was largely seasonal, the development of trade and marketing facilities encouraged hill merchants to invest in land in the Terai, though they were usually absentee landlords, their land being cultivated by indigenous labourers.

In addition, the government from the late eighteenth century had placed much emphasis on land reclamation and settlement (Regmi 1976, 1978). Initially, settlement was encouraged from India and Tibet, and subsequently also from the Hills (Rana and Thapa 1974). Regmi (1978) commented that population pressure in the Hills was not great enough to produce migration to an area such as the Terai, with a very different environment and climate to that of the Hills. Most migration was from India, and concentrated near the Indian border, though unofficially people had started moving slowly to the Inner Terai. Official settlement schemes had little success, apparently because people were afraid to attempt settlement because of malaria.

There were other reasons, however, for the limited success of government settlement policies. Regmi (1976, 1978) argued that incentives for settlement were limited because governments in the eighteenth and nineteenth centuries took in tax at least half the produce of the land. Large-scale conscription and forced labour were further disincentives to migration. However, since land tenure across the border was very insecure, settlement in Nepal was attractive, and there was considerable movement of people from India into the Outer Terai. Other areas of the Terai remained sparsely populated, for a variety of reasons. Blaikie *et al.* (1980) commented that the fertile and flat, though forested, areas along the northern edge of the West Central Terai remained uncleared, unlike the Terai further south, because their remoteness increased the risk of banditry and wild animals. Regmi (1978) noted malaria as one reason for the underpopulation of the Inner Terai, though commenting that malaria did not inhibit settlement elsewhere because it was a familiar illness to settlers from India. He also argued that the Inner Terai was deliberately left undeveloped in the eighteenth and nineteenth centuries for reasons of national security: it was seen as a barrier to invasion.

Several case studies of the Far West Terai shed further light. Both Dahal *et al.* (1977) and McDougal (1968) noted the remoteness of the Far West Terai, its relatively poor-quality land, and its distance from centres of population in the Hill. In the nineteenth century Tharus from Dang in the West Inner Terai moved to the Far West Terai, but few wealthy Hill farmers bought land in the Far West Terai for investment, preferring instead to invest in Hill land. In contrast, Dang was more accessible from the Hills, and land was acquired on quite a large scale by Hill farmers for around forty years prior to malaria control. As the forest was cleared and the valley became more open, the danger from malaria is said to have been less (McDougal 1968), though until recently few Hill people stayed in the valley throughout the year. This and other information confirms that before malaria control there was heavy settlement of people from the Hills in the West Inner Terai, mainly in the Dang Valley, with a spill-over from the West Inner Terai to the Far West Terai. There was very little immigration into these areas from India.

A special migration survey (Population Commission 1983) presented information on the date of migration for 10 sampled Outer Terai districts. It supports the evidence of considerable migration into the Terai, particularly in the East but also elsewhere, before malaria control. The greatest increase in settlement seems to have taken place in the late 1960s in the more central districts, and in the early 1970s in outlying districts. By the early 1980s, migration was still continuing, though at a lower level.

Once the malaria eradication campaign was under way, population statistics were collected that can be used to track the change in population in hyperendemic and hypoendemic areas (Mills 1988). The population growth-rates of previously hyperendemic areas clearly exceeded those of hypoendemic areas, confirming the picture from the censuses of the sparser population – and thus greater potential for immigration – in hyperendemic areas.

Evidence from anthropological investigations and settlement schemes indicates that whatever the reasons for the initial neglect of the sparsely populated areas, malaria control had a major impact on people's perception of the desirability of settlement. Elder *et al.* (1976), in a study of planned resettlement, reported that initially anyone who applied got land, but that within four years there were long queues. Migration, both temporary and permanent, had for centuries been a solution to the economic problems of the Hills: malaria control and settlement schemes channelled it to areas in the Terai, though no one migrated unless they had to (Dahal *et al.* 1977).

Once the fear of malaria had been removed and news spread that land was available, a complex pattern of factors influenced migration patterns. Sainju and Ram (undated) concluded that the economic reasons for migration were the strongest. Push factors were declining economic conditions in the Hills because of high population to cultivated land densities; disasters such as floods and landslides, which led to loss of land; limited employment opportunities; low income and income inequalities; debt; food shortages; and relative government neglect in terms of development activities. 'Pull' factors were primarily the availability of land and better economic conditions in the Terai – more land and thus a higher income per household – as well as the availability of employment in agricultural, industrial, and trading activities, and better social and economic infrastructure. Contributing causes were institutional – the resettlement and land distribution programme; and social – many migrants moved to join relatives and neighbours in the Terai.

A particularly important factor, operating to a considerable extent independently of malaria control, was road construction. The East-West highway and north-south roads stimulated movement, trade, and the development of commercial centres (Blaikie *et al.* 1980). The development of communications and increasing agricultural production in the Terai also stimulated urban development. A comparison of population increase in some town *panchayat* localities (Gurung 1982) showed that most of the increase was in Terai and Inner Terai towns. Large towns emerged out of modest Inner Terai hamlets; border towns expanded significantly.

In order to complete the picture of population distribution since malaria control, a further piece of information is needed: the origin of the migrants. The special survey on migration (Population Commission 1983) showed that in the districts experiencing the greatest immigration, migrants were largely from the adjacent hills. However, the East Terai itself provided the greatest proportion of immigrants in three Terai districts, and a significant proportion in two others. Taking the 10 survey districts as a whole, 65 per cent of immigrants were from the Hill, 30 per cent from the Terai, and 4 per cent from the Inner Terai.

To what extent are these proportions likely to be representative of all migration into the Terai? Only two Far West districts were included in the survey, although the Far West experienced considerable migration from the Hills. Inner Terai districts were also excluded; and again these migrants were most likely to be from the Hills. Therefore Hill-dwellers are likely to have made up a larger proportion of migrants for the whole Terai, including the Inner Terai, though the figures presented above are a useful warning that not all migrants were from the Hills.

Immigration from India also contributed to the growing population of the Terai. In the 1961 census 10.8 per cent of the total population of the Terai was born outside the country (98.9 per cent of these in India). This proportion declined in subsequent censuses, but is thought to be unreliable because of the sensitivity of the issue. Immigration also contributed to urbanization: immigrants make up a higher proportion of the urban than of the rural population (Population Commission 1983).

The volume of migration. From the point of view of further analysis, it is necessary to translate percentage changes in population distribution into absolute numbers. Because of the difficulties in comparing regional populations over time, two estimates were made: the first based on CBS (Central Bureau of Statistics) data, using consistent boundaries but not distinguishing the Inner Terai from the Terai; and the second based on the Tuladhar *et al.* (1977) and Gurung (1982) figures, which do distinguish the Inner Terai (though regional boundaries are not necessarily consistent between these two sources).

The population growth-rates for 1961–71 and 1971–1981 were applied to the regional populations for 1961 and 1971, the difference between the resulting population estimates for 1971 and 1981 and the census figures then being attributed to migration. The two estimates of numbers migrating, shown in Table 2.4, are reasonably consistent, except that the outmigration from the West Hills is considerably greater in the CBS-based estimate. In terms of absolute numbers, the majority of migrants settled in the Outer rather than the Inner Terai. The East Terai gained between 700000 and 750000 people, and the Far West Terai around 360000. The Central Inner Terai gained considerably more people than the West and – even more so – the East Inner Terai. In total, the Terai and Inner Terai gained 1.56–1.74 million people as a result of migration, and the Hills lost between 1.34 and 1.62 million. These numbers suggest that migration is likely to have had major economic and social consequences.

The pattern displayed by the Tuladhar *et al.* and Gurung data was checked by using data for the period 1961 to 1971 from ESCAP (1979). The resulting migration numbers were very similar, except that the Central Inner Terai appeared to gain about 100000 less, and the Western Terai about 70000 more.

Changes in land cultivation and crop production in the Terai

Despite malaria, the Terai before malaria control was by no means unproductive. In the southern parts, large open stretches of arable land had existed for centuries, producing paddy, oilseeds, cotton, jute, tobacco, and sugar-cane (Regmi 1976), and the Terai provided large amounts of revenue for the ruling classes in Kathmandu from the export of forest products and grain (Blaikie *et al.* 1980). Two districts in the West Terai were said by an official of the East

Table 2.4 *The volume of migration, 1961 to 1981*

Population by region based on CBS regional population estimates

	1961	1971	1981	1981 pop. assuming pop. growth-rates	Change due to migration (4)–(5)
	(2)	(3)	(4)	(5)	(6)
Nepal	9412996	11555983	15022839	14860967	161872
East Hill	1886722	2036240	2287173	2978702	(691529)
Kathmandu Valley	459990	618911	766345	726219	40126
East and Inner East Terai	2406948	3234181	4585162	3800020	785142
Central Terai	244236	493958	811810	385593	426217
W., Mid-W., Far W. and Inner W. Terai	770515	1041624	1746777	1216467	530310
West Hill	3644585	4131069	4825572	5753966	(928394)

Population by region based on Tuladhar *et al.* (1977) and Gurung (1982) regional population estimates

	Change due to migration 1961–71	1971–81	Total change 1961–81
Nepal	126154	39127	165281
Eastern Hills	(258016)	(378364)	(636380)
Eastern Inner Terai	23618	4825	28444
Eastern Terai	274638	431316	705954
Kathmandu Valley	58738	(20830)	37909
Central Inner Terai	221533	41146	262678
Western Hills	(211863)	(487410)	(699273)
Western Inner Terai	47798	54156	101954
Western Terai	(38748)	139075	100327
Far Western Terai	94078	262249	356327

India Company in the mid-eighteenth century to be 'as nearly as well cultivated as Bihar or Benares' (Regmi 1976). Land-revenue statistics suggest that there was a significant expansion in land cultivation in the mid-nineteenth century in both the East and Far West Terai (Regmi 1978).

The pattern of land-ownership and employment before malaria control is indicated by information from the 1952–4 census on the employment status of the economically active population. In the

Hills and the East and Central Inner Terai own-account subsistence farming appears to have been the norm. In all parts of the Outer Terai and in the West Inner Terai over 40 per cent of economically active men, and almost the same proportion of women, worked as employees (virtually all in agriculture). This suggests the predominance of large-scale land-ownership in the Outer Terai before malaria control (and before land reform in the 1960s).

The earliest agricultural statistics for Nepal date from 1961/2 and are therefore of little use for charting changes prior to malaria control, but do provide a baseline for charting subsequent changes. In 1961 a surprising 63 per cent of the cultivated land of Nepal was in the Terai (mainly the East Terai), with a further 9 per cent in the Inner Terai (Table 2.5); 59 per cent of total paddy and maize production came from the Terai, and 8 per cent from the Inner Terai.

Analysis of the change in land cultivated and in production since 1961/2 should ideally encompass all areas of production: crops, livestock, forestry, fishing, mining, and agro-industries. Since comprehensive information is not available, and the Terai economy

Table 2.5 *Total cultivated land and paddy and maize production by region, 1961*

Region	Cultivated land (ha)	% by region	Paddy & maize prod. (m tons)	% by region
East Hills	175923	10.2%	356193	12.1%
West Hills	274448	16.0%	519747	17.6%
Kathmandu Valley	27175	1.6%	83667	2.8%
Hills	477546	27.8%	959607	32.5%
East Inner Terai	47027	2.7%	85358	2.9%
Central Inner Terai	53331	3.1%	69869	2.4%
West Inner Terai	58157	3.4%	87265	3.0%
Inner Terai	158515	9.2%	242492	8.2%
East Terai	749613	43.6%	1301125	44.1%
West Terai	170397	9.9%	255717	8.7%
Far West Terai	162107	9.4%	191349	6.5%
Terai	1082116	63.0%	1748191	59.3%
Nepal	1718177	100.0%	2950290	100.0%

Source: Ministry of Economic Planning (1962)

is based on agriculture, the following indicators were studied: total land area cultivated by region; reduction in forested area; total land area cultivated by region and type of crop; crop production by region and type of crop; and the economic circumstances of farmers.

Total land area cultivated by region. Complete time-series data using consistent regional boundaries are unavailable, so information from a variety of sources was used. All sources show that the cultivated area grew steadily from the early 1960s, at over 2 per cent per year (Pant and Jain 1969; IBRD 1974; Khadka and Lohani 1981; Lal Das 1982). However, its regional distribution, and the relative growth of the various regions, is unclear. Land cultivated in the Inner Terai appears to have grown particularly fast between 1961 and 1971, but cannot be distinguished after 1971, being incorporated in Terai statistics. Over the period 1969/70 to 1980/1, the cultivated land area of the East Hill grew fastest, followed by the Far West Terai (Khadka and Lohani 1981). Overall, between 1965 and 1980 the rate of expansion of land in the Hills (on average 2.2 per cent per year) slightly exceeded that in the Terai (on average 1.9 per cent per year), maintaining the Hills' share of total cultivated land (Lal Das 1982).

Given the change in population distribution over this period, the slowness of growth in the area cultivated in the Terai and Inner Terai is surprising. Part of the explanation may be that the migrants cultivated areas of land that were smaller than the average: thus a given percentage increase in population would not result in an identical percentage increase in land cultivated. Another part of the explanation may lie with faulty data. Statistics of total cultivated land are based on sample surveys, and may thus be prone to error. Moreover, much of the settlement in the Terai and Inner Terai in the 1960s and 1970s was illegal. It must be questionable, therefore, whether land area (and production) statistics fully took into account the rapidly changing settlement and cultivation patterns.

Reduction in forested areas. Evidence on the decline in forested areas is also of poor quality. The survey of migration (Population Commission 1983) gave a total of 1.03 million ha lost in the Terai (excluding the Inner Terai) between 1964 and 1981. The statistics on land cultivated suggested the cultivated area in the

Terai increased from 1.17 million hectares in 1965/6 to 1.50 million in 1980/1, an increase of 0.33 million ha. Not all the loss of forest area would represent a gain in cultivated area: however, even allowing for other uses, there seems to be a considerable discrepancy between the area lost to forests and the area gained for cultivation.

Total land area cultivated by region and type of crop. From knowledge of changing settlement patterns it might be expected that growth in land cultivated with staple crops such as paddy and maize between 1965 (when regional crop statistics start) and 1980 would have been faster in the Terai and Inner Terai than in the Hills. This does not appear to have been the case (Lal Das 1982). For the main crop, paddy, land area cultivated changed only slowly in the Terai, at an average of between 0.3 per cent and 1.2 per cent per year. Land cultivated in the Inner Terai showed a marked increase only for crops which took up a small proportion of the cultivated land (Ministry of Food and Agriculture 1972). Average regional growth rates in land cultivated by crop did not show any very consistent differences between different periods. Since the data start in 1965/6, they may have missed the substantial increase in cultivation that is said to have followed malaria control in the Central Inner Terai in the late 1950s, though they should reflect most of the changes that occurred following malaria control in other regions.

Crop production by region and type of crop. Statistics on crop production by geographical region for the period 1965/6 to 1970/1 showed a slight growth in paddy and maize production throughout the Terai, with greater growth in the Hills for paddy but a reduction for maize (Ministry of Food and Agriculture 1972; Lal Das 1982). In the period 1974 to 1979 it is striking how many of the regional growth-rates were negative for paddy and maize: only the East Terai for maize and the East Hill for paddy had positive growth-rates. Wheat production increased sharply through the whole period, especially in the Terai, where by the end of the period it had overtaken maize as the most important crop after paddy.

Declining growth-rates of crop production and slowly growing land areas were reflected in declining yields: for maize and paddy, yields were largely static between 1966 and 1971, and then fell universally for paddy and in everywhere except the East and West Terai for maize. Wheat yields declined sharply in the early period, but recovered slightly in the later period.

Information on yields can be used to see whether there was any change in yields that might be associated with malaria control. Coverage was achieved by 1962 in the Central and West regions, and by 1964 in the East, so for these regions the available data may be too late to pick up any effect. However, farmers may have adapted to malaria by adopting cultivation practices that were less vulnerable to temporary shortages of labour; if so, it may have taken a number of years for farmers to change these practices, and for gains in productivity to become apparent. The evidence does not suggest any major effect on yields in the Far West Terai, nor any delayed adaptation to malaria control in the rest of the Terai and Inner Terai. If any improvement in productivity did occur as a result of malaria control, it was obscured by other influences.

Economic circumstances of farmers. What changes were there in the economic circumstances of farmers in the Terai? There was a marked change in employment status. Those regions and districts which had a high proportion of employees in 1952–4 showed a much lower proportion by 1981. The most likely explanation is the influx of settlers, though land reform may have changed the status of part of the indigenous population. Average farm size was, and continues to be, greater in the Terai than in the Hills (McDougal 1968; IBRD 1980; Ministry of Food and Agriculture 1971). Average income per holding is also greater in the Terai, though less so than might be expected from average size (Ministry of Food and Agriculture 1971; National Planning Commission 1978). In the Hills 75 per cent of this income was derived from agriculture, and in the Terai, 55 per cent, reflecting the greater availability of non-agricultural employment (National Planning Commission 1978). The same survey estimated that the proportion of the population below the poverty line (defined as a minimum level of income) was 68 per cent in the Mountains, 34 per cent in the Hills, and 33 per cent in the Terai.

Thus, despite the larger farm size in the Terai and greater off-farm employment opportunities, average income is only slightly higher than in the Hills. It is clear that Terai land is on average farmed much less intensively. In addition, the Terai has to a greater extent than the Hills a considerable number of marginal farmers with low incomes who are dependent to a major extent on wage-labour for survival. Around 1980, 23 per cent of the Terai population were landless, but only 1 per cent of the Hill population (IBRD 1980). This reflects not merely the poverty of sections of the Terai population, but also the availability of non-farm employment, which attracts the landless from their home districts.

Economic changes in the Terai and Inner Terai, 1961 to 1981. What conclusions can be drawn on the extension of cultivation and increase in production following malaria control? A major concern is the reliability of the evidence: the Terai and Inner Terai cultivated land area increased by 0.33 million hectares between 1961 and 1981, or 28 per cent, compared to an increase in population (due to both natural increase and immigration) of 109 per cent. In addition, the forested area decreased by at least 1.03 million hectares. There must be a strong suspicion that the land area cultivated was underestimated.

The increase in land area increased production, though yields generally declined from the early 1970s, owing to the cultivation of increasingly marginal soils and to low levels of investment. This tended to reduce the production gain from malaria control. One notable feature, however, was the change in cropping patterns. The area under wheat grew markedly, as did that for cash crops such as sugar-cane, jute, and oilseeds.

The discussion here has focused on crop production as the main potential source of economic gain from malaria control, given the predominantly rural nature of Nepal. There were, however, other economic changes in the Terai. For example the livestock population increased, and thus meat and milk products. Indeed, IBRD (1974) estimated that livestock production made up 21 per cent of total agricultural gross domestic product. The increase in grain and also oilseed production, together with an increased urban population, stimulated the development of agro-industries, primarily rice-milling and oilseed processing, though there was also some sugar-cane processing. There was also a limited development of other industries, particularly brick and tile manufacturing and stone-quarrying and crushing, to meet the demand for construction materials in the growing towns.

Part 2: Economic gains and losses associated with malaria control

Analytical approach

Before attempting to quantify and evaluate the economic gains and losses associated with malaria control, it is first necessary to consider how extensive were the probable ramifications of the changes induced by malaria control. Were they so wide-reaching that the entire Nepali economy was affected, or were the changes less massive and more localized?

Temporarily setting aside the issue of the extent to which malaria control alone was responsible for the observed changes, the magnitude of population migration between 1961 and 1981 suggests that major economic changes would have resulted. Between 1961 and 1981 it was estimated above that the Terai gained between 1.56 million and 1.74 million people as a result of migration, and the Hills lost between 1.34 million and 1.62 million. Relative to a total population in 1961 of 9.4 million and in 1981 of 15 million, these were sizeable changes. Surprisingly, statistics on increases in land area cultivated and crop production show less change than might be expected from these population movements. Indeed, the average annual growth-rate in land cultivated in the Hills between 1965 and 1980 actually exceeded that of the Terai. The presumption must be that data-collection did not manage to keep pace with the changing population-distribution patterns in the Terai.

At the same time, there are grounds for believing that the economic impact of population migration may have been less major than might have been predicted from its volume. Firstly, population growth-rates (reflecting both natural increase and migration) varied considerably between different areas of the Terai and Inner Terai (see Tables 2.2 and 2.3). There was considerable growth in some districts (for example the extreme east and the extreme west), and less drastic change in others.

Secondly, economic studies of organized and illegal settlement suggested that much of any increase in the area cultivated would have been used primarily for subsistence farming. Subsistence farming is less likely than commercial farming to have a major impact on the population at large, for instance through large increases in the production of food surpluses, in marketed produce, or in exports.

Further, it is probably unreasonable to view Nepal as a single economy, where changes in one geographical region will have ramifications throughout that economy. Particularly in the earlier periods reviewed here, communications difficulties were such that it is probably more accurate to view Nepal as a set of loosely connected local economies. This view is supported by evidence in the 1960s on paddy and maize prices, which showed considerable price differences between areas (Lal Das 1982). No clear tendency existed for the Hill price to be higher, although the great majority of Hill districts produced less grain than they consumed, in contrast to surpluses in most Terai and Inner Terai districts (Pant and Jain 1969), and although transport was costly. This suggests that trade in grain was insufficient to even out prices, and that a surplus or deficit in one area had limited effects elsewhere. By 1980 Hill-Terai price levels reveal a differential that might be expected from a knowledge of grain surpluses and deficits and transport costs, but still suggest that transport difficulties prevented the emergence of a national market.

What implications do these conclusions have for the evaluation of gains and losses associated with malaria control? In some districts there was considerable change, in others less. Even where there was considerable change, it is difficult to predict how this will have affected the rest of the economy. The practical approach adopted here is to list the likely gains and losses, and to estimate a value where feasible. Since the balance of the evidence suggests (as is discussed further below) that malaria control had greater effects on the supply of land than on the productivity of already cultivated land in malarious areas, values are expressed per hectare of land rather than in terms of national gains and losses. This sidesteps the issue of the total magnitude of gains and losses, yet still provides a clear indication of whether or not there is likely to have been a net gain. The discussion concentrates on identifying the magnitude of changes in the quantity of inputs, and discusses probable changes in their quality. Most evidence is available on changes in land and labour inputs, and so the discussion concentrates on these, thus neglecting the contribution of other inputs (for example animal labour, tractors, or irrigation). Various accounts suggest that the new land available for settlement often could not be easily irrigated, because of its distance from water sources (Kansakar 1979), and that labour and land are by far the most important inputs in small-scale traditional farming

(Pudasaini 1976), so this emphasis is considered justified. A guide to the discussion is provided in Table 2.6, which lists the main gains and losses.

In those districts where malaria control and migration resulted in only marginal changes to the supply of factors of production, the gains can be valued in terms of the existing marginal products per hectare of the main agricultural inputs (conventionally classified as land, labour, and capital). In districts where major change occurred, this approach is questionable, because increases in the quantity and quality of factors of production were so great that they were likely to have affected marginal products. However, known marginal products still have some value, if only as a baseline which can be adjusted upwards in the light of what is known about changes in the main agricultural inputs. Yet these changes are likely

Table 2.6 *Types of economic gains and losses associated with malaria control*

Gains	Losses
1. Marginal product of land brought into cultivation	Loss of marginal product of land in source area of migrants Loss of marginal product of forested land Ecological damage from loss of forests, e.g. erosion, climatic change Cost of rendering new land productive
2. Marginal product of new settlers: — agricultural — non-agricultural	Loss of their marginal product in their source areas
3. Protection for indigenous population from banditry, wild animals	Loss of income for indigenous population from — loss of forest products, grazing areas — effects of increased labour supply on wages.
4. Increased output and productivity of indigenous population because of reduction in malaria morbidity and mortality	Costs associated with a larger population, e.g. costs of social services, environmental damage, reduced rate of public and private saving
5. Increased income for service industries	Loss of income for service industries in source areas

to have been quite complex and varied. For example, it is possible to envisage all the following situations:

- previously uncultivated areas where the supply of land, labour, and capital all increased (for example, settlement schemes);

- previously uncultivated areas where the supply of land and labour increased, but settlers had relatively little capital (illegal settlement);

- previously cultivated areas where settlers were forced to occupy increasingly marginal land; and

- cultivated areas where the supply and productivity of labour increased through a reduction in malaria, but the supply of land and capital remained the same.

These are all relatively short-term changes. In the longer term, changes may be brought about by the effect of malaria control on fertility and mortality rates, and thus on population growth: these latter effects are not quantified below.

Gains and losses from new land

The first (two-part) question to be addressed is as follows: what would have happened to land cultivation in the absence of malaria control; and how much of the gains in land area cultivated can be attributed to malaria control? In hypoendemic areas, the evidence available suggested that malaria was not a major barrier to settlement. Much of the Terai before malaria control was already heavily settled and productive, and land-tenure systems, heavy taxation, and the climate (for Hill dwellers) were of greater importance than malaria in deterring further settlement.

In hyperendemic areas, the evidence of Phillips (1925) suggested that malaria was a considerable deterrent to settlement. On the basis of changes in population distribution and in cultivated land by region, it seems that the greatest expansion of cultivation took place in these previously sparsely populated areas rather than in the already settled, hypoendemic Outer Terai, and that the success of the expansion was due in considerable part to malaria control. Yet evidence from the West Inner Terai, where migration occurred before malaria control, suggested that settlement was possible in hyperendemic areas, though at the cost of considerable morbidity and mortality in the early years. Once the forest had been cleared, the land cultivated, and the vector habitat changed, a measure of control was probably achieved purely through these environmental changes.

The Inner Terai is unfortunately not identified in land-area statistics after 1970/1. In that year, hyperendemic areas accounted for 35 per cent of all land cultivated in the Terai, as compared with 26 per cent in 1961. In terms of the growth in land cultivated that occurred in the Terai between 1961 and 1970/1, 71 per cent occurred in the Inner Terai and the Far West Terai. After 1970/1 this fast rate of expansion seems not to have continued, though growth in the Far West and the West Terai still exceeded that in the East and the Central Terai. Malaria control, therefore, appears to have provided an important stimulus to increased cultivation in hyperendemic areas.

So, in summary, probably the greater part of the *growth* in land cultivated in the Terai from the late 1950s resulted from the stimulus provided by malaria control, though the influence of malaria control is likely to have been important in only a minority of the entire land area of the Terai. In the absence of malaria control, given continuing population pressure in the Hills, it is likely that migration would still have occurred in hyperendemic areas, but at a slower rate, and at considerable cost to the settlers in terms of morbidity and mortality.

But, more precisely, what were the gains and losses associated with the expansion of cultivation; and how worthwhile was malaria control? On the positive side, at least 256 000 hectares of land have been gained in the Terai and Inner Terai since malaria control started. In other countries, it has been assumed that this land is more fertile (i.e. provides a higher marginal product) than already-cultivated land. In Nepal, there is reason to believe that this was not always the case. Certainly, the initial land cultivated in the Central Inner Terai was said to have been very productive, though cultivation was later extended to marginal, non-irrigated land (Khadka and Lohani 1981). A number of other sources commented that the good-quality land in the Terai and Inner Terai was already cultivated by indigenous settlers or the labourers of absentee landlords (Kansakar 1979; IBRD 1978). Further, the Far West, where considerable expansion of cultivation occurred, is drier and less fertile than the rest of the Terai. Thus much of the new land may not have been particularly productive, even though net returns must have been positive, since cultivation persisted.

There are virtually no empirical estimates available of the marginal product of land in different parts of Nepal. Only one study on this was located (Pudasaini 1976), and this attempted to assess the marginal product of different inputs using a Cobb-Douglas production function; but its sample was extremely limited (102 farmers in Bara district in 1974/5). The marginal value product of crop land was estimated at Rs 810–840 per hectare. Bara, a relatively fertile district, is likely to represent the upper limit of the marginal product of new land, so to approximate better the value of land of average fertility, the equivalent of Rs 810 in 1980 prices is taken, namely Rs 1300.

On the negative side, the losses associated with opening up new land were fourfold: loss of the marginal product of land in the source area of the migrants; loss of the marginal product of the forested lands; ecological damage from the loss of forests; and the opportunity cost of the resources required to open up the land. The magnitude of the losses is now considered.

There are good reasons for supposing that the loss of marginal product of land in the source area of the migrants was not very great. In the first place, some migrants moved because they had lost some or all of their land in the Hills in floods or landslides; others were not farmers (being, for example, political refugees). In the second place, population pressure in the Hills was sufficient to ensure that land cultivated continued expanding, but into more and more marginal land (as is implied by the declining yields). Migration does not appear to have caused an absolute decline in the cultivated area in the Hills, though possibly it caused a slower rate of expansion. Yields declined at a faster rate in the Hills than in the Terai (Chapagani 1976), suggesting that the land being gained in the Terai was more productive than the land that remained to be exploited in the Hills. Moreover, slowing down the rate of expansion in the Hills may actually have been beneficial if it reduced the risk of environmental damage from the cultivation of marginal land subject to erosion.

The loss of the marginal product of forests took the form of the loss of timber products and grazing for animals from the estimated 1.03 million hectares of forest lost between 1964 and 1981. The value of the yearly harvest of wood, if properly exploited, was estimated at Rs 70 and Rs 95 per hectare of all forest land (Dixon

1975; UNDP 1972). A gain of one hectare of agricultural land was likely to have resulted in a loss of more than one hectare of forested land (allowing for loss due to grazing, collection of firewood, etc.). Assuming a hectare of agricultural land was gained at the cost of 2 hectares of forest, this gives a cost per hectare of agricultural land gained of Rs 140–190 (Rs 220–400 in 1980 prices). Additional costs arose from loss of grazing for animals (Rana (1971), for example, commented that the ghee (clarified butter) industry in the Hills was badly affected by deforestation in the Far West Terai, because it was dependent on winter pasturage in the Terai forests) and loss of the indirect benefits of forested land (watershed and catchment protection, protection of steep slopes from erosion and landslides, wild life habitats and recreation, and scientific study (Willan 1967)). These losses from the removal of forests may have been compensated for, to some extent, by a slower increase in deforestation in the Hills than would otherwise have occurred.

Finally, both malaria control and the infrastructure development required to open up new land entailed 'losses' or costs. Approximately 85 per cent of malaria-control costs can be attributed to the Terai (Mills 1987), resulting in a cost up to 1980/1 of Rs 815.58 million, or Rs 37.07 million per year. In order to compare this cost with the gains from cultivation, it was divided by the total land cultivated in the Terai in 1981 (a convenient end-point, providing a sufficient period of time for any changes resulting from malaria control to have taken place) giving a total cost of Rs 545 per hectare. The great majority of malaria-control costs are recurrent, not capital, so this total is simply averaged over the years of the control programme, giving an annual average cost of Rs 25 per hectare. This cost is an overestimate to the extent that land cultivated is underestimated.

In terms of infrastructure development costs, 29 per cent and 50 per cent were taken as the lower and upper limits of the proportion of the agricultural expenditure of development plans that was spent in the Terai, and these figures were divided by the total Terai land cultivated in 1981, giving a cost per hectare in the range Rs 980 to Rs 1700. By 1980, assuming an average length of life for development projects of 20 years, on average half of the 1960–1980 investment would still be productive, and on average this would have a 10-year life-span. This implies an average annual equivalent cost (at 5 per cent real rate of interest) of agricultural investment in the period 1960 to 1980 of Rs 63 to Rs 110 per hectare.

To allow for all investment in the Terai, total plan expenditures 1960/1 to 1979/80 (at 1980 prices) were multiplied by 0.29 (representing the Terai share), and divided by total hectares cultivated in 1981, to give Rs 3800 per hectare, or an annual equivalent cost of Rs 246 per hectare. This is very much an upper limit, since it distributes all development expenditure, including that more closely related to industrial and urban infrastructure, to the expansion of cultivation in the Terai.

It should be noted that these figures represent an average over the whole Terai. It seems likely that investment was biased towards the already settled Terai (especially the East), so that the figures overestimate the share of the newly settled areas except for official settlement scheme areas. These latter areas provide some data on the magnitude of investment costs in areas of intensive development. The forestry and settlement costs of a World Bank-funded scheme amounted to Rs 3462.2 million (1976/7 to 1980/1) and made available 18600 hectares (IBRD 1983). This represents an investment cost of Rs 1860 per hectare, and an annual cost, assuming a 20-year life-span, of Rs 149. This, as would be expected, is higher than the Rs 63–110 annual equivalent costs of agricultural investment per hectare estimated above from the development plans, but less than the highest figure of Rs 246, and provides some confirmation that the range calculated above is correct.

Gains and losses from labour migration

Some 1.56 to 1.74 million people, or 270000 to 300000 families, migrated and settled in the Terai and the Inner Terai between 1961 and 1981. Taking the proportion of the population aged 10 and over who were economically active, namely 85 per cent of men and 46 per cent of women (1981 census), and a ratio between male and female labour of 1:1.5, this implies that migration led to a gain of productive manpower equivalent to 629000 to 714300 units of labour. Since labour moved to previously unexploited land and, on average, cultivated more land than in the Hills, the supply of labour expanded along with the supply of land (so marginal workers are unlikely to have been unemployed or underemployed).

Certainly, evidence from settlement schemes suggested that migrants improved their level of income by migrating; though how well they did in the Terai depended on a number of factors, not least the quality and size of the land they obtained, the presence or absence of irrigation, and the capital they brought with them. A survey of 7 settlement schemes in the Terai indicated that while the migrants interviewed felt they were better off, most were doing poorly in terms of both incomes and yields relative to the indigenous population, usually because they had poorer-quality and non-irrigated farms (Kansakar 1979). Though agriculture was usually the main source of income, non-farm income was an important supplement, and also a protection against bad harvests.

Gains in income for settlers were achieved at the cost of the work required to establish themselves. Organized settlers received considerable help; but illegal settlers bore the costs themselves. Even in organized schemes many settlers were in debt; this is likely to have been true also for illegal settlers. None the less, the overall balance appears positive for most settlers: they were surviving, if at a fairly low standard of living.

Pudasaini (1976) estimated the marginal value product per man day amongst the sampled farmers in Bara to be around Rs 11 in 1974/5. Taking this as a rough approximation of the marginal value product of labour in fertile areas of the Terai in 1974/5, its equivalent in 1980 prices was Rs 18. This figure is arbitrarily reduced by 50 per cent to take account, firstly, of the predominance of poor-quality, non-irrigated land in new settlements; and secondly of declining yields in recent years. The resulting figure of Rs 9 per day seems plausible when compared to an average wage per day in the West Terai in 1984 of Rs 15 per day (Mills 1985); furthermore, this latter wage would have been lower in areas which were more remote and had a less active labour market, and would not have been available throughout the year.

In order to relate the figure of Rs 9 to the gains from the expansion of cultivated land, it is convenient to express it in per hectare terms. Assuming four labour units per household, an average farm size of 2 hectares (Ministry of Agriculture 1981/2), and 150 days of work a year, this gives a gain in the marginal product of labour per hectare of Rs 2700 per year.

Against this figure has to be set the corresponding *loss* of marginal product in the areas from where the migrants moved. The data suggest that most came from adjacent hill areas. The size of the loss of their marginal product depends firstly, on the proportion who were landless or virtually landless; and secondly, on the extent to which their labour was surplus to requirements on their family farm.

Studies of migration have suggested that it was a decision not easily taken: this implies that economic circumstances had to be bleak before households would decide to re-locate. While the very fact of settlement indicates that net private benefits were positive, the question for society is how positive? Some reports argued that the Hills were drained of people with leadership qualities and skills; agricultural pursuits were left unattended; cottage industries and handicrafts were depressed; construction work in some Hill areas had to employ imported labour from India (Ministry of Food and Agriculture 1981). In addition, there was some loss elsewhere, because settlers did not previously spend all their time working in the Hills, but migrated temporarily for work in the Terai and in India. Yet this gloomy picture does not match well with continuing reports of population pressure in the Hills, surplus labour looking for employment opportunities elsewhere, and expansion of cultivation to marginal land. Other interpretations are possible. For example, employment of Indian labourers has been attributed to the contracting system, which favoured large, external contractors (Rana 1971).

Several reports in the 1960s and 1970s suggested a high level of underemployment in the rural work force. For example, Pant (1983) quoted estimates for 1967 that 48 per cent of the total agricultural labour force was surplus; for 1974 that the average farm-worker was employed for only 55 days in the Hills and 180 days in the Terai; and for 1977 that 64 per cent of available days were unused in rural areas. More recent studies have tended to take a rather different view, partly because of a greater appreciation of seasonal labour needs, and partly because of a broader definition of what constitutes employment. Labour-force definitions, particularly for women, do not fit well the pattern or nature of work in the rural subsistence sector. If the tasks of maintaining the household are included as 'work', a substantial number of hours per day are spent working, and women tend to work longer hours than men. For example, a study of a number of village communities in Nepal found mean hours of work per day per person in each village to vary between 6.20 and 10.06 hours for men, and 8.46 and 12.50 hours for women (Acharya and Bennett 1982).

It is therefore unwise to assume that withdrawal of labour

through migration caused no loss, though available evidence on the shortage of labour opportunities in the Hills suggested that the returns to marginal workers were less in the Hills than in the Terai. A World Bank appraisal (IBRD 1978) estimated that the opportunity cost of settlers, based on employment opportunities in their source areas and former areas of temporary migration, was Rs 532 per year for men (1980 prices). Multiplying this by the four labour units per household assumed earlier gives Rs 2128, equivalent to Rs 1214 per hectare.

In contrast to the position of migrants, it is likely that the indigenous population in settlement areas lost more than it gained. On the benefit side was increased protection from banditry and wild animals, resulting from the greater density of population; and increased income for indigenous traders and service industries. On the cost side were losses of timber products and grazing. The Tharus, in particular, were losers because they were primarily hunter/gatherers, living off the forests. In addition, wages fell in some settlement areas because of the increased labour supply (Elder *et al*. 1976; Sainju and Ram, undated). The converse of this was the gain experienced by those who hired labour.

Increased productivity and survival of the indigenous population

The evidence reviewed earlier did not take the discussion of the contribution of malaria control to raising the productivity of the indigenous population much further. On the basis of evidence from elsewhere (Mills 1989), an assumption seems reasonable that the settled population in a hyperendemic area does not suffer major effects on productivity as a result of malaria, because of immunity. In hypoendemic areas, the parasite rates quoted earlier are sufficiently low to suggest that a significant effect on productivity was not likely there either, except when epidemics occurred. It is true that malaria transmission peaks coincide with peak agricultural labour demands. However, it is likely that, except in years of epidemics, there was a sufficient supply of household labour to cover for those ill. If productivity has improved as a result of improved health status, this is most likely to be attributable to a range of health interventions, rather than to a single disease-control programme.

The other major question is the effect that malaria control had on population growth. Nepal has certainly already experienced costs associated with population growth, and faces more severe costs in the future (IBRD 1980). Population density in relation to cultivated land is denser than in Pakistan, Bangladesh, or India. Agricultural production has not kept pace with population growth in recent years. Stagnant or declining yields per hectare have been attributed to practices made necessary by dwindling resources per capita of the population, such as the use of increasingly marginal land for agriculture. However the extent to which population pressure is due to malaria control alone is questionable. It was calculated above that before malaria control 9 per cent of the population lived in hyperendemic areas, and 25 per cent in hypoendemic areas. On the basis of this information, it seems unlikely that malaria control was *the* major factor in population growth. Indirectly, it may have influenced population growth by enabling households to obtain more land and to improve their nutritional status. And by assisting in the exploitation of new land it may have helped to postpone the conflict between a growing population and a limited supply of land.

Overall gains and losses from malaria control

The estimates of the gains and losses resulting from malaria control can now be summarized (see Table 2.7). The values in Table 2.7 represent the approximate values of the gains and losses for an 'average' hectare of land gained. While the losses in the source area of migrants and the costs of malaria control would remain the same regardless of the quality of the land brought under cultivation, the returns to land and labour would be higher (or lower), the more (or less) fertile the land.

The figures in Table 2.7 suggest that the cost of malaria control was insignificant in relation to the returns from settlement. It was also considerably less than the cost of other investments required to open up the new land. Even if the cost of malaria control is added to the costs of agricultural investment, the gains from settlement still greatly exceed the cost of opening up the land. This conclusion is strengthened by the probable underestimation of investment costs: costs are divided by a figure of hectares cultivated which is probably too low, thus exaggerating unit costs per hectare. The most crucial estimates affecting the balance of gains and losses would appear not to be the resources invested, but rather the projected losses in the source areas of migrants. Several appraisals

Table 2.7 *The value of gains and losses associated with malaria control (1980 prices)*

Category	Gains	Losses
Marginal product of land	Max. of Rs 1300 per ha and probably rather less	
Marginal product of settlers	Approx Rs 2700 per ha	
Loss of marginal product of land in source areas of migrants		Unknown but probably small
Loss of marginal product of settlers in source areas		Approx Rs 1200
Loss of marginal product of forested land		Minimum of Rs 220–400 per ha of agricultural land gained
Cost of malaria control		Average of Rs 25 per ha per year of control programme
Cost of agricultural investment		Rs 63–110 per ha per year
Ecological damage		Unknown
Gains and losses of indigenous population in settlement areas	Unknown	Unknown
Increased output and productivity of indigenous population	Small	
Costs associated with larger population		Only to a small extent attributable to malaria control

and evaluations of agricultural settlement, while varying in the estimated rate of return, confirm that net returns from settlement (allowing for losses in source areas) were positive (UNDP/FAO 1974; IBRD 1978; IBRD 1983).

Hence, on efficiency criteria, Nepal clearly gained from the new land. However, several authors have commented on its adverse equity effects, both between the Terai and the Hill and within the Terai. Those who gained sufficient land in the Terai prospered in comparison with Hill families. Within the Terai, migrants who failed to obtain land, or who obtained land but were forced to sell through indebtedness, produced an increase in the group of landless labourers. In some of the older settlement schemes, land ownership has intended to become increasingly concentrated (Elder *et al.* 1976). In addition the indigenous population, particularly the Tharus, were affected adversely.

Conclusions

The overall conclusions of this study can now be stated. Before malaria control, large parts of the Terai were well-settled and productive, supporting approximately 25 per cent of the population of Nepal, and producing surpluses for export and consumption elsewhere in Nepal. In these areas, malaria was hypoendemic, and the predominant parasite species was *P. vivax*, resulting in a background of relatively minor illness punctuated by occasional severe epidemics. The Inner Terai, the Far West Terai, and the extreme East Terai were heavily forested and sparsely settled (possessing around 9 per cent of Nepal's population), and experienced hyperendemic malaria, principally from *P. falciparum*. The indigenous population developed immunity to the extent that adults probably experienced only mild bouts of fever, but at the cost of a relatively high infant mortality. Migrants to these areas were extremely vulnerable to malaria, and thus malaria inhibited further settlement.

In both hypoendemic and hyperendemic areas there were important influences, other than malaria, that inhibited greater settlement. In hypoendemic areas these included unfavourable land-tenure systems and heavy taxation; as for the hyperendemic areas, the government valued their inaccessibility as a barrier to invasion.

The main economic effect of malaria control measures was to encourage migration to the Inner Terai and the far East and West Terai. The experience of the West Inner Terai suggests that settlement was possible even in the absence of malaria control, and that clearing the land for cultivation itself produced some measure of environmental control. However, the malaria control programme removed the risk of malaria, and thus made settlement easier, and also had an important psychological effect on potential Hill migrants, since malaria had been much feared.

Estimates of the probable value of gains and losses from land settlement suggest that expenditures on malaria control were a relatively minor component of the overall cost of making the new land productive. The total gains from land settlement seem to have outweighed the total losses, though the size of the net gains from settlement depended crucially on the extent to which the returns to land, labour, and capital were greater in the newly settled areas than in the source areas of the migrants.

To a considerable extent, the expansion of the land area culti-vated has enabled Nepal to cope with her expanding population. Yet most of the gains in terms of land area have now been realized, with little further land remaining suitable for cultivation. The intensity of land use is considerably less in the Terai than in the Hills, suggesting that it may still be possible to increase production by increasing labour inputs, though the lack of capital available to subsistence farmers is a major hindrance to increased output.

In already settled areas, it seems unlikely that malaria control led to major increases in productivity, since parasite rates before control had been relatively low. It is also difficult to attribute to malaria control a major role in reducing mortality rates and in increasing fertility rates and thus population growth. Mortality rates were falling before malaria control, and their continued decline was more likely to have been due to a complex mix of factors, including a number of disease-control programmes and improved nutritional status, than to a reduction in malaria alone.

Changes in the Terai over the last twenty to thirty years have drastically changed the environment, and thus vector habitats: *A. minimus*, formerly the main vector in hyperendemic areas, has apparently disappeared. The relative success of the control programme means that the human population is now presumably more vulnerable to malaria; an additional threat comes from recent identification of chloroquine-resistant strains of parasite in Nepal. It would be unwise, therefore, to conclude that because malaria probably did not have severe adverse effects on labour productivity in the past, it might not affect labour productivity in the future. However, as important from the point of view of human welfare are the morbidity and mortality consequences of malaria epidemics. It is vital, therefore, that policy-makers should assess not merely the issue tackled in this chapter, the economic benefits of control, but also the efficient mix of control measures.

References

Acharya, M. and Bennett, L. (1982). *Women and the subsistence sector. Economic participation and household decision making in Nepal*, World Bank Staff Working Papers No. 526. World Bank, Washington DC.

Banister, J. and Thapa, S. (1981). *The population dynamics of Nepal*, Papers of the East-West Population Institute, No. 78. East-West Centre, Honolulu.

Blaikie, P., Cameron, J., and Seddon, D. (1980). *Nepal in crisis: growth and stagnation at the periphery*. Oxford University Press.

Cassen, R.H. (1981). Population and development: a survey. In *Recent issues in world development*, (ed. P. Streeten and R. Jolly), pp. 1–51. Pergamon Press, Oxford.

CBS (Central Bureau of Statistics) (1985). Data users' seminar on 'Intercensal changes of some key census variables, Nepal 1952/4–81'. Kathmandu, Nepal.

Chapagani, D.P. (1976). Agricultural productivity pattern in Nepal and its regional variations. In *Research, productivity and mechanization in Nepalese agriculture* (ed. B. Dhungana), pp. 20–35. Centre for Economic Development Administration, Kathmandu.

Dahal, D.R., Rai, N.K., and Manzardo, A.E. (1977). *Land and migration in far-western Nepal*. Institute of Nepal and Asian Studies, Tribhuvan University, Kathmandu.

Dixon, J.A. (1975). Report on the agricultural sector in Nepal with an emphasis on irrigated and forest land in the Terai. (Mimeograph.)

Elder, J.W., Ale, M., Evans, M.A., Gillespie, D.P., Nepali, R.K., Poudyal, S.P., and Smith, B.P. (1976). *Planned resettlement in Nepal's Terai*. Institute of Nepal and Asian Studies, Tribhuvan University, Kathmandu.

ESCAP (Economic and Social Commission of Asia and the Pacific) (1979). *Population of Nepal*. ESCAP, Bangkok.

Gurung, H. (1982). *Population increase in Nepal 1971–81*, New Era Occasional Paper No 004. New Era, Kathmandu.

IBRD (International Bank for Reconstruction and Development) (1974). *Nepal Agricultural Sector Survey*. World Bank, Washington DC.

IBRD (International Bank for Reconstruction and Development) (1975).

A review of major issues related to Nepal's development prospects.
World Bank, Washington DC.
IBRD (International Bank for Reconstruction and Development). (1978).
Nepal Forestry Sector Review. World Bank, Washington DC.
IBRD (International Bank for Reconstruction and Development) (1980).
Agricultural Sector Review. World Bank, Washington DC.
IBRD (International Bank for Reconstruction and Development) (1982).
Kingdom of Nepal. Report on Population Strategy. World Bank,
Washington DC.
IBRD (International Bank for Reconstruction and Development) (1983).
Nepal Settlement Project, Project performance audit report No 4567.
World Bank, Washington DC.
Jamison, D.T. (1980). *Notes on human resources and development in
Nepal.* The World Bank, Washington DC.
Kansakar, V.B.S. (1977). *Population censuses of Nepal and the problems
of data analyses.* Centre for Economic Development and Administra-
tion, Tribhuvan University, Kathmandu.
Kansakar, V.B.S. (1979). *Effectiveness of planned resettlement pro-
grammes in Nepal.* Centre for Economic Development and Admin-
istration, Tribhuvan University, Kathmandu.
Khadka, K.R. and Lohani, I.R. (1981). *Effects of population pressure on
land tenure, agricultural productivity and employment in Chitwan and
Tanahun districts.* Centre for Economic Development and Administra-
tion, Tribhuvan University, Kathmandu.
Kirkpatrick, W. (1811). *An account of the Kingdom of Nepal.* Reprinted
1969, Manjusri Publishing House, New Delhi.
Lal Das, A.K. (1982). *An analysis of total factor productivity in Nepalese
agriculture.* Centre for Economic Development and Administration,
Tribhuvan University, Kathmandu.
Landon, P. (1928). *Nepal.* Constable, London.
McDougal, C. (1968). *Village and household economy in Far West Nepal.*
Tribhuvan University, Kathmandu.
Mills, A. (1985). Economic evaluation of health programmes. Application
of the principles in developing countries. *World Health Statistics Quar-
terly,* **38** (4), 368–82.
Mills, A. (1987). *Economic study of malaria in Nepal. The cost-
effectiveness of malaria control strategies.* Evaluation and Planning
Centre, London School of Hygiene and Tropical Medicine.
Mills, A. (1988). *The impact of malaria control on the economic devel-
opment of Nepal.* London School of Hygiene and Tropical Medicine.
Mills, A. (1989). The application of cost-effectiveness analysis to disease
control programmes in developing countries, with special reference
to malaria control in Nepal. Unpublished Ph.D. thesis, University
of London.
Mills, A.J. and Colbourne, M.J. (1985). *Economic study of malaria
in Nepal: analysis of data collected by the NMEO and ICHSDP.*
Evaluation and Planning Centre, London School of Hygiene and
Tropical Medicine.
Ministry of Agriculture (1981/2). *Farm management study in the selected*

districts of the Hills and Terai of the Central Development Region
of Nepal. Economic Analysis Division, Department of Food and
Agricultural Marketing Services, Kathmandu.

Ministry of Economic Planning (1962). *Sample census of agriculture.* The
Ministry, Kathmandu.

Ministry of Food and Agriculture (1971). *Farm management study in the
selected regions of Nepal, 1968–9.* Economic Analysis and Planning
Division, Kathmandu.

Ministry of Food and Agriculture (1972). *Agricultural statistics of Nepal.*
The Ministry, Kathmandu.

Ministry of Food and Agriculture (1981). *Nepal's experience in hill
agricultural development.* The Ministry, Kathmandu.

National Planning Commission. Secretariat (1978). *Employment, income
distribution and consumption patterns in Nepal. 1976/7.* The Commission, Kathmandu.

NMEO (Nepal Malaria Eradication Organization) (1966). *Revised plan
of operations for malaria eradication.* NMEO, Kathmandu.

NMEO (Nepal Malaria Eradication Organization) (1970) *Global Strategy
Review.* NMEO, Kathmandu.

Pant, Y.P. (1983). *Population growth and employment opportunities in
Nepal.* Oxford and IBH Publishing Co, New Delhi.

Pant, Y.R. and Jain, S.C. (1969). *Agricultural development in Nepal.*
Vora and Co. Bombay.

Phillips, J. (1925). A preliminary report on a malarial survey carried out
in the valley between the Churria and Mahabharat ranges of Hills.
(Unpublished.)

Population Commission (1983). *Report of a survey on migration.* The
Commission, Kathmandu.

Prescott, N.M. (1979). *The economics of malaria, filariasis and human
trypanosomisasis,* Paper prepared for the Special Programme for
Research and Training in Tropical Diseases. WHO, Geneva.

Pudaisani, S.P. (1976). *Resource productivity, income and employment in
traditional and mechanized farming: an empirical evidence from Bara
district, Nepal.* Centre for Economic Development and Administration,
Tribhuvan University, Kathmandu.

Rana, R.S.J.B. (1971). *An economic study of the area round the alignment
of the Dhanagadi-Dandeldhura Road, Nepal.* Centre for Economic
Development and Administration, Tribhuvan University, Kathmandu.

Rana, R.S.J.B. and Thapa, Y.S. (1974). *Population migration in Nepal.
Seminar on population and development.* Centre for Economic Development and Administration, Kathmandu.

Reejal, P.R. (1979). *Integration of women in development. The case of
Nepal.* Vol. 1, part 5 of *The status of women in Nepal.* Centre for
Economic Development and Administration, Tribhuvan University,
Kathmandu.

Regmi, M.C. (1976). *Landownership in Nepal.* University of California
Press, Berkeley.

Regmi, M.C. (1978). *Thatched huts and stucco palaces. Peasants and
landlords in 19th century Nepal.* Vikas Publishing House, New Delhi.

Sainju, M.M. and Ram, B.K.C. (undated). *Hill labour migration: issues and problems*. Centre for Economic Development and Administration, Tribhuvan University, Kathmandu.

Sakiyama, T. (1971). *International assistance to Nepalese agriculture. Subsectoral and project analysis (1951–70)*, EADP Staff Paper No 4. Ministry of Food and Agriculture, Kathmandu.

Seddon, D. (1984). *Nepal – a state of poverty*, Monographs in Development No 11. School of Development Studies, University of East Anglia.

Taylor, C.E. (1965). Health and population. *Foreign Affairs*, **43**, 475–86.

Tuladhar, J.M., Gubhaju, B.B., and Stockel, J. (1977). *The population of Nepal: structure and change*. University of California Center for South and Southeast Asian Studies Research Monograph No 17. University of California, Berkeley.

UNDP (1972). *Nepal country background paper*. UNDP, New York.

UNDP/FAO (1974). *Forest development, Nepal. Land use*. UNDP, New York.

White, G.B. (1982). *Malaria receptivity stratification and projections for malaria vector control in Nepal*, Assignment Report, 1 September – 29 October 1980, and 24 August – 21 October 1981 SEA/MAL/144. WHO, SEARO, New Delhi.

Willan, R.G.H. (1967). Forestry in Nepal. (Unpublished report.)

Author's note

The study reported here formed part of a larger study on economic aspects of malaria control in Nepal, funded by the Overseas Development Administration of the British Government. The information for this study was collected in a visit to Nepal by the author and Dr M. Colbourne, Department of Tropical Hygiene, London School of Hygiene and Tropical Medicine. Dr Colbourne reviewed the history of malaria control and the records of the National Malaria Eradication Organization (NMEO) on population change: his vital contribution is gratefully acknowledged. Staff of the NMEO were most helpful in searching out their library material and in supplementing written evidence with their personal recollections. Thanks are particularly due to Dr M.B. Parajuli, formerly Chief of the NMEO, and Mr S. L. Shrestha, formerly Deputy Chief of the NMEO. I am also most grateful to my colleagues in the Health Policy Unit for commenting on earlier drafts. The last phase of this study was completed when the author was head of the ODA-supported Health Economics and Financing Programme.

3

Health-sector disparities in Peru

Dieter K. Zschock

Introduction

This chapter summarizes some of the major findings of a comprehensive study, the Health Sector Analysis of Peru (HSAP),
carried out in 1985–6 by a team of Peruvian and international
researchers (HSAP 1986). The HSAP was designed to test the
premiss – shared by Peruvian health-sector authorities and foreign
aid officials – that current patterns of resource-allocation in the
country's health sector were inappropriate for the implementation
of the Peruvian government's major health-sector policy goal: to
make primary health care (PHC) and essential hospital services
geographically and financially accessible to all Peruvians within the
five-year term of the government elected in 1985. The HSAP also
examined the impact of the previous government's reduction of its
financial commitment to health care in response to Peru's serious
economic recession of 1982–3. This reduction came at a time when
the need for health services was greater than ever before, and
as foreign donors were attempting to assist the government in
implementing its policy of expanding primary health care (PHC)
coverage.

In examining the disparity between the health sector's resource-
allocation and its policy mandate, it became clear to HSAP
researchers that virtually no information existed on the organization, expenditure, and coverage of the private health sector in
Peru, or on its interaction with the public sector. Thus agreements
were reached to undertake the extensive data-gathering efforts
required for a comprehensive health-sector analysis.

The HSAP differed from other health-sector assessments, of
the type carried out at the initiative of the World Bank or
the US Agency for International Development (USAID), in
its organization, backing, and participation. Expenditure and
coverage of health services were analysed for all three major
components of the health sector: the Ministry of Health (MOH),

the Peruvian Institute of Social Security (IPSS), and private health-care organizations. The HSAP therefore contrasts with many previous health-sector studies which have focused on ministries of health (partly because of data limitations in the other two components of the sector, and partly because most public international aid is channelled through health ministries). The HSAP was designed to be carried out primarily for the direct benefit of Peruvian health-sector policy-makers, and with the full participation of Peruvian health-sector institutions and professionals. The study was planned jointly by the State University of New York at Stony Brook and the Pan-American Health Organization (PAHO), which together provided technical assistance and administered the study's funds. Its design and implementation were approved by the Peruvian MOH and IPSS. Professionals who participated in the study were drawn primarily from these four organizations, as well as from two Peruvian institutions of higher education and a US consulting firm (see Author's note).

The design of the HSAP drew upon several health-care financing guides (see Cumper 1986), and reflected the recommendations for health-care financing analysis synthesized by the World Bank (1987). The HSAP's concern for the impact of economic recession on health-sector expenditures was foreshadowed by PAHO research on this issue (PAHO 1986), and the in-depth studies of social security and private-sector financing and coverage drew upon the author's work (Zschock 1986) and a report prepared by the Group Health Association of America (GHAA 1985).

But the HSAP, as a study of organization and resource-allocation rather than merely financing, was more broadly conceived than even these references might suggest. It compared the expenditure and coverage of the health sector's three main components – MOH, IPSS, and private – with their respective allocation of physical, human, and pharmaceutical resources. It also related financial and real resource-allocation to the geographical distribution of the Peruvian population. It is these supply-side elements of the study that are summarized in this chapter, although the HSAP also produced in-depth studies of the population's health status and of household and community demand for health services.

The project involved an exhaustive inventory and review of Peruvian and international primary databases and reference materials, now available in a computerized documentation base in PAHO's offices in Lima, Peru. All primary datasets used in the HSAP were created from raw data provided by Peruvian health-sector institutions and the country's national statistical institute.

Aggregate health-sector spending

In 1984 health care – including all public- and private-sector services – comprised 4.5 per cent of GDP. Between 1981 and 1984, a period of steadily worsening economic conditions in Peru, the country's aggregate health-sector expenditure remained stable in relative terms, but declined in absolute terms from US $813 million to $732 million, a 10 per cent reduction over four years (Table 3.1). During the same period, the per capita income of Peruvians declined 16 per cent. While the health sector as a whole inevitably suffered the consequences of the country's economic recession, in general it appears to have maintained its standing relative to other sectors of the economy.

The decline in aggregate health expenditures would have been more precipitous had it not been for an increase in spending on private health services as the Peruvian population, increasingly disenchanted with public health care, turned in greater numbers to the private sector. The expenditure of the MOH and IPSS declined by 16 and 26 per cent respectively, with an overall

Table 3.1 *Sectorial composition of health expenditures, 1981–1984 (totals in millions of US dollars)*

Sector	1981 Total	%	1982 Total	%	1983 Total	%	1984 Total	%
Public sector:								
MOH	238	29	213	27	201	28	201	27
IPSS	304	37	301	38	229	32	240	33
Other	53	7	52	7	45	7	46	6
Subtotal	595	73	566	72	475	67	487	66
Private sector	218	27	227	28	236	33	245	34
Health-sector total	813	100	793	100	711	100	732	100

decline in public spending of some 20 per cent. However, this fall was partially offset by a 12 per cent increase in expenditure on private care. The effect of these 1981–1984 trends was a reduction in public expenditure from 73 to 66 per cent of the health-sector total, and a corresponding increase in the private share from 27 to 34 per cent.

Since the mid-1970s, public-sector health expenditure in Peru has declined relative to central government expenditure, suggesting that public health has declined in importance among government priorities – most sharply during the economic crisis of the early 1980s. MOH expenditure was reduced from 4.9 per cent to 4.2 per cent between 1981 and 1984, and had still not recovered by 1985. IPSS spending declined from 6.3 per cent to 5.0 per cent of central government expenditure (Table 3.2). The somewhat offsetting increase in private health-care spending suggested that household demand for health care may have been stronger than the government's commitment to this sector.

Foreign aid represented only about 2 per cent of total Peruvian health-sector expenditure in 1984. However, it accounted for one-third of the total MOH financial commitment to primary health care (PHC), estimated at US $50 million for 1984. Since Peru's return to democratic government in 1980, the World Bank, USAID, and the German Technical Assistance Agency had contributed a total of about US $40 million in loans and grants for health care in Peru. Although most of the World Bank loan and some USAID funds remained unspent by mid-1985, foreign donor support increased in four years from almost nothing to about 5 per cent of total MOH revenues annually. At the same time, MOH transfer payments to private-sector voluntary organizations (PVOs) declined from 12 per cent to only 1 per cent of the MOH

Table 3.2 *MOH and IPSS expenditures on health care, 1981–1984 (as percentages of central government expenditures (CGE))*

Year	(1) MOH/CGE	(2) IPSS/CGE	(1) + (2)
1981	4.95	6.34	11.29
1982	4.58	6.47	11.05
1983	4.46	5.09	9.55
1984	4.19	5.02	9.21

annual budget. PVOs, which operated many primary health-care facilities in Peru, were typically affiliated with – and supported by – international, church-related charities. The reduction in MOH transfer payments thus demonstrated that the balance of primary health care financing in Peru had shifted from the private to the public sector.

Ministry of health expenditure

Of a total of about 19 million Peruvians, 11 million were medically indigent, meaning that they were unable to pay for anything beyond food, clothing, and shelter – if indeed they could afford even these most basic needs. The MOH was responsible for providing health care to these impoverished Peruvians, for exercising regulatory control over and providing policy guidance for the health sector as a whole, for promoting preventive health care, and for constructing potable water and basic sanitation facilities in rural areas. Yet the greater part of MOH resources were allocated not to these tasks, but to the delivery of curative medical care in urban hospitals.

The MOH accounted for about 27 per cent of total Peruvian health-sector expenditure (Table 3.1), a proportion that declined only modestly over the 1981–4 period. In absolute terms, however, the MOH had only about US $200 million to spend in 1984, compared with some US $238 million annually in 1981. Moreover, while the Ministry's financial resources were shrinking, Peru's population was increasing. Average per capita expenditures for the MOH target population thus dropped from about US $24 in 1981 to US $20 in 1984. MOH services, however, were accessible to less than half of the country's medically indigent, which meant that the actual per capita expenditure for the five million people the Ministry did reach was twice this average, or about US $40.

But, because of the onerous financial burden that its hospital services placed on the Ministry, only about one-quarter of total MOH expenditures were used to provide primary health care outside hospitals. This meant that actual MOH expenditure on PHC amounted to only about US $10 per capita for the estimated five million urban and rural poor for whom it provided health care. To compound the problem, much of this care was ineffective, since many MOH health centres and posts were poorly maintained, understaffed, and undersupplied. In 1984, in an attempt to alleviate this problem, the MOH created a new budget category, earmarking close to 10 per cent of its total expenditure for medicines, training, and transport in support of PHC. Most of the expenditure in this new category was financed with foreign donor support, buffering what might otherwise have been a much greater decline in MOH expenditure between 1981 and 1984.

In addition to the elimination of transfer payments to PVOs, there was a reduction in MOH expenditure for physical facility investment and supplies, including essential medicines, whose availability in public health services declined drastically. In absolute terms, between 1981 and 1984, MOH investment in physical facilities declined by 56 per cent, and expenditure for medical supplies by 83 per cent. Spending for wages and pensions, on the other hand, increased over the period, both in relative and absolute terms. For the MOH as a whole, including both national-and regional-level expenditure, the wage share increased from 58 to 70 per cent of recurrent expenditure, and pension payments rose from 4 to almost 9 per cent. In absolute terms, these increases represented a rise of almost 9 per cent in wage payments, and a near-doubling of pension disbursements, in a period of overall decline in financial resource availability. Medical personnel were thus the main beneficiaries of MOH spending priorities.

Regional-level expenditure (for 16 health regions, covering 25 states) represented over 80 per cent of total MOH recurrent spending in 1984, compared to 75 per cent in 1981. At the regional level, the wage share rose from 70 to 79 per cent of expenditure, while supplies declined from 19 to 15 per cent, and services such as maintenance remained a very low proportion. The regional distribution of MOH expenditure reflected the heavy concentration of public hospital facilities and medical personnel in Peru's major urban states. The metropolitan areas of Lima/Callao, Ica, and Arequipa, with 39 per cent of the population, accounted for 59 per cent of all MOH regional expenditure in 1984. To the rest of the country, with 61 per cent of the population, the MOH allocated a mere 41 per cent of its total financial resources. The major urban states received an even more disproportionate 63 per cent of total MOH expenditure on medicines.

Institute of Social Security expenditure

IPSS, which provided health care for about 18 per cent (3.5 million) of the Peruvian population, spent considerably more than the MOH – US $240 million in 1984, or US $68 per capita. But annual expenditure exceeded the revenue of the Institute's medical care fund from 1977 to 1984, resulting in deficits that were financed by fiscally unsound internal transfers from the IPSS pension and invalidity funds. The roots of these annual deficits lay in two continuing problems: the government's failure, as an employer, to pay the full contribution for its employees covered by the IPSS medical care programme, and extensive evasion of social security payments by private-sector employers. In 1984/5 the Government increased its contributions, and IPSS improved its private-sector collections. In 1985, for the first time in a decade, the IPSS medical care programme had an annual surplus.

Medical care under IPSS has been one of the most expensive and least efficient programmes of its kind in Latin America. The Institute's internal debt may never be repaid; nor was it likely that the Government would make good on the contributions it owed as an employer. The result was that pensioners and invalids may suffer reductions in compensation from the funds to which they have contributed. Moreover, the Institute's medical coverage has been quite restrictive; until the early 1980s, dependants of workers were provided only with maternal and infant care. Legally mandated coverage was then extended to all dependent children up to the age of fourteen, but very few actually enrolled in the programme and held the identity card necessary to obtain medical services. Spouses' benefits were still limited to maternal care.

IPSS coverage was concentrated amongst urban wage-earners with stable employment. Fully 58 per cent of its beneficiaries lived in Lima/Callao, and the capital region accounted for 64 per cent of the Institute's total medical care expenditure. The composition of IPSS spending was similar to that of the MOH, in that wages represented about three-quarters of the total, although supplies, including medicines, accounted for about 20 per cent – a higher proportion than the MOH's meagre expenditure on this category. IPSS expenditure data revealed almost no capital outlays: construction and equipment purchases were financed by long-term, low-interest loans from the pension and invalidity funds, but these were not shown in IPSS medical programme accounts.

Reasons why the IPSS spent considerably more per capita on medical care than the MOH included its even greater reliance on hospital-based care, its very high administrative costs, and its wages, which were substantially higher than those paid by the MOH to employees with comparable qualifications.

Private health-care financing

Expenditures for private health care in Peru, estimated separately for medical services and pharmaceuticals in the HSAP, totalled approximately US $245 million in 1984, or about one-third of total health-sector expenditure. Only four million Peruvians obtained most of their medical services from private providers; but most purchased the majority of their pharmaceuticals directly from private pharmacies. Although the private sector operated only 18 per cent of all hospital beds and less than 5 per cent of all primary health centres and posts, it employed over half the medical doctors in the country, and accounted for 72 per cent of all pharmaceutical sales.

Among the four million Peruvians who relied primarily on private health services, about half a million paid for them directly. Another 400000 were covered by various risk-sharing mechanisms, 900000 belonged to co-operatives, and 2.2 million were beneficiaries of PVOs. While these estimates were derived from supply-side information, they were substantiated on the demand side: in 1984, the private health sector accounted for 37 per cent of all ambulatory visits in Lima and for 62 per cent in the urban areas of the mountain states.

Private health insurance had not existed in Peru until the mid-1970s, and prepaid health care managed by employers or providers was an even more recent development. The emergence and evolution of these risk-sharing mechanisms in the private health sector were intricately bound up with the country's declining economic situation and its effect on publicly-financed health services provided through the MOH and IPSS. Private risk-sharing mechanisms were attractive to a small minority of the population whose real income was relatively high, and also to a somewhat larger number of middle-class Peruvians whose real incomes had probably declined over the previous ten years but for whom the poor quality of public-sector services had made these no longer acceptable as the primary source of their ambulatory health care.

The risk-sharing market was developed and dominated by insurance companies and brokers working with major employers; but since 1982 prepaid plans offered by several large clinics had emerged as an important new private financing alternative. Four clinics in Lima offered prepaid family plans, with an estimated total of 40000 members. The subscription fees and services provided under these plans suggested that they primarily catered for middle-income families. The principal source of revenue for the clinics, however, remained user fees, paid directly by individuals or by insurance companies for those registered with them.

Co-operatives and PVOs together provided medical services for some 3.1 million Peruvians, the equivalent of about 24 per cent of all modern health-care coverage in Peru. They were therefore a major element in the Peruvian effort to provide basic health services at reasonable cost; but their economic viability may have been undermined during the country's severe recession.

Of 2000 co-operatives identified in a 1981 census, only 172 reported providing some form of health services to their members. In the urban areas, savings and loan associations were most likely to offer such services, while a number of agricultural co-operatives provided some health services in rural Peru. Urban co-operatives offering such services primarily benefited middle-income residents who belonged to savings and loan associations, especially workers' dependants, since household heads were typically covered through IPSS. Agricultural co-operatives, which accounted for over half of all co-operatives providing health services in 1982 (91 of 172), had smaller memberships, on the average, than savings and loan associations. Their financial resources, largely derived from levies on the sales of members' products, had always been very limited. Under these conditions, rural co-operatives' health services were restricted to some ambulatory health care and the purchase of medicines for their members. The only exceptions were the several sugar co-operatives that provided hospital services.

While co-operatives were indigenous entities receiving almost no external support, most PVOs providing health care were organized by international religious and other charitable groups. Moreover, while co-operatives charged members little or nothing in user fees, most PVOs charged patients substantial user fees. In 1982, 270 PVOs were in operation – most of them in co-operation with the MOH. It should be recalled that in 1982 the MOH was still providing substantial subsidies to the PVOs; these transfers started their precipitous decline in 1983. Whether, or to what extent, PVOs were able to offset the decline in MOH support for their operations, either from increased international donations or through increased user fee revenues, was not known.

In 1982, when PVOs served an estimated 2.2 million beneficiaries, close to 60 per cent of their expenditures and coverage were concentrated in the coastal cities. It was likely that PVOs did not primarily serve the medically indigent in the cities, since the user fees they charged required at least a lower-middle-class income. It was therefore safe to conclude that most PVOs operated at the borderline between the public and private health sectors in the coastal urban areas, and had average per capita expenditures similar to those estimated for PHC provided by the MOH (i.e., approximately US $10). Judging from field observations, however, the quality of their services might have been generally better than PHC services at MOH facilities.

In sum: the combined expenditures on modern medical care by households – both directly and indirectly, through various prepaid plans, co-operatives, and PVOs – totalled an estimated US $100 million in 1984. This included household expenditures for traditional health care by six million very poor Peruvians who were beyond the current reach of MOH services, estimated at US $34 million. Finally, private-sector pharmaceutical purchases totalled US $145 million in 1984, bringing the private health-sector expenditure total to US $245 million, as is shown in Table 3.1.

Supply of health services

Complementing its analysis of health-care financing, the HSAP analysed the supply of health services in Peru separately for physical facilities, medical personnel, and pharmaceuticals, emphasizing the relationship between both financial and real resource-allocation and population distribution. The heavy concentration of hospitals and medical doctors in the Lima/Callao metropolitan region was particularly striking. Since no comparable distribution data were available for pharmaceuticals, the HSAP examined why the government's efforts to promote the use of low-cost essential medicines in the public sector were largely unsuccessful.

Physical facility distribution

The sector-wide distribution of health facilities in 1985, compared with population distribution by states, revealed a severe imbalance: the heavily-urbanized states, representing 39 per cent of the population, accounted for 65 per cent of all hospital beds, and while these states' share of health centres equalled their population shares, they had only 18 per cent of all health posts in the country (Table 3.3). Conversely, the rest of the country had a less than proportional share of hospital beds, but a considerably larger than proportional share of health posts.

In accordance with its strong policy orientation toward primary health care expansion, Peru had, over the previous ten years, significantly increased the number of its health centres and posts. Without a corresponding superstructure of hospital facilities, however, the process of referring patients from lower levels of care could not work. On the other hand, with too few health posts in the major urban areas, urban residents necessarily had to use hospitals as a source of primary health care.

An analysis of the adequacy of health-care facilities should also include data on equipment inventories and the physical condition of buildings, public utility services, and equipment. Since such information was virtually non-existent in Peru, the HSAP undertook a survey of all MOH hospitals, health centres, and posts in two largely rural states, Cusco and Cajamarca. The results revealed that about half of all the utilities and items of equipment at those facilities were inoperative through disrepair.

Furthermore, the distribution of health-care facilities in the public sector was uneven. The MOH played a major role as a

Table 3.3 *Population and facility distribution, 1984*

States	Population Total (000)	%	Hosp. beds Total (000)	%	Health centres Total (000)	%	Health posts Total (000)	%
Urbanized states*	7566	39	19448	65	304	39	336	18
Rest of country†	12132	61	10536	35	481	61	1589	82
Total	19698	100	29984	100	785	100	1925	100

* Arequipa, Ica, Lima/Callao
† Twenty-two other states

provider of health care at all levels, administering 34 per cent of all hospitals and 54 per cent of all hospital beds (which shows that MOH hospitals tended to be relatively large); but these MOH facilities were located predominantly in the Lima/Callao metropolitan area. At the primary-care level, the MOH operated 78 per cent of all health centres and 89 per cent of all health posts. Referrals from health posts to hospitals were difficult, however, since most of these primary-care facilities were located in the disadvantaged rural states, and most hospitals in the more advantaged urban states.

The number of MOH hospital beds decreased somewhat over the 1980s as some of the oldest facilities were taken out of service, although the number and distribution of health centres and posts greatly improved. At the same time, the state of repair of most facilities seems to have worsened. Paradoxically, there was an excess supply of hospital beds in Lima/Callao, whereas more hospitals may have to be built in the predominantly rural states. Yet health centres and posts in these states – still insufficient in number – were in such bad repair that renovation, re-equipment, and the establishment of a well-organized maintenance programme may have been of higher priority than the construction of new facilities.

Medical personnel distribution

Human resources are, of course, the most important element in the delivery of health care. According to the 1981 census, Peru had a total of 52350 trained medical personnel for a population of 17 million. This total included 12500 doctors, 10200 nurses, 27000 paramedical workers, and 2650 pharmacists.

In order to estimate health-service accessibility, the HSAP calculated the ratios of medical personnel to population by states and provinces, and related these ratios to the presence or absence of medical schools or hospitals in state and provincial capitals (Table 3.4). This comparison clearly showed that medical personnel tended to concentrate where hospital facilities were located, leaving a large proportion of the Peruvian population beyond the normal reach of medical personnel and hospital facilities. The major urban areas (particularly Lima/Callao) not only enjoyed the highest ratios of doctors, nurses, and pharmacists to population, but also the highest concentration of paramedical personnel

Table 3.4 *Medical personnel – population ratios, 1981*

	Percentage of national population	Numbers of trained personnel per 10000 inhabitants			
		Doctors	Nurses	Paramedics	Pharmacists
Lima/Callao	27.1	17.0	10.7	27.8	3.3
State capitals with medical school	7.1	11.2	10.5	20.3	2.7
State capitals without medical school	18.9	4.0	5.5	15.4	1.0
Provincial capitals with hospital	30.9	2.1	2.4	10.7	0.6
Provincial capitals without hospital	16.0	0.5	0.8	3.7	0.1
National total or average	100.0	6.9	5.6	15.8	1.5

(mostly auxiliary nurses and health promoters), who were theoretically the principal staff of primary health-care delivery facilities in smaller towns and rural areas.

While health sector analyses in developing countries often focus on auxiliary nurses and health promoters because of their importance to primary health care, the HSAP focused on medical doctors. They accounted for over half of Peru's recurrent health-care expenditure, provided close to four-fifths of all medical care consultations, and were the main decision-makers in the health sector, directly or indirectly affecting all levels of health-care delivery.

In 1984, the distribution of doctors by subsector was decidedly unbalanced: 43 per cent worked in the public sector, and 57 per cent in the private sector. (Many MOH and IPSS doctors also worked in the private sector; but the data did not reflect this information.) The geographical maldistribution of doctors was even more pronounced. Some 67 per cent of all doctors were concentrated in Lima/Callao, and if the other state capitals with medical schools were added in, the concentration of doctors in state capitals climbed to 80 per cent. Only about one-third of the Peruvian population, however, had access to these doctors – a finding made all the more disturbing by the fact that 71 per cent of all doctors who worked primarily for the MOH were located in one urban area: Lima/Callao.

The analysis of why doctors chose to practise where they did was constrained by lack of information on compensation – surely an important determinant of doctors' location. Among the variables for which data were available, birthplace and place of professional training turned out to be significant determinants of where doctors practised. While the same type of analysis was not pursued for the other three categories for which comparable data were available, the descriptive evidence shown in Table 3.4 suggested that nurses, paramedical personnel, and pharmacists also preferred to locate themselves in the major urban areas, even though training institutions for these occupations tended to be more widely distributed in Peru than were medical schools.

The pharmaceuticals market

Appropriate medication, in adequate quantity and at affordable prices, is the third critical resource in the delivery of effective health care. Peru has tried since the early 1960s to develop an essential medicines programme in the public sector using generic drugs, but with little success. Medicines were usually in short supply in the health-care programmes of the MOH and IPSS. These two organizations, which together provided health care for close to half the Peruvian population, accounted for less than 20 per cent of total pharmaceutical expenditure; and less than half of this expenditure was for generic drugs.

Unlike other Latin American countries, Peru largely relied on the private sector to supply essential medicines for the public sector, rather than producing them through state enterprises. But the social objectives of the public sector have been in conflict with the economic motives of the private sector ever since the government began to experiment with essential medicines programmes. This experiment coincided with the emergence and relatively rapid expansion of domestic pharmaceutical production and distribution in the private sector.

Government price-controls on pharmaceutical sales through private pharmacies kept the prices of many brand-name ethical and over-the-counter pharmaceutical products not much higher than those of generic products sold to the public sector. However, the most significant result of price-controls, especially as these coincided with a notable decline in purchasing power, was a sharp reduction in the volume of pharmaceutical production and importation in Peru from 1980. The share of total sales represented by essential medicines, in terms of both volume and expenditure, remained small. Moreover, essential medicines programmes were directed by the MOH, but the main users of the available supplies were the IPSS, the armed forces, and the police. In MOH health-care facilities essential medicines and other supplies were usually in very short supply, because the Ministry's budget allocated only about 5 per cent of its revenue to pharmaceuticals.

The result was a policy contradiction. Health care for the majority of Peruvians was a public-sector responsibility, but pharmaceutical production and distribution was largely a private-sector activity subject to severely inhibiting government control – a situation that contributed significantly to the ineffectiveness of Peruvian public-sector health care. While distribution data for medicines were lacking, it was quite apparent that the MOH had a serious shortage of medicines for its primary health-care programmes. The population outside the major urban centres may have had access to private pharmacies, but, without access to medical doctors for prescriptions or even to qualified pharmacists for advice, many Peruvians were left without appropriate guidance in buying medicines.

Conclusions and recommendations

The disparity in Peru between health-sector resource allocation and population distribution was most clearly evident in the following conclusions of the HSAP. Firstly, the MOH, with 27 per cent of total health-sector expenditure, might at first glance seem adequately financed in relation to its population coverage of 26 per cent. But three-quarters of MOH resources were spent on urban hospital services, while a third of the population had no access whatsoever to modern health care.

Secondly, IPSS expenditure for medical care – 34 per cent of the health-sector total for an 18 per cent population coverage – was much higher, on a per capita basis, than that of the MOH. The difference was primarily due to higher IPSS wage-rates, better equipment, and more medicines; but it was by no means clear that these added up to more satisfactory services. Indeed, the increase in private insurance coverage suggested growing dissatisfaction with IPSS services.

Thirdly, the private health sector, which provided ambulatory services for between one-third and two-thirds of the urban population, accounted for one-third of total health-sector expenditure. A more serious imbalance in private health care, however, was that it administered only 18 per cent of all hospital beds, but accounted for over half of all medical doctors. Since physicians tended to practise near hospitals, it was likely that many of them provided ambulatory care privately, but treated patients in the public sector when hospitalization was needed, thus contributing to the financial burden of the public sector.

These conclusions suggested the following recommendations. Both the MOH and IPSS should significantly improve the quality of their existing services before greatly expanding their health-care coverage. Public-sector financial resources were insufficient for the achievement of both quality and coverage objectives in the short run. The new government's intention to expand coverage through the construction of more PHC facilities, with no apparent increase in the MOH operating budgets, would not help to increase the confidence of the public. Significant expansion of coverage was unlikely to be effective as long as public health services did not enjoy the confidence of the population they were intended to serve.

More specifically, the MOH should work to improve the quality of its primary health care. This required reallocating some expenditure from hospitals to health centres and posts, and could be accomplished in a number of ways: by closing more of its most antiquated hospitals; by improving the maintenance of buildings and equipment at the remaining hospitals and primary health-care facilities; by turning over the operation of some hospitals to private-sector health-care providers (including PVOs); by reassigning medical personnel from public hospitals to primary health-care facilities; and by providing all public health services with adequate quantities of essential medicines. There was no indication in the new government's stated health-sector policy that these priorities were being attended to, other than to limit public hospital investment to the completion of several facilities under construction.

The medical care programme of IPSS should implement its recent mandate to provide health care to insured workers' children – an estimated 2.5 million of them. Coverage for these children would significantly reduce pressure on MOH services in urban areas. IPSS efforts to reduce employer-contribution evasion, together with an agreement by the government as employer to pay its required contribution in full, should make this expansion of coverage possible. IPSS should also implement its intended expansion of coverage in rural areas, under an agreement with rural co-operatives. Policy statements issued by the IPSS president in 1985 indicated that all of these measures were to be implemented.

The potential for expansion of the still-small private health-insurance industry in Peru should not be overlooked in sector-wide health planning. In particular, those who could afford to pay for private health care should be excluded from publicly-funded services, or public services should be made available to those who could afford to pay at fees equivalent to those charged by private health care providers. Either alternative would help stimulate demand for private health insurance and other types of prepayment arrangements.

In order to achieve better co-ordination between public and private health services, major private-sector institutions (such as insurance companies, the health funds of large employers, urban and rural co-operatives, and private voluntary organizations) should be invited to join the MOH and IPSS in comprehensive health-sector planning. The more affluent groups of the population should have their IPSS coverage co-ordinated with supplementary private insurance and employer health funds. Access to MOH hospital services for the middle-and lower-level income groups, whose employment may not provide IPSS coverage, should depend on referral from the ambulatory care they may receive from co-operatives or PVOs.

The HSAP differed from other health-sector analyses in two major respects. First, in terms of process, its extensive host-country participation not only facilitated access to information but also guaranteed that the study would be accepted as an indigenous effort rather than rejected as a foreign one. Indeed, the equal participation of host-country and international institutions and individual professionals might profitably be emulated in other health-sector analyses. Second, in terms of product, the HSAP's focus on three relationships – between health-sector performance and the country's general economic situation, between financial and real resources, and between resource-allocation and the population's distribution – resulted in a much more comprehensive analysis than a primary focus on financing could have provided. It is strongly recommended that future analyses should enlarge their focus from health-care financing alone to these three important relationships.

References

Cumper, G. (1986). *Health sector financing: estimating health expenditure in developing countries.* Evaluation and Planning Centre for Health Care, London School of Hygiene and Tropical Medicine.

GHAA (Group Health Association of America) (1985). *Managed prepaid health care in Latin America and the Caribbean: a critical assessment* (Vols. I–III). Group Health Association of America, Inc., Washington, DC.

HSAP (Health Sector Analysis of Peru) (1986). *Health sector analysis of Peru technical reports.* Department of Economics, State University of New York at Stony Brook, New York.

  (a) Zschock, D.K. *Health sector analysis of Peru: summary and recommendations.*
  (b) Gomez, L.C. *Health status of the Peruvian population.*
  (c) Gertler, P. Locay, L., and Sanderson, W. *The demand for health care in Peru: Lima and the urban sierra, 1984.*
  (d) Davidson, J.R. *Health and community participation in Peru.*
  (e) Carrillo, E.R. *Health care facilities in Peru.*
  (f) Locay, L. *Medical doctors in Peru.*
  (g) Gereffi, G. *Pharmaceuticals in Peru.*
  (h) Mesa-Lago, C. *Coverage and costs of medical care under social security in Peru.*
  (i) Zschock, D.K. *Health care financing in Peru.*

PAHO (Pan-American Health Organization) (1986). *Health conditions in the Americas, 1981–1984* (Vol. I). Pan-American Health Organization, Washington, DC.

World Bank (1987). *Financing health services in developing countries: an agenda for reform.* World Bank, Washington, DC.

Zschock, D.K. (1986). Medical care under social insurance in Latin America. *Latin American Research Review*, **XXI**, (1), 99–122.

Author's note

The HSAP, directed jointly by the author and a Peruvian study co-ordinator (initially Dr Julio Castaneda and subsequently Dr Walter

Torres), was carried out under a grant from the US Agency for International Development. Co-operating institutions included the State University of New York at Stony Brook; the Pan-American Health Organization; the International Resources Group, Ltd., of Stony Brook, New York; and the Universidad Peruana Cayetano Heredia and Escuela de Administración de Negocios para Graduados, both of Lima, Peru. These five institutions provided the services of 70 professionals – 47 Peruvians and 23 others – who collectively carried out the research for the study. The author is indebted to all these participants for a magnificent collaborative effort, but absolves them from any responsibility for the contents of this chapter.

4

The development, growth, and distribution of public and private medical resources in the Philippines

Charles C. Griffin and Vincent B. Paqueo

Introduction

A striking feature of primary health programmes, and more generally of government health planning, is a failure to realize that the government is one among many providers of health services in developing countries. Even if we disregard the 'informal' parts of medical systems – traditional healers and midwives, private drug-sellers, and after-hours practices of government physicians – in most countries, sizeable numbers of modern allopathic providers and facilities operate fee-for-service, charitable, or mission facilities outside the government's system.

Although a few governments in Africa do co-ordinate their health activities with mission facilities, and South American countries depend partially on the private sector to deliver health services for their social security systems, for the most part governments and the international health community have neglected these other providers and how people use them. The private sector is often ignored in developing countries because it is assumed to be small and to serve only an urban élite clientele. Recently, the debate over the public and private medical sectors in developing countries has intensified. Some seek to assert more control over it; others see its growth as a natural reaction to the government's inability to provide adequate services; and still others continue to view it as largely irrelevant to health policy.

Few countries have collected detailed data on private health-providers, so there is almost no information about the size, distribution, and service characteristics of the private sector. A review of the limited information and available literature on service-utilization patterns in developing countries suggests extensive use of non-government providers in both urban and rural areas (Akin *et al.* 1985). Aggregate expenditure estimates indicate that private spending as a proportion of total health expenditure is highest among the poorest countries (World Bank 1987). Household expenditure surveys in a number of developing countries suggest that the poorest households may spend a higher percentage of their income on health care than do high-income households, even when free government care is available (Griffin 1987).

Such utilization and expenditure patterns indicate that the non-government sector is a significant part of many countries' health systems, and may indeed serve a broader spectrum of the population than was hitherto believed. This possibility raises a number of health-policy questions, including the proper role of government in providing and financing curative care; whether governments duplicate or complement other service-delivery systems; which income-groups actually do benefit from public subsidies intended for the poor; the relative efficiency of government and private systems; and whether public systems perform better than private systems in achieving desired health-sector goals. For the most part, these issues cannot be evaluated until information about the private sector is collected.

This chapter is primarily a descriptive analysis illustrating – for the Philippines – the types of information that can be collected, and what such data can reveal about the health-care system. The historical development of public and private medical services in the Philippines is summarized as a preliminary to then analysing the size, distribution, and growth of those services. Survey data describing the availability of services in the public and private sectors in one region are presented. The chapter concludes with a description of the geographical distribution of personnel and lower-level facilities in the Philippines.

International comparisons

Table 4.1 contrasts aspects of the Philippines' health system with those of its sister countries in the Association of Southeast Asian Nations (ASEAN) and two high-income countries, Japan and the United States, for the period relating to the data presented in this study. Life-expectancy figures for Malaysia, Thailand, and the Philippines were broadly comparable with each other, although some 10 to 12 years lower than in the US and Japan. Singapore had achieved parity with the two high-income countries on most measures of health, but at a much lower level of per capita income. Indonesia's mortality statistics were considerably worse than those of its neighbours.

In relation to most ASEAN countries other than Singapore, population densities were high, with a high proportion of the Philippine population living in urban areas. Although physicians-to-population rates in the Philippines were average for the region, such settlement patterns meant that even urban-based physicians were accessible to a relatively high percentage of the Filipino population. One notable aspect of these statistics is the low ratio of physicians to nurses in the Philippines, a situation which will be discussed in more detail later. Private hospitals, including both charitable and profit-making institutions, accounted for at least a third of the hospital facilities for those countries included in this table.

Historical development of the Philippine medical system

The Government sector

Under American colonial rule, the first nine government hospitals were opened between 1898 and 1923, and provincial and municipal boards of health established. Between 1923 and 1957 – a period spanning both the Japanese occupation during the Second World War and the end of American colonial rule in 1946 – over seventy additional hospitals were built. Thus, by the early 1950s, a substantial public hospital infrastructure was in place. It continued to expand, reaching 506 hospitals and 35334 beds by 1983.

Rural Health Units (RHUs), government-run clinics providing general outpatient, maternal, and preventive care, began to be established in 1953. By 1954 there were 81 RHUs, expanding to 1991 RHUs by 1983. In 1978, as part of the Philippines' primary health-care strategy, the health system was restructured and the term *RHU* redefined to encompass not only the clinic itself (the Main Health Centre) but also Barangay Health Stations staffed by trained midwives. Each midwife supervised several Barangay Health Workers, who were the main practitioners in the Philippines' primary health-care strategy. By 1981 over 7000

Table 4.1 *Comparison of Philippine medical statistics with those of other ASEAN Nations, Japan, and the United States*

	Government Expenditure		Income	Demography		Facilities and personnel				Measures of health	
	Central gov't expenditure to health (percentage of total)	Central gov't expenditure (percentage of GNP)	GNP per capita (US dollars)	Pop. density (per square kilometre)	Urban pop. (percentage of total)	Pop. per doctor (no.)	Pop. per nurse (no.)	Pop. per bed (no.)	Gov't hospitals (percentage of total)	Infant mortality rate (per 1000 live births)	Life expectancy at birth (years)
Year	1981	1980	1982	1977	1982	1980	1980	1977	1977	1982	1982
Indonesia	2.5	27	580	75	22	11530	2300	1560	55	102	53
Malaysia	4.4	41	1860	38	30	7910	940	270	28	29	67
Philippines	5.0	13	820	150	38	7970	6000	640	37	51	64
Singapore	7.2	25	5910	3973	100	1150	320	280	—	11	72
Thailand	4.3	19	790	86	17	7100	2400	800	58	51	63
Japan	—	19	10080	306	78	780	240	100	—	7	77
United States	10.7	23	13160	23	78	520	140	150	36	11	75

Source: World Bank 1984 various tables.
Golladay 1980, pp.67–83.

Barangay Health Stations and more than 30000 Barangay Health Workers had been deployed.

The overwhelming problem within the government's rural health system was that of staff vacancies. In 1974, 15 per cent of physician posts and 38 per cent of nursing posts were unfilled (Valenzuela *et al.* 1981). From 1976, medical and nursing-school graduates were required to work in the rural health system as part of the licensing procedure. From 1979 to 1981 an annual average of 1391 underboard doctors and 18000 underboard nurses, as they are called, were rotated through the rural health system (ROP, NEDA 1979, 1980, 1981).

The private sector

At the end of Spanish rule, in 1898, there were 13 independent non-government hospitals in the Philippines (Adorna 1976). By 1954 there were 222 private hospitals (compared to 80 government hospitals). Thirty per cent of these private hospitals were in Manila, with the rest in the provinces (Human Relations Area Files 1955). The private system expanded more rapidly than the government system, reaching 1192 hospitals and 43625 beds by 1983.

A 1948 tally counted a total of 3478 physicians (Human Relations Area Files 1955). Given that 668 physicians were reported to be employed by the government in 1963 (Chaffee 1969), a backward extrapolation suggests that the 1948 statistic contained a high proportion of private physicians.

The first medical school began operating in 1871; by 1960, there were 6 private medical schools, 1 government-supported medical school (Chaffee 1969), and 30 nursing schools (Valenzuela *et al.* 1981). An average of over 1400 new physicians were registered each year from 1956 to 1967 (ROP, NEDA 1984), indicating a vigorous medical education sector and a rapidly increasing potential supply of private physicians during the post-war years. By the mid-1980s there were 23 medical schools and 132 nursing schools. All the nursing schools and most of the medical schools were operated either privately or by non-profit institutions (Paqueo 1985; Valenzuela *et al.* 1981).

Emigration provides an incentive for students to enter medical education in the Philippines, although what little data are available suggest that many medical personnel do not in fact leave. It is estimated that 20 per cent of medical school graduates emigrated between 1962 and 1967 (Ghosh 1984). Between 1967 and 1969, 2041 physicians emigrated to the US, which would be about half of all new graduates. From 1975 to 1981, 1642 physicians were placed overseas by government overseas placement agencies (Valenzuela *et al.* 1981), which is a substantial subset of the total number trained.

Output of private medical services (measured by value added) increased at an annual average rate of 16 per cent from 1970 to 1983. Although real GNP fell between 1981 and 1985, output in the private medical sector continued to grow, and the proportion of all health expenditure accounted for by the private sector increased from 68 to 76 per cent.

Interface between public and private sectors

As far back as 1925, Puericulture Centres, which were forerunners of Rural Health Units, provided mother-and-child care in the main towns of many municipalities. Although partially funded by the public sector – principally by local government – Puericulture Centres have historically depended on voluntary private contributions and the services of local private physicians and nurses (ROP, DOH, NEDA 1975). By 1955, when the RHU system was just getting started, there were already 531 Puericulture Centres (Human Relations Area Files 1955), and their numbers stabilized at about 774 over the last decade.

An important public-private initiative, which had far-reaching implications for the future of the medical system, was the establishment in 1972 of Medicare, a national health-insurance programme. The Medicare system covered about half the working population for inpatient care, functioning as a co-insurance plan financed by a payroll tax. Beneficiaries were free to choose public or private providers, with the Philippine Medical Care Commission – a semi-autonomous unit of the Ministry of Health – regulating the system.

Accounting data indicated that about 90 per cent of Medicare benefits were spent on care from the private sector (Griffin and Paqueo 1985). In order to provide services to beneficiaries in rural areas, and in anticipation of eventually expanding coverage to the whole population, the Medicare system built 81 10-bed Community Hospitals and Health Centres in rural municipalities during the

1970s. It also provided construction loans for some private hospitals (Sen 1975).

Organization of the system

Each public hospital operated under one of several government agencies – the Ministry of Health, the Office of the President, the Ministry of Justice, the Ministry of National Defence, and city governments. The Ministry of Health operated 90 per cent of the public hospitals in 1978 (ROP, NEDA, NCSO 1979). Private hospitals were licensed by the Ministry of Health. Licensing was a legal requirement, but also carried a pecuniary incentive (i.e. it was required in order for hospitals to receive Medicare payments).

Public hospitals had a three-tier fee structure – free or low prices for ward patients, Medicare reimbursable prices for Medicare patients, and somewhat higher prices for private accommodation in pay wards. In 1979, 65 per cent of public hospital patients were accommodated in charity wards, 22 per cent were Medicare patients, and 13 per cent were in pay wards (Azurin 1980). In areas where public charity wards were not readily accessible, charity beds in private hospitals were underwritten. Charity ward patients accounted for about 7 per cent of private hospital patients in 1980 (Azurin 1980).

The public sector was formally, albeit loosely, organized into a pyramidal referral network, with Barangay Health Workers at the bottom and the Philippine General Hospital in Manila at the top. Hospitals were differentiated by their status as primary, secondary, or tertiary facilities, according to the complexity of care they offered. This is a typical organizational pattern, with the bottom of the pyramid recently broadened by village-level primary health-workers.

The charitable sector – most of which received some government funds – included the Philippine Tuberculosis Society, the Philippine National Red Cross, and the Philippine Heart Centre for Asia. In addition, there were many other government programmes that have not been mentioned, such as a mental health hospital, malaria-control units, chest clinics, schistosomiasis units, leprosaria, immunization drives, and family-planning clinics. Furthermore, the government required private businesses, schools, and other large institutions to provide certain medical services to their employees or students. Finally, there were the most ubiquitous of the private practitioners, traditional healers and midwives.

Provincial Distribution of Hospital Beds, 1971 and 1983

To understand the public and private sectors better, this section explores the provincial distribution of hospitals and hospital beds in 1972 and 1983. Our provincial-level data on public and private hospitals for 1972 come from the *Philippine Yearbook*. For 1983, we obtained from the Ministry of Health's licensing bureau a list of public and private hospitals with their locations by municipality, number of beds, and classification (tertiary, secondary, or primary). The 1983 data were matched with published census data, which allowed us to determine urban/rural location and population per bed at the provincial level. We concentrate on hospitals, even though we also assembled data on personnel and clinics. The hospital data are more reliable and disaggregated, and can be compared for two different time-periods.

If we combine both public and private hospital beds in 1972, there were an average of 751 people per bed. Figure 4.1 shows how provinces ranked in terms of population per bed in that year. The map shows the 10 provinces with the fewest people per bed (horizontal lines), the 10 provinces with the most people per bed (solid), and the 46 provinces that lay between (clear). We use this simple comparative approach because there is no predetermined standard for people per bed against which to judge these statistics.

Urbanized provinces (Manila and Cebu) did relatively well, as would be expected; but so too did a number of relatively sparsely populated northern Luzon provinces. The provinces which were poorly endowed with beds in 1972 were concentrated in Central Mindanao and in a band spanning Southern Luzon and the Eastern Visayas. Only 7 out of 66 provinces did better than the national average of 751 people per bed, because the national average was strongly weighted downward by Manila's 166 people per bed.

Figure 4.2 displays 1983 population-to-bed ratios using the same cut-off points as in 1972 to illustrate the dramatic changes in hospital coverage that took place over the 11-year interval. By 1983, and despite a 31 per cent increase in population, the national

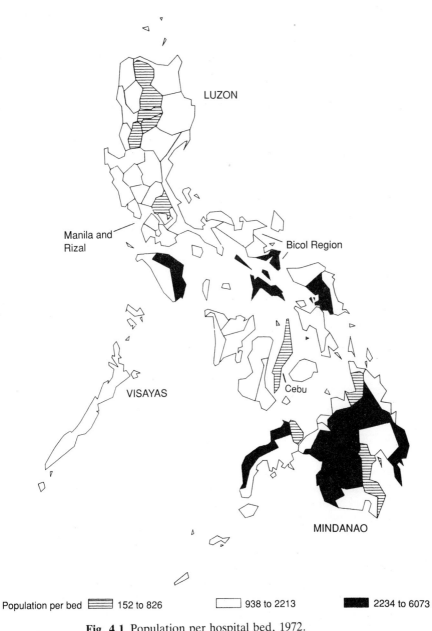

Fig. 4.1 Population per hospital bed, 1972.

Population per bed ▤ 152 to 826   ☐ 938 to 2213   ■ 2234 to 6073

average dropped by 20 per cent to 609 people per bed, and all but one province achieved a population-to-bed ratio of less than 2000. The delimiter for the ten best-endowed provinces in 1972 was low enough to include 38 provinces in 1983. The bottom province in 1983 had half the population-to-bed ratio of the bottom province in 1972, and the gap separating the best from the worse was cut in half.

Figure 4.3 shows the top and bottom 10 provinces in terms of the change in hospital bed coverage over the 11-year period (horizontal lines signify provinces with the largest improvement; solid, the smallest). Generally, the patterns in Fig. 4.3 are the opposite of those in Fig. 4.1, indicating that hospital bed expansion tended to occur in places where it was most needed, particularly in Mindanao. An example is Agusan del Sur, where the population grew by 52 per cent, but the number of beds increased by 891 per cent. It moved from the bottom 10 in 1972 to the top 10 in 1983. In Manila, in contrast, the total population grew by 55 per cent, but the number of beds actually fell by 1 per cent, owing to a decrease in government beds.

These trends show up clearly in the national averages. As mentioned earlier, there was an average of 751 people per bed in 1972. This statistic dropped by 19 per cent to 609 in 1983. If each province is weighted equally in calculating that average (to remove the strong effect of Manila's extremely low people-per-bed ratio and large population), there was a national average of 1657 people per bed in 1972, and it dropped by 51 per cent to 816 in 1983. The divergence between the two calculations narrowed in 1983 (751, weighted by population, versus 1657, weighted by province, in 1972; compared to 609 versus 816 in 1983) because of the gains made by the provinces relative to Manila.

These statistics demonstrate the problem of evaluating and planning programmes on the basis of highly aggregated national statistics. While the national people-per-bed average changed only slightly from 1972 to 1983, that ratio obscures the fact that the proportion of hospital resources accounted for by Manila dropped significantly, despite an absolute increase in the number of beds there. It also masks the fact that availability of those resources improved dramatically all over the country but especially in several provinces which were the worst off in 1972. This was a remarkable shift in the distribution of health infrastructure toward

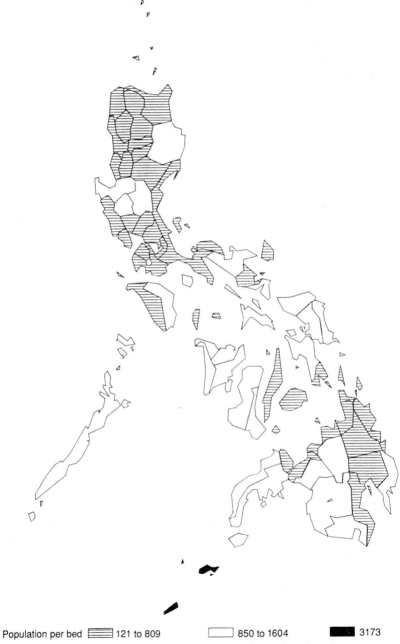

Population per bed ▤ 121 to 809   □ 850 to 1604   ■ 3173

Fig. 4.2 Population per hospital bed 1983 (groupings based on
1972 data).

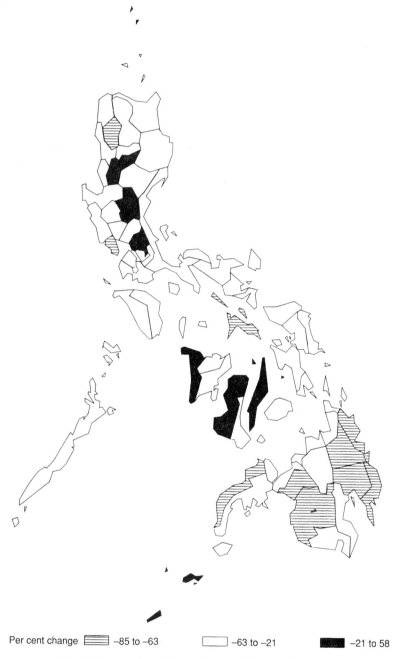

Fig. 4.3 Percentage change in population per hospital bed, 1972 to 1983.

Per cent change 〰️ −85 to −63   ▢ −63 to −21   ■ −21 to 58 those provinces most in need of additional investment, especially as it was accomplished in only one decade.

Public versus private distribution of hospital beds

Was the government responsible for these changes, or was it the private sector, or both? In trying to answer this question, we discuss a number of measures of growth, coverage, and dispersion of hospitals.

Growth

Over the 1972–83 period, the number of public hospitals rose nationally by 81 per cent, while private hospitals proliferated at twice that pace, by 167 per cent. Similarly, public beds increased by 29 per cent, and private beds by 104 per cent. Overall, about 77 per cent of the growth in numbers of hospitals and 74 per cent of the growth in beds originated in the private sector.

Relative size and level of care

Although most large hospitals expanded over the period, the bulk of new construction consisted of smaller hospitals in both the public and private sectors. The average number of beds per government hospital actually fell by 29 per cent from 1972 to 1983, and the average size of private hospitals fell by 23 per cent. This decline in average hospital size is desirable in the sense that it means a more dispersed system of curative care delivery that is probably more appropriate to the health problems of rural areas. However, if smaller hospitals are more costly to operate on a per-patient basis, there may be an offsetting loss in terms of reduced economic efficiency in the health sector. Evidence from the US suggests that hospitals up to a limit of about 200 beds may indeed experience declining unit costs as size increases. From a social standpoint, however, such cost-efficiencies must be weighted against higher travel costs for patients and a less equal distribution of health services implicit in a more centralized pattern of infrastructure. Thus it is difficult to judge whether smaller hospitals are better or worse from a standpoint of pure efficiency.

Outside Manila, average beds per hospital were 51 in the public sector and 25 in the private sector in 1983. Private hospitals offered a more basic level of care, with 59 per cent (compared to 38 per cent of public hospitals) classified as primary-level facilities capable of supporting only minor surgery and a few basic laboratory tests (ROP, PMCC 1984).

Distribution: Manila versus the provinces

In 1972 Manila accounted for 55 per cent of all government beds, 47 per cent of all private beds, and 11 per cent of the population. In 1983, it contained 31 per cent of all government beds, 31 per cent of the private beds, and 13 per cent of the population. Although the mix of beds in the capital changed, owing to a 26 per cent decrease in the number of government beds and a 35 per cent increase in the number of private beds, growth in both sectors was primarily outside the capital.

Distribution: what happened in the 'worst 10' provinces?

The 'worst 10' provinces on the basis of population-per-bed ratios in 1972 (see Fig. 4.1) might reasonably have been targeted for additional allocations of public resources. This appears to have been the case. While nationally the number of public hospitals and beds increased by 81 and 29 per cent respectively, they increased by 167 and 141 per cent in the worst-off group. However, private hospitals, which increased nationally by 167 per cent, increased by 555 per cent in the worst-off group. Private beds increased by 104 per cent nationally, but by 465 per cent in the bottom group. To illustrate the phenomenon, in Lanao del Sur, the province at the bottom of the people-per-bed rankings in 1972, the public sector grew from 75 beds in 2 hospitals in 1972 to 115 beds in 3 hospitals in 1983. The private sector, starting with no beds in 1972, expanded to 183 beds in 9 hospitals.

Although new public and private facilities were built or expanded in the best-off group in 1972, it was at a slower rate than elsewhere. The differences in new hospital-bed provision nationally, and for the best-off and worst-off group, are shown clearly in Fig. 4.4. In every group, private provision accounted for over 70 per cent of all new beds. By 1983, only two provinces, the islands of Romblon and Camiguin, had no private hospitals, compared with a figure of nine provinces in 1972.

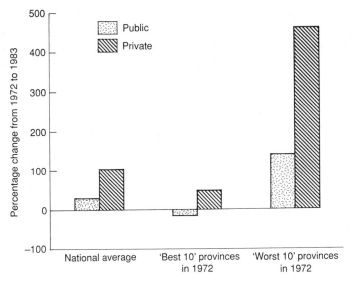

Fig. 4.4 Distribution of new public and private beds in the Philippines, 1972 to 1983.

Access and urban/rural distribution

'Population per bed' is commonly used as a measure of the adequacy of bed supply. However, it is an imperfect measure in that it does not take economic efficiency into account: an unused bed by this measure is preferable to no bed. In this section, we discuss other measures that add detail to our understanding of how hospital resources were distributed in the country.

Geographical coverage

One measure of geographical coverage is the size of catchment area (i.e. number of square kilometres) per hospital. Whilst insensitive to hospital location, this measure does provide additional information when considered in conjunction with the population-to-bed ratio. Figure 4.5 displays the top and bottom 10 provinces ranked by the square kilometres-per-hospital ratio. Three provinces rank in the bottom group both for people per bed and size of catchment area per hospital, and another 12 are in the bottom group for one or the other measure. These 15 provinces would be obvious candidates for additional allocations of public resources, because they had relatively many people per available bed, but each hospital also served a relatively large geographical area. From 1972 to 1983, the government did increase its presence in those provinces; but the private sector made an even stronger showing. Over the period, the private share of total beds actually rose at a faster rate than it did nationally.

In the solid-filled provinces, beds were 3 to 7 times more concentrated in urban areas than were people; they were provinces in which the hospitals tended to be in a few cities, while the people lived in the countryside. It is interesting to note that, for this group of 10 provinces, 42 per cent of public hospitals and 54 per cent of private hospitals were urban, which was not much higher than the national averages. The problem, therefore, was greater dispersion of the people. From a planner's perspective, these provinces would be prime targets for government or private investment in rural clinics.

Proportion of beds in largest provincial city

An alternative to the 'degree of urban concentration' measure is to calculate the proportion of hospital beds located in the largest provincial city. Thirty-five per cent of public beds (16 per cent of hospitals) and 43 per cent of private beds (28 per cent of hospitals) fell into this category in 1983. In other words, slightly over a third of all beds and about a fifth of hospitals were located in the largest town in each province, with the public system being slightly less concentrated in the main city than the private sector. While the 'urban' measure discussed in the previous section suggests that two-thirds of beds were in urbanized areas, the 'largest city' measure indicates that these hospitals were dispersed among a number of cities, and not all concentrated in the same place.

Costs and services in the public and private sectors

This provincial-level analysis provides much more detail than is usually available on the distribution of the public and private sectors, yet it still does not give an idea of differences in the

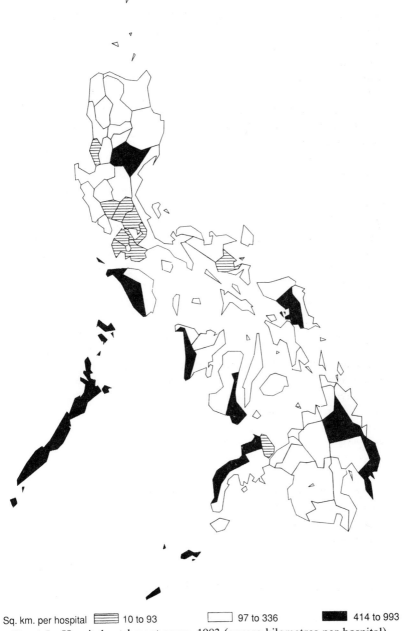

Sq. km. per hospital [10 to 93]   [97 to 336]   [414 to 993]
Fig. 4.5 Hospital catchment areas, 1983 (square kilometres per hospital).

two sectors in terms of accessibility, quality, prices, and services. This information must be culled from facility-level surveys, which are rare indeed. One representative sample of facilities and practitioners in three provinces of the Bicol region (see Fig. 4.1 for its location) in 1981 provides a glimpse of the type of information that could be collected (Griffin *et al.* 1981). This survey made an inventory of medical facilities available to a representative sample of 100 villages by asking officials to identify the practitioners, clinics, and hospitals used by local people. Each facility was visited to collect price and service data, a subset of which is displayed in Table 4.2. Although 66 public facilities and 103 private facilities were visited, the private sector was actually under-sampled because of cost constraints: 75 per cent of public hospitals, but only 44 per cent of private hospitals were surveyed.

The data indicate that the public and private sectors were approximately equally accessible in geographical terms to the sample villages. Staffing patterns were quite different, with private clinics providing primarily physician services rather than the services of nurses and midwives. Outpatient visit costs were much higher in the private sector (about US$2 in 1981), although paying for care in the private sector did assure attendance by a physician. Moreover, over 75 per cent of private physicians adjusted their fees to patients' ability to pay, and accepted in-kind payment. Indeed one problem in administering the survey lay in eliciting any one single response on prices from private physicians, who not only adjusted prices, but also treatment, length of care, and choice of drugs to patients' ability to pay.

Urban versus rural

Another measure of access is the percentage of beds located in urban areas. An urban area in the Philippines is not a city – any municipality in which more than 28 per cent of the people are located in towns is classified as urban. By this definition 61 per cent of public, and 67 per cent of private *beds* were urban in 1983, compared to 31 per cent of the people. However, 31 per cent of public, and 46 per cent of private *hospitals* were in urban areas. That beds were more concentrated than hospitals is not surprising if one assumes that larger hospitals are built in urban areas for economic reasons. Smaller hospitals, especially smaller public-sector hospitals, were more dispersed.

A summary urban measure is provided by the ratio of the percentage of urban beds to the percentage of urban people in a province. A value of 0 indicates no urban beds; a value of 1 indicates equal percentages of beds and people in urban areas; and larger values indicate higher and higher concentrations of hospital beds

Table 4.2 *Characteristics of Public and Private Health Facilities, Bicol Region, Philippines, 1981*

	Public clinics	Private clinics	Public hospitals	Private hospitals
Average distance to sample barangay — urban (km)	3.4	3.7	19.0	10.1
Average distance to sample barangay — rural (km)	9.2	10.0	19.1	15.4
Physicians	58	69	91	92
Nurses	108	22	188	165
Midwives	376	18	73	158
Outpatient services				
Availability (%)	98	100	100	100
Cost (pesos)	0	13.90	2.53	14.93
Physician usually attends (%)	46	100	100	98
Sliding fee scale (%)	0	81	53	77
In-kind payment (%)	8	76	0	50
Average hours open per week	43	70	168	168
Service available after hours (%)	6	73	NA	NA
Open on holidays (%)	10	96	100	100

Note: NA means 'not applicable'. Units are shown in parentheses. The per cent signs refer to the percentage of facilities. For example, in 98 per cent of the public clinics, outpatient services were available.

Source: Griffin *et al.* (1981).

relative to people. For the Philippines in 1983, the values ranged from 0 to 7, with the highest value indicating that hospital beds were 7 times more concentrated than people. Figure 4.6 displays this measure in a slightly different manner from previous figures. Provinces filled with horizontal lines have ratios from 0 to 1.4 and have bed distributions that are roughly consistent with the urban – rural distribution of people. This category contains a large group of provinces – the most urban, where both beds and people were urban, and the most rural, where both beds and people were rural.

While both public and private hospitals were open 24 hours a day during a typical week, public clinics were open for business only 61 per cent of the hours that private clinics were. Private clinics also tended to provide services after hours and on holidays, which was rare in public clinics.

The Bicol region was one of the poorest in the Philippines in terms of per capita income, and over 80 per cent of the population lived in the countryside. However, in terms of population-per-bed statistics and public-private mix of hospitals, it was near the national average. It was certainly not a wealthy urbanized area; yet this survey suggested a wide availability of private clinic and hospital services. Analysis of other data from the Bicol region has shown high use of the private sector by both the poor and the rich (Akin *et al.* 1985). The distinct differences in service characteristics between the public and private sectors indicated that people faced a broad range of choices and amenities in the private sector that may have made it an attractive alternative to free public care for households in a wide range of income-groups.

Provincial distribution of personnel

Physicians

Several different tallies of physicians are available: an apparently exhaustive inventory of physicians in 1970 by the Association of Philippine Medical Colleges (Adorna 1976); a Department of Health (DOH) inventory from 1973; and the membership of the Philippines Medical Association (PMA) from 1974 until 1983. However, none of the tallies allowed one to discern the public and private distribution of physicians, nor did they allow reliable comparisons between two points in time.

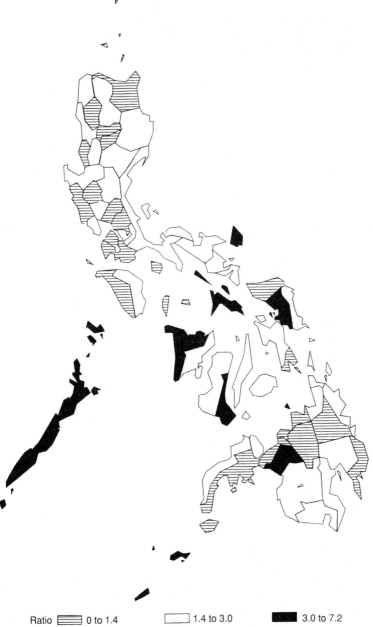

Fig. 4.6 Ratio of percentage of urban beds to percentage of urban people, 1983.

Ratio ▦ 0 to 1.4   ☐ 1.4 to 3.0   ■ 3.0 to 7.2

Nationally, there were 2694 people per physician in 1973. If provincial averages are given equal weight, to remove Manila's heavy influence, the ratio rises nearly two-thirds, to 4301. Extrapolating from the three different data-sources, we estimate that the number of physicians rose at an annual average rate of between 4.3 per cent and 8.4 per cent over the period 1972 to 1983. This implies population-to-physician ratios of between 2580 and 2000 in 1983, a 22 per cent improvement over 1973.

Figure 4.7 shows the top and bottom 10 provinces, and those in between, ranked by population per physician in 1973. Although Manila itself accounted for 31 per cent of the nation's physicians, the shaded area on the map around the capital accounted for 42 per cent of the total. About 64 per cent of the doctors lived in urban municipalities, although, if the provinces are equally weighted with Manila, some 46 per cent of physicians would be classified as urban. While physicians were about twice as likely as the general population to live in urban municipalities in 1973, the proportion in rural areas was considerable.

The worst-off provinces in Fig. 4.7 include the same few in southern Luzon and the Visayas that did poorly for hospital coverage (see Fig. 4.1). However, fewer of the provinces in Central Mindanao were in the bottom category. The relative abundance of doctors in the region in the early seventies may help to explain its strong performance in private hospital construction during the decade.

Nurses and midwives

The DOH inventory of medical personnel in 1973 indicates that the Philippines had more active physicians than nurses or midwives. Figures 4.8 and 4.9 present the data for population per nurse and per midwife using the same cut-off points as for physicians. Comparing the three personnel maps demonstrates how much worse was the availability of these auxiliary personnel in relation to that of doctors. Population per nurse and per midwife put the majority of provinces in what would be the worst group for population per physician.

Other surveys confirm these low ratios of nurses and midwives to physicians. In 1978 there were 3821 physicians, 6585 nurses, and 224 midwives in MOH hospital employment, yielding ratios of 1.4 nurses and 0.06 midwives per physician in government employment

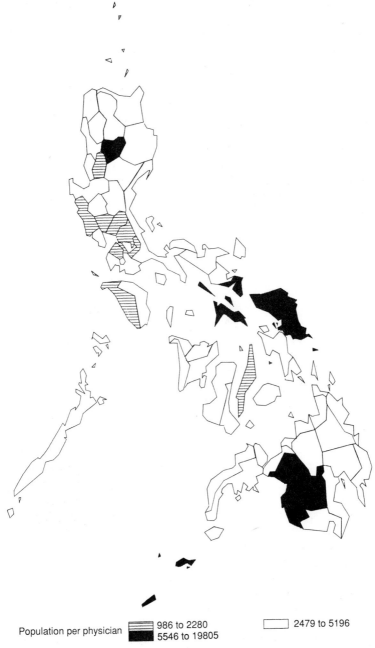

Population per physician — 986 to 2280 / 5546 to 19805 — 2479 to 5196

Fig. 4.7 Population per physician, 1973.

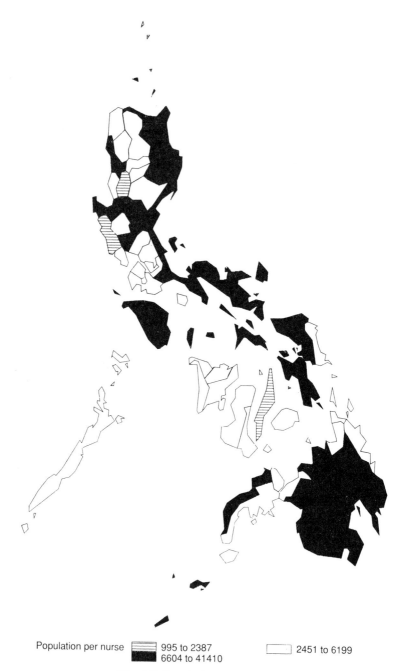

Population per nurse ▦ 995 to 2387 ▢ 2451 to 6199
■ 6604 to 41410

Fig. 4.8 Population per nurse, 1973.

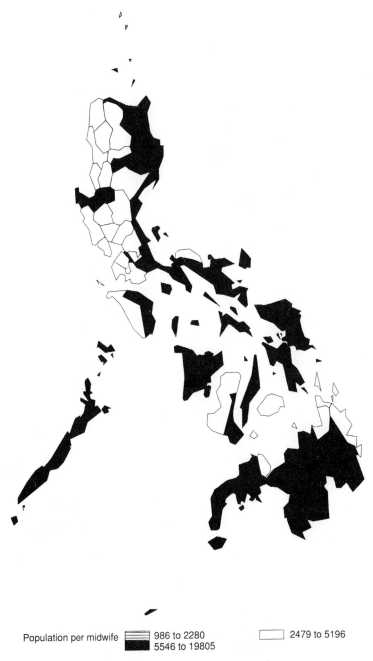

Population per midwife   ▦ 986 to 2280   ☐ 2479 to 5196
                    ■ 5546 to 19805

Fig. 4.9 Population per midwife, 1973.

(ROP, NEDA, NCSO 1979). The previously mentioned survey in the Bicol region counted about 1.5 nurses and 2.0 midwives per doctor (Griffin *et al.* 1981). A similar survey in Cebu City found 1.8 nurses, but only 0.4 midwives per doctor (Akin *et al.* 1982).

A notable aspect of the nurse and midwife data is that so few were employed relative to the numbers trained (at their own expense). From 1977 to 1981 an annual average of 12188 graduates passed the nursing examination, and 4540 passed the midwifery examination (Valenzuela *et al.* 1981). In 1980, 51750 nurses renewed their licences. Although at least 11586 nurses were placed overseas between and during 1975 and 1979, that figure was not even equivalent to one year's graduating class. One might reasonably interpret the available data to conclude that the Philippines had a huge reservoir of trained nurses and midwives who were not working in their chosen professions, and who had not figured in the government's primary health-care strategy over the last decade.

Primary care facilities

As with personnel, data on clinics are unreliable and not readily available. Table 4.3 presents the available clinic statistics by region. The private sector accounted for 69 per cent of all clinics in 1974. Nearly 100 per cent of private clinics were general practice offices (ROP, DOH, NEDA 1975). About 41 per cent of private clinics were in the environs of Manila in 1974, compared to 20 per cent of RHUs (public clinics). Excluding these clinics in Manila, both systems were fairly evenly distributed across regions.

The RHU system expanded by 58 per cent from 1974 to 1981, an 8.3 per cent annual average rate which is slightly greater than the 7.4 per cent annual average for public hospitals. However, an extraordinary 70 per cent of the growth in RHUs took place in an area surrounding, and just to the north of, Manila (Central Luzon and Southern Tagalog) that was already well covered by hospitals, public clinics, private clinics, private physicians, and private hospitals. From 1974 to 1981, the area around Manila increased its share of RHUs from 20 to 38 per cent of the national total! This odd expansion pattern of public clinics was inconsistent with the stated goals of the health system, and markedly different from the changes in the hospital sector. Unfortunately, we cannot compare

Table 4.3 *Primary health care clinics, Philippines, 1974, 1981, and 1983*

Region	RHU 1974	RHU 1981	RHU % change	Pueri culture 1974	Pueri culture 1983	Pueri culture % change	Barangay Health Station 1981	Private Clinics 1974
Ilocos	130	205	58	48	95	98	759	29
Cagayan Valley	116	116	0	44	40	−9	567	292
Central Luzon	88	179	103	131	116	−11	881	1112
Southern Tagalog	161	578	259	202	192	−5	964	775
Bicol	96	115	20	46	36	−22	658	452
Western Visayas	106	127	20	94	72	−23	767	787
Central Visayas	129	138	7	67	73	9	638	215
Eastern Visayas	120	150	25	43	38	−12	504	190
Western Mindanao	64	87	36	10	7	−30	130	357
Northern Mindanao	106	124	17	62	51	−18	609	293
Southern Mindanao	77	82	6 }	47 }	39 }	−17	508 }	128
Central Mindanao	70	90	29 }		15 }		368 }	
National	1263	1991	58	794	774	−3	7353	4630

Note: City health offices and separate family planning clinics are not included.
Sources: ROP, DOH, NEDA (1975); ROP, TFHS, DAP (1975); Puericulture League (1984).

it with changes in the distribution of private clinics because no data are available. Quite obviously, from Table 4.3, government resources in the rural sector during the late 1970s were devoted to creating Barangay Health Stations, which were non-existent in 1974, and deploying the associated personnel.

Conclusion

Generalizations from the Philippine experience are often discounted by international health experts because the country has substantial medical resources and because it also exports medical personnel. However, the apparent abundance of facilities and personnel have not prevented those same planners from advocating an enormous volunteer-based primary health policy for the country. Moreover, the Philippines is not so atypical as is usually claimed. Its aggregate health statistics are similar to those for other countries in Southeast Asia, and, except for its much higher population densities, are also comparable to South American statistics. Thus, the findings in this research might be instructive for many other countries in similar circumstances.

Our hospital data suggest a huge improvement in the availability and distribution of Philippine medical resources between 1972 and the early 1980s. The private sector played a much larger role than the public sector in the expansion and geographical equalization that took place in the 1970s.

Both sectors built many smaller hospitals instead of concentrating resources in large centralized institutions. However, the private sector was far more successful in targeting new construction to provinces that needed it most. This is a surprising finding, since it is usually believed that the government must compensate for the urban and high-income orientation of the private sector. Moreover, public investment decisions were a highly centralized, planned activity, while growth in the private sector was the result of many small, uncoordinated decisions. By every supply measure we were able to develop (urban location, largest city location, area covered), the private sector performed as well as or better than the public sector.

For clinic facilities, growth in the government's RHU system seems to have been concentrated around Manila, which is a very odd pattern. In addition, however, huge numbers of Barangay

Health Stations were constructed all over the country. We cannot compare these changes with private investment in clinics, but if our data from the Bicol region are an indication, and if private clinics expanded at a pace anywhere near that of private hospitals, it would seem likely that the number and distribution of private clinics improved over the period.

In terms of personnel, we can only make an informed guess that there was considerable growth in the supply of physicians. Thousands of nurses and midwives were trained from 1970 on, yet the Philippines was nowhere near the international average of about 4 or 5 working nurses to a doctor. As a consequence, the country appeared to have huge reserves of untapped medical resources in the form of people who had financed their own training at the college level but were not yet working in their chosen professions. Yet there was a shortage of nurses and midwives in the government's rural health units. We can speculate on the causes of this mismatch – low pay, exit from the labour force due to marriage or childbearing, or a bias in favour of physicians in government hiring practices; but without better data, we can do little more than guess.

The data suggest that the government could have been more effective in planning its own sector if it had taken account of private-sector growth and better targeted its curative-care investment on the few provinces which consistently ranked at the bottom of our measures. Nevertheless, simply by reducing the concentration of public beds in Manila, the government improved the distribution of its resources, although the concentration of new rural health clinics near the capital offset the improvement.

Without the type of information discussed in this chapter, health planners can only be guided by 'stylized facts' about medical systems. They are also bound by preconceived notions about the services people should have, notwithstanding what those same people may already be purchasing for themselves or what other providers are already delivering. Even the poorest countries generate epidemiological, demographic, and census data, but little is known about the economic dimensions of the medical system in poor and rich countries alike.

Although our data are not adequate to analyse rigorously the determinants of the situation we describe or the effects of the organization and financing of the medical system on health outcomes, even such basic descriptive information can provide useful insights and a number of surprises. One of the more tantalizing issues that we cannot yet answer is the role of income distribution in the observed development process – how did the level and variation in incomes (within and across provinces) affect the distribution of public and private investment in medical facilities? More detail on other issues would also be helpful for planning, such as what information might enable us to predict where the private sector will develop; whether private expansion into under-served areas was permanent or led to bankruptcies; and how road-construction affected access to and use of urban-based facilities.

References

Adorna, C. L. (1976). The distribution of health resources in the Philippines. Unpublished Master's thesis, Quezon City, University of the Philippines.

Akin, J. S., Flieger, W., Guilkey, D. K., and Popkin, B. H. (1982). Survey of health facilities [Mimeo]. Office of Population Studies, University of the Philippines, Cebu, Philippines.

Akin, J. S., Griffin, S. C., Guilkey, D. K., and Popkin, B. H. (1985). *The demand for primary health services in the Third World*. Rowman and Allanheld, Totowa, New Jersey.

Azurin, J. C. (1980). *A profile of Philippine hospital system*. Ministry of Health, Manila.

Chaffee, F. E. (1969). *Area handbook for the Philippines*. US Government Printing Office, Washington, DC.

Ghosh, P. K. (ed.) (1984). *Health, food and nutrition in Third World development*. Greenwood Press, Westport, Connecticut.

Golladay, F. L. (1980). *Health: sector policy paper* (2nd ed). World Bank, Washington, DC.

Griffin, C. C. (1987). *User charges for health care in principle and practice*, PHN Technical Note 87–16. World Bank, Washington DC.

Griffin, C.C. and Paqueo, V. B. (1985). *Description and analysis of the Philippine Medical Care Plan*. Carolina Population Center, University of North Carolina at Chapel Hill, Chapel Hill, NC.

Griffin, C. C., Hamilton, S., Popkin, B. H., and the Ateneo de Naga Research and Service Center (1981). *The Bicol Multipurpose Supplemental Survey*. Carolina Population Center, University of North Carolina at Chapel Hill, Chapel Hill, NC.

Human Relations Area Files (1955). *Subcontractor's monograph HRAF-16 Chicago-5, The Philippines, Volume III* [Mimeo]. Human Relations Area Files, New Haven.

Paqueo, V. B. (1985). *Risk sharing and health care in a developing economy: towards a community health maintenance system*. World

Bank, Department of Population, Health and Nutrition, Policy and Research Division, Washington, DC.

Puericulture League (1984). *List of active puericulture centers.* The League, Manila.

ROP, DOH, NEDA (Republic of the Philippines, Department of Health, National Economic and Development Authority) (1975). *National Health Plan 1975–1978.* The Authority, Manila.

ROP, NEDA (Republic of the Philippines, National Economic and Development Authority) (1979). *Philippine Development Report 1979.* The Authority, Manila.

ROP, NEDA (Republic of the Philippines, National Economic and Development Authority) (1980). *Philippine Development Report 1980.* The Authority, Manila.

ROP, NEDA (Republic of the Philippines, National Economic and Development Authority) (1981). *Philippine Development Report 1981.* The Authority, Manila.

ROP, NEDA (Republic of the Philippines, National Economic and Development Authority) (1984). *Statistical Yearbook of the Philippines 1984.* The Authority, Manila.

ROP, NEDA, NCSO (Republic of the Philippines, National Economic and Development Authority, National Census and Statistics Office) (1979). *Journal of Philippine Statistics*, **30** (3), 50, Table 3.9.

ROP, PMCC (Republic of the Philippines, Philippine Medical Care Commission) (1984). *Guidelines for Medicare accreditation.* The Commission, Manila.

ROP, TFHS, DAP (Republic of the Philippines, Task Force on Human Settlements, Development Academy of the Philippines) (1975). *Social services development in the Philippines*, Part II, Health. The Academy, Manila.

Sen, P. (1975). Financing of medical care insurance in the Philippines. *International Social Security Review*, **28**, 139–50.

Valenzuela, A. V., Pardo, O. D., Tadiar, F. H., and Raynes, D. N. (1981). *Health sector study: Philippines.* University of the Philippines, Institute of Public Health, Health Sciences Center, Quezon City.

World Bank (1984). *World Development Report 1984.* Oxford University Press, New York.

World Bank (1987). *Financing health services in developing countries: an agenda for reform.* World Bank, Washington, DC.

Authors' Note

This chapter was written while both authors were economists at the World Bank. An earlier draft was written while Griffin was a postdoctoral fellow at the Economic Growth Center, Yale University, and Paqueo was at the University of the Philippines. It is a shortened version of a report written for the United States Agency for International Development (USAID) under contract OTR-0082-C-00–3353–00. We appreciate the support of those institutions, Joy Riggs-Perla of USAID, Maureen Lewis, the Carolina Population Center (CPC), and our colleagues at the CPC: John Akin, David Guilkey, and Barry Popkin. We thank Cynthia Miguel in Manila for an extraordinary effort in tracking down data. We also appreciate the efforts of Noni Jose and Georgette Winther, who prepared the chapter for publication.

5

A study of hospital fees in the Dominican Republic

Maureen A. Lewis

Background

Most public health systems in the developing world have been built in the belief that health care is a fundamental right; that the state must meet the health needs of the population; and that public services should be free at the point of use. Concerns over equal access and affordability have further enhanced the appeal of free-services policies. Yet despite the desirability of ensuring access to health services, recent economic events have made it clear – for the foreseeable future at least – that such policies are unaffordable for much of the developing world. The World Health Organization's 1987 World Health Assembly concluded as much.

Public health systems can be costly because of the inherent inefficiencies in public health-care delivery (Lindsay 1975; PPSS 1984), and especially where the subsidy encompasses the entire population. Where services are free, there are no built-in incentives to discourage utilization other than the patients' own time and travel costs. Building a health-care infrastructure is costly enough; the cost of operating a free, open system can be staggering, especially for a high recurrent-cost sector such as health.

The financial crisis facing the health sector in many developing countries is not only due to a commitment to costly and broad social service coverage, however. The world-wide recession of the early 1980s, falling prices for primary products, and the persistent debt problems of developing countries have also been significant factors. Requirements to reduce government spending in order to reschedule debt repayments have forced governments to cut back on expenditures in all sectors, including health. Indeed, between 1972 and 1983, government allocations to health dropped to 4.5 per cent of total budgets (Griffin 1987).

Despite the fiscal crisis, a commitment to subsidized health services for those unable to pay for care remains in many countries, including the Dominican Republic. However, reductions in resources mean that unless alternative sources of funds can be identified, facilities will deteriorate or resources must be concentrated on a few facilities or services. The need for additional resources due to both decreases in funding and growth in demand, has led a number of governments to examine alternative methods for sharing costs with patients.

Cost-sharing can take several forms: it may involve private third-party payers (insurance companies), government insurance, health services as an employee benefit, or user payments. Costs can also be reduced through improvements in productivity, but that option is not addressed here (see Lewis, *et al.* 1990 for an analysis of efficiency and productivity in a Dominican hospital). User fees have many attractions: they are conceptually simple; require minimal administration and regulation; and can demonstrate their effectiveness in a short time (see Bekele and Lewis 1986). User charges are becoming of increasing interest to governments wanting to subsidize care but unable to afford free health care for all services or for all citizens. User fees are not without problems. Difficulties emerge with regard to what services should have charges; how prices should be set; who should pay for them; how they should be administered; how revenues should be allocated; and how to develop mechanisms for identifying and exempting those patients who cannot afford to pay.

While a number of countries have implemented user fees in public hospitals, some have been more successful in raising revenues than others. Typically the percentage of recurrent costs recovered through user fees ranges between 2 per cent and 17 per cent, with the vast majority of countries at the lower end of this range (Ainsworth 1984; de Ferranti 1985). Detailed evidence from Sudan (Bekele and Lewis 1986), Rwanda (Shepard *et al.* 1987), Ethiopia (Dunlop and Donaldson 1987), Honduras (Overholt 1987), Ghana (Waddington and Enyimayew 1989) and Jamaica (Lewis and Parker 1991) suggests that fees can generate significant resources at all levels of the health-care system even without an expressed policy or a centrally imposed user fee system. Furthermore, the revenues generated from such fees can raise quality significantly. For instance, if fee revenues are allocated to purchasing simple inputs such as bandages, syringes, or X-ray film, or can allow the hospital to fix a leaking roof, the marginal value of these inputs is extremely high. Stagnant or falling overall budgets often produce a reduction in operation, maintenance, and asset-replacement funds. As the proportion of government budgets allocated to salaries rises or remains constant, the marginal benefit of the user fee revenue may be of great value, even where revenues are modest. It may permit fundamental improvements either to the physical environment or in the availability of supplies – two areas of particular need in the public health facilities of most developing countries that are known to affect productivity. In effect, fee revenues can serve as an incentive for workers by upgrading their working conditions or enhancing their productivity by making complementary inputs such as equipment and supplies more consistently available.

The success of user fee systems in generating revenues for the health system depends upon the incentives hospitals face in collecting fees. Clearly, it is essential that central governments either endorse or at least do not prohibit fees at public health facilities. Moreover, fee collection must be in the interests of the hospital, otherwise it will be expending its own scarce resources in order to raise general government revenues. This is increasingly acknowledged as a problem. In order to enhance incentives Jamaica, for example, has experimented with modifications to its traditional system of remitting revenues to the central government to allow hospitals to retain some part of the revenues collected, and hospital revenues have risen (Lewis and Parker 1991).

The equity implications of user charges remain an issue for many governments which perceive the target groups of public services as unable to pay for health care. However, the poor may be willing to pay much more for private care than the fees at public facilities (de Ferranti 1985). Despite this, governments have historically preferred to ensure free access for those whose income is sufficiently low by providing free care to all comers.

There are numerous other means by which free or subsidized services for the poor may be organized. For systems that do have means tests, the income cut-off and the method of exemption vary by country. In the Sudan, free services were supplemented by various subsidized fee-for-service alternatives for those able to pay something (Bekele and Lewis 1986); in Jamaica food stamp recipients, some preventive services, high-risk pregnancies, and some children's dental care services are exempt (Lewis and Parker 1991); a number of Latin American and Caribbean countries have social workers who screen patients for their ability to pay. While cumbersome and often highly porous, such systems do allow governments both to apply charges and yet to meet the needs of a narrower target group. How effective such systems are is not known, but they represent an attempt at segmenting the market and narrowing the eligibility for subsidies. *Ceteris paribus*, they should therefore reduce costs.

This study examines many of these issues with reference to the Dominican Republic's experience of user fees in public hospitals between 1984 and 1986. The study describes the background and context to user fees; the different systems operated; the resources generated by fees and how they were used; and the means devised to accommodate patients unable to pay.

The Dominican Republic

From the late 1970s, the economy of the Dominican Republic rapidly deteriorated. Between 1968 and 1975, per capita GDP growth-rates approached 7 per cent, and foreign-exchange earnings grew by over 25 per cent. In contrast, the 1977–1984 period saw per capita GDP growth fall below 1 per cent, and export growth slow to less than 2 per cent a year. Projections of GDP growth and foreign exchange earnings promised further deterioration (Ceara-Hatton 1987).

Not surprisingly, the recession adversely affected government expenditures. The IMF stand-by agreement further reduced real government spending, particularly in those sectors with high recurrent costs. For example, in 1985, the Dominican government allocated DR $131 million (US $42.2 million), or 5 per cent of the budget, to public health services: down from 8 per cent in 1982. Despite modest growth in the public health budget in nominal terms between 1981 and 1985, it fell by about half in real terms.

When the central government attempted to cut its health budget after 1981 by freezing hospital operating budgets at their 1981 levels (Bartlett, undated), hospitals were forced to adjust to fewer budgetary resources. Some hospital directors responded by cutting back on services, while others aggressively pursued additional sources of income. Charging for health services was possible because hospitals in the Dominican Republic enjoyed a high degree of autonomy, and because of the ambiguities in government policy towards user fees.

The constitution of the Dominican Republic promised 'adequate protection against . . . illness' and 'free medical assistance and hospitalization to those whose economic resources require it.' This pledge was the foundation for continuing disagreement and controversy over pricing policies in government facilities, in particular whether all health care had to be free to all citizens or only for some citizens or for some services. While government policy stipulated that charges for all inpatient services were prohibited, policy toward outpatient care was ambiguous. The lack of guidance provided a conducive environment for experimentation by individual hospitals, and resulted in a diverse range of practice.

The public health system

The Secretariat for Public Health and Social Welfare (SESPAS) owned and operated 101 hospitals, health centres, and subcentres in seven regions and in the national capital area. The 46 public hospitals provided the full range of primary, secondary, and tertiary care, although some rural hospitals provided only limited services. Specialty hospitals in Santo Domingo and the regional hospital in Santiago provided specialized diagnostic and treatment services such as dialysis, incubators, and cancer treatment. Hospital operating budgets were allocated and regulated by SESPAS. All services were meant to be free, especially for those who could not afford to pay. Indeed, central government allocations to hospitals were aimed at allowing facilities to extend free care.

Hospital budgets were in two parts. The first of these was the personnel budget. Personnel were recruited by competitive examination and assigned and paid by the central government. Since there was no established civil service system, staff composition tended to shift with changes in administration, which in practice meant every four years. Moreover, there was no system of programme budgeting, so personnel allocations were unsystematic with regard to numbers, type, and specialty. In 1984, personnel captured about 68 per cent of the total budget, compared with 50 per cent in 1975 and 58 per cent in 1980. The 1984 proportion was to remain constant over subsequent budget periods. The SESPAS ratio of expenditures on materials and supplies to spending on personnel decreased by 36 per cent between 1980 and 1983 (Bartlett, undated).

The second part of the budget comprised the operating funds for all non-personnel costs. In the past this was based largely on historical allocations, although recent reforms were meant to establish a systematic budgeting process for health facilities. Individual facilities could supplement government allocations through revenue from patients or through a group of friends of the facility, the 'Patronato', that raised money through outright gifts, charity functions, or international donor contributions of materials.

SESPAS had a set formula for allocating hospital operating budget expenditures: drugs 50 per cent, food 30 per cent (to feed both patients and staff), maintenance 5 per cent, staff education and professional development 1 per cent, and the remainder for other items. Government auditors oversaw expenditure of central funds, but were not responsible for reviewing the books of internally generated revenues, nor were hospitals required to report the sources or amounts of revenue raised. Thus these monies became a source of discretionary expenditures for hospitals.

Methods

The facilities in this study included nine regional or specialty hospitals and the Dr Defillo National Laboratory. The nine hospitals were selected from four of the seven regions and the capital city, with a bias toward facilities in Santo Domingo. Hospitals included both regional and general hospitals and three specialty hospitals. The National Laboratory was included because of its extensive and successful experience with user fees. Chronic care facilities were excluded.

Data were collected from each individual hospital through the examination of accounting and patient records, and discussions with hospital directors, administrators, and social workers. Data quality was very high, although incomplete due to irregular bookkeeping and changes in key personnel following the changed administration in 1986.

The facilities included in the sample and some salient characteristics for each are presented in Table 5.1. The largest hospital was José Maria Cabral y Báez in Santiago, the Dominican Republic's second largest city. The hospital provided a broad range of services

Table 5.1 *Summary characteristics of public facilities in the sample*

Facility	Type of facility	Location	No. of beds (1986)	No. of inpatients (1986)	No. of outpatients (1986)
Carl George	Region V hospital	San Pedro de Macoris	48	4926	21700
Dr Dario Contreras	Trauma hospital	Santo Domingo	233	4014	49465
Jaime Mota	Region IV hospital	Barbados	90	4673	32117
José Maria Cabral y Báez	Region II hospital	Santiago	414	21099	119700
Juan Pablo Pina	Region I hospital	San Cristobal	234	10706	70947
Maternidad, Nuestra Señora de la Altagracia	Maternity hospital	Santo Domingo	252	19224	79232
Dr Luis E. Aybar	General hospital	Santo Domingo	225	5045	69383
National Laboratory Dr Defillo	National laboratory	Santo Domingo	n.a.	n.a.	n.a.
Dr Padre Billini	General hospital	Santo Domingo	148	2981	40257
Robert Reid Cabral	Children's hospital	Santo Domingo	268	7632	112143

Source: SESPAS statistics.
Note: n.a. means data are not available.

– both general and specialized – and was a unique institution in the Dominican Republic. The other regional hospitals were of varying size, but each represented the main facility in that region. The number of inpatients and outpatients per facility also varied widely. The ratio of inpatients to outpatients ranged from about 7 to 24 (Maternidad Hospital), with the lower ratios more common in the specialized hospitals in Santo Domingo where lengths of stay may have been longer, and hence the numbers of inpatients smaller. If this was the case, then it suggests the system was operating as planned, with specialized care providing more intensive care and regional hospitals providing more general care. Unfortunately, data on case-mix, average lengths of stay, or occupancy rates were not available. These kinds of measures would have allowed a more meaningful comparison of costs and utilization across facilities.

User fees in hospitals

Outpatient services

Because there was no clear policy from the central government on outpatient charges at public hospitals, fees evolved in an *ad hoc* fashion in response to perceived needs and the initiative of hospital directors. All of the ten facilities in the sample had some fees for outpatients. A number of hospitals referred to fees as 'donations' to indicate the optional nature of these charges. Facilities varied widely in respect of the services charged and the amount they charged. Table 5.2 summarizes the fee schedules for the ten facilities, showing only selected services. Few facilities published fee schedules that indicated charges on a service-specific basis. The National Laboratory and Cabral y Báez Hospital had the most extensive and complete fee systems.

Juan Pablo Pina, Dario Contreras, and Maternidad Hospitals had fee schedules, but included only some services; however, this was not surprising in Contreras Hospital, the trauma centre, and in the maternity hospital, which treated only a certain range of problems. The others had charges for some select services, but their fee systems were less comprehensive.

Outpatient fees were based on a fraction of private-sector prices, the average costs of supplies, and the perceived ability and willingness of patients to pay. Fees rarely exceeded 10 per cent of private-sector prices for similar services, and in most cases were less. The Cabral y Báez Hospital set charges according to cost estimates of the chief medical officer in each department or 10 per cent of private prices, and their prices were on average higher than those at other hospitals, which suggests that fees were well below market levels. The National Laboratory used rough estimates of the cost of personnel, equipment, and supplies to determine prices. Most facilities, however,

Table 5.2 Outpatient fee schedule for selected services at ten hospitals, 1986 (Dominican Pesos)

Hospital	Laboratory		Pap smear	Blood typing	Haemo gram	X-ray[a]		Electro cardio-gram	Consul-tation
	Min. Fee	Max. Fee				Min.	Max.		
Carl George[b]	5.00	5.00	N/A	2.00	2.00	8.00	16.00	N/A	none
Dr Dario Contreras	1.50	10.00	N/A	1.50	1.50	5.00	20.00[c]	N/A	0.50
Jaime Mota	0.05	3.00	5.00	3.00	3.00	6.00	6.00	N/A	none
José Maria Cabral y Báez	5.00	[d]	1.00	5.00	5.00	10.00	40.00[e]	2.00	0.50[f]
Juan Pablo Pina	0.50	5.00	10.00	0.50	1.00	20.00	20.00	10.00	0.25
N.S. de la Altagracia	1.00[g]	40.00	3.00	2.50	2.00	30.00	60.00[e]	N/A	0.10[h]
Dr Luis E. Aybar	1.00	5.00	N/A	3.00	3.00	10.00	75.00	N/A	none
National Laboratory	3.00	35.00[i]	6.00	6.00	5.00	N/A	N/A	N/A	none
Dr Padre Billini	2.00	12.00	5.00	n.a.	n.a.	10.00	45.00	5.00	0.50
Robert Reid Cabral	1.00	1.00	N/A	1.00	1.00	5.00[i]	40.00	10.00	0.25[k]

[a] Price was per X-ray film taken unless otherwise indicated. [b] Pregnant women, children, and students were not charged. [c] X-ray services ranged from a picture of a child's thorax (DR$ 5.00) to simple abdominals (DR$ 20.00). [d] Routine tests such as tests for creatinism and haemoglobin levels were charged the minimum price. Sophisticated tests were not included in the price list, but all tests had fees attached. [e] Charged inpatients and outpatients for record card on first visit. [f] For a first outpatient visit, a set of five tests were provided for a flat fee of DR$ 5.00. Tests included a pap smear, a blood typing, and urine, blood, and STD tests. [g] Upper range covered glucose tolerance tests and hormonal radioimmunoassays. [h] For the first paediatric visit. [i] X-ray charges varied according to ability to pay and were assessed by the nun in charge of the X-ray department. Roughly 50 per cent of patients paid the minimum. [k] Charge for receptacle for medication.

Notes: N/A indicates not applicable. n.a. indicates data are not available. Exchange rate 8/87 US$ 1.00 = DR$ 3.70.

set charges that typically covered the marginal cost of supplies (for example, X-ray film, chemical reagents, and EKG paper), since government allocations were insufficient to cover these expenses. Indeed Robert Reid Cabral Hospital estimated that the Government budget allocation only covered one quarter of X-ray supply costs. Consideration of cross-subsidization or utilization incentives was not typically included in fee-setting decisions.

Some hospitals charged per test, others had a flat fee for all laboratory (Carl George Hospital) or X-ray (Jaime Mota Hospital) services, regardless of how many or how complex these tests were. Contreras Hospital charged per X-ray for simple services and a flat fee for a series of more complicated X-rays. The National Laboratory and Cabral y Báez Hospital charged separately for each service. Expensive procedures and drugs were borne by the hospital whenever possible, but typically patients were asked to contribute toward the cost as well. About half the facilities in the sample levied a consultation fee.

The differences between hospitals in the range and level of prices for specific services were considerable. For example, some hospitals had a flat fee for laboratory work and others had no upper limit, since prices were a function of average costs. The differences were striking also also for X-ray charges. Some of the differences in the maximum X-ray price reflected the limited availability of more sophisticated and costly services.

Inpatient services

In accordance with the constitution, most inpatient services were provided free of user charges, although there were a few exceptions. Some hospitals sent patients to other facilities for tests (for example to the National Laboratory), and patients were required to pay any associated fees there. Cabral y Báez Hospital charged DR$ 0.50 for a record card. Aybar Hospital had a nominal charge of DR$ 25.00 for eye-bank surgery because of the specialized nature of the service. Contreras Hospital charged for physical therapy, starting at DR$ 1.00 per session. Otherwise, hospitalization was free.

Cabral y Báez Hospital had a private wing of 24 beds where patients received improved hotel and additional nursing services at prices below the private-sector charges. Patient services were recorded on their charts, and charges imposed for all goods and services. A 20 per cent fee was added to the total to compensate the hospital for the enhanced services, and the attending physician charged the patient separately. Separate accounting methods for private patients led to minimum abuse of the system, although the net earnings to the hospital from private inpatients had never been assessed.

The only other charges associated with inpatient care at some hospitals were for blood. Each hospital handled its own blood needs. Patients either brought their own blood supplies with them or paid to have the hospital acquire it. Charges were remarkably uniform, suggesting that fees were based on cost.

If user fees are to discourage over-utilization and reflect the true resource cost of services provided, charges should be linked to the costs of providing services. All curative services should be charged for, with the price of inpatient care set higher than outpatient services, and with more costly diagnoses and treatments reflected in higher fees. A counterweight to these efficiency criteria are the political ramifications associated with fees and their levels, and the costs and difficulty of administration. In the fee structures described here the latter considerations predominated. Only Cabral y Báez Hospital and the National Laboratory attempted to set fees according to hospital costs (and the fee levels at Padre Billini suggested a similar strategy in past years). Thus while the system as a whole attempted to raise revenues, most hospital directors did not try to do so in an efficient manner.

The cost of collecting fees was not seen as a big problem, though data on collection costs were not available. Hospitals had seen some increase in emergency outpatient demand after cashier hours, and while they were considering extending cashier and social worker hours, this would raise the costs of collection and would have to be balanced against increased revenue. In Sudan, Bekele and Lewis (1986) found that user fee collection costs ranged between 5 and 7 per cent of gross earnings, which was not inconsistent with the perceptions of hospital directors in the Dominican Republic.

A major impediment to more rational charging was the inability to charge for the high cost of hospitalization. Inpatients require a much broader set of services than outpatients, and outpatients subsidized inpatients. Outpatients were expected to pay for tests which were free to inpatients, and inpatient consultations were free, whereas outpatients paid a fee to see a physician at some hospitals. Such practices provided inappropriate incentives to patients to seek admission to hospital. Moreover, since outpatients are much more likely to be seeking preventive services (for example, pap smears or prenatal care) than are inpatients, there was a greater incentive to seek curative rather than preventive care. If government perceives that preventive services are merit goods and therefore warrant subsidies to increase their use above what they would otherwise be (Roth 1987; de Ferranti 1985), the subsidy to preventive care should be greater than that for curative care, where demand is high and the benefit to the individual exceeds that to society.

In short, pricing practices promoted inpatient over outpatient care, and curative care rather than preventive care. By charging inpatients, especially at specialized hospitals where inpatients could often pay, more revenue would be generated, and, more importantly, fees would then better reflect resource use. Hospitalization should not and need not be free for everyone.

Sources of medical facility resources

Government operating budgets for most hospitals remained largely static during the first half of the 1980s. This same period saw high inflation rates (130 per cent between 1980 and 1985), recession, and a relatively high population growth-rate of 2.5 per cent per annum (Ramirez *et al.* 1986). The incentives for hospital directors to seek operating funds elsewhere, or to expand their debt by delaying payment of bills, were therefore very strong. Hospital financing was achieved through a combination of government transfers, mounting hospital debt (supplier credits), and facility revenues, supplemented in some instances by the 'Patronatos' and other donor and charitable contributions.

The two budgets for personnel and operating costs, hospital debt, and the outpatient revenues of the ten facilities are shown for 1986 in Table 5.3. There appears to be no clear relationship between the personnel and operating budgets.

Cabral y Báez Hospital had the largest budgets, the highest supplier credits, and the greatest revenues. The National Laboratory's outpatient revenues were almost twice its operating budget, while

Table 5.3 *Personnel and operating budgets, debt burden, and outpatient revenues for selected facilities, 1986 (Dominican pesos)*

Facility	Personnel budget	Operating budget	Hospital debt	Outpatient revenues*	Average outpatient revenue
Carl George	831054	180000	88784	27914	1.29
Dr Dario Contreras	1261548	960000	326342	178163	3.60
Jaime Mota	785450	126000	n.a.	6420	0.20
José Maria Cabral y Báez	6174230	2190000	792271	257118	2.15
Juan Pablo Pina	1782168	540000	50823	59290	0.84
Maternidad, Nuestra Señora de la Altagracia	2551612	840000	177238	85400	1.08
Dr Luis E. Aybar	1739038	900000	254253	35443	0.51
National Laboratory	n.a.	132000	13427	238660	n.a.
Dr Padre Billini	n.a.	315000	n.a.†	52495	1.30
Robert Reid Cabral	1967350	840000	0	24121	0.22

* Excludes donor and charitable contributions as well as the donations of the 'Patronato' where these apply. Includes José Maria Cabral y Báez Hospital's inpatient receipts.
† Records cannot be located, but according to the previous director of the Robert Reid Cabral Hospital, Dr Padre Billini Hospital was the only other debt-free public hospital in 1986.

Jaime Mota, Robert Reid Cabral, and Aybar Hospitals raised only 3 to 4 per cent of their operating budgets. Padre Billini Hospital raised about 17 per cent of its budget. The rest clustered at around 10 to 12 per cent. Clearly evident is the importance of fees in relation to operating budgets at Contreras, Padre Billini, and Cabral y Báez Hospitals and the National Laboratory. The prices at these facilities were slightly higher than average for comparable services, and they charged for each service even if the fee was modest (for example, consultation fees). The last column of Table 5.3 suggests the consistency of collection across patients (implicitly assuming equal ability to pay) for these four facilities. User fees in Jaime Mota and Robert Reid Cabral Hospitals, on the other hand, were almost incidental: far below those of other public hospitals.

Deficit financing of operating costs had become increasingly popular in public hospitals, and in 1986 only Robert Reid Cabral Hospital (and reportedly Dr Padre Billini) were debt-free. Supplier credits as high as 50 per cent of operating budgets were evident (Carl George Hospital), although most hospitals were closer to 30 per cent of their operating budgets. The National Laboratory and Juan Pablo Pina Hospital had a modest debt of roughly 10 per cent of their SESPAS operating budgets.

In the short term, supplier credits may be used as a source of low (or zero) interest loans. Indeed, the National Laboratory expanded its facility, raised significant amounts of funds, and yet maintained a modest debt balance. In the longer term, given budget projections, hospitals will have to rely more on user contributions or charity. There is a limit to the amount of credit that can be accumulated, since providers will terminate their services to non-paying hospitals.

Table 5.4 puts the scope for cost recovery into perspective, showing the composition of operating funds (personnel costs are excluded) for the ten facilities in the sample. Excluding the National Laboratory, hospitals received the bulk of their funding from SESPAS. Outpatient fees were the single largest non-budget source of funds for all but Robert Reid Cabral Hospital. Inpatient fees were significant only for José Maria Cabral y Báez Hospital, which had a functioning private wing. Robert Reid Cabral and Maternidad Nuestra Sra de la Altagracia Hospitals had active 'Patronato' efforts that raised considerable amounts, which exceeded and equalled, respectively, the proportion that fees contributed to resources in these facilities. A number of the hospitals also had volunteer groups within the hospital that raised money, assisted needy patients, and generally contributed to the overall functioning of the hospital. No estimates were available of the value of these services.

In some facilities, consultation fees probably brought in the largest amount of revenue: although the fee was modest, the volume of patients ensured considerable revenue. Both laboratory and X-ray services had considerable revenue potential. The results in the table reflect a combination of how much was charged, how frequently services were needed, and the overall patient load of the facility.

Table 5.4 *Sources of funds for selected facilities, 1986 (Percentage breakdown)*

Facility	Operating Budget	Donors	Patronato	Outpatients			Inpatients	Other
				Lab	X-ray	Total*		
Carl George	80.5	0	7.0	9.1	2.1	12.5	0	0
Dr Dario Contreras	83.8	0	0	1.0	13.0	15.6	0.6	0
Jaime Mota	95.2	0	0	4.8	0.0	4.8	0	0
José Maria Cabral y Báez	69.9	0	0	1.9	3.4	8.2	12.1	9.8
Juan Pablo Pina	89.4	0.8	0	N/A	N/A	9.8	0	0
Maternidad, Nuestra Señora de la Altagracia	79.3	2.4	8.1	3.9	N/A	8.1	0	2.1
Dr Luis E. Aybar	94.0	0.4	0	N/A	N/A	3.7	1.9	0
National Laboratory	34.2	3.9	0	61.9	0.0	61.9	0	0
Dr Padre Billini	85.3	0†	0	0.0	3.6	14.2	0	0.5
Robert Reid Cabral	73.3	12.6	12.0	0.6	0.4	2.1	0	0

* The total also included consultation fees, special charges, health cards and other payments; hence the percents do not add up to the outpatient percent total.

† Donations were received from various sources but neither the donor nor the amount or value were recorded.

Trends in medical facility resources

In most instances, fee revenue was rising rapidly. The trends in outpatients, outpatient revenues, government budgets, and debt are shown in Table 5.5. Although trend data on fee levels were not available, it would appear that, in nominal terms, either charges had increased, new fees had been introduced, or hospitals were collecting revenues more consistently.

Around 6 of the hospitals experienced declining outpatient attendances, and yet revenues rose sharply, typically outpacing inflation. Only Jaime Mota experienced a modest downturn in

Table 5.5 *Growth in outpatients, operating budgets, and debts for selected facilities, 1984 to 1986*

Hospital*	Percentage change in number of outpatients	Percentage change in government budget	Percentage change in debt	Percentage change in outpatient revenues
Carl George	12.2%	0.0%	15.5%	21.4%
Dr Dario Contreras	–12.4	0.0	2611.5	6.3
Jaime Mota	–13.5	0.0	0.0	–1.3
José Maria Cabral y Báez	–14.7	18.1	2.8	103.4
Juan Pablo Pina†	–14.2	12.5	–32.3	29.7
N.S. de la Altagracia	–14.2	0.0	–13.3	24.8
Dr Luis E. Aybar	13.3	12.5	31.4	185.8
National Laboratory	n.a.‡	0.0	36.8	6.7
Robert Reid Cabral†	17.2	27.3	–100.0	90.6

* Trend data not available for Dr Padre Billini Hospital.
† Changes are between 1982 and 1986
‡ Although outpatient data were not available for the National Laboratory, the annual number of tests performed rose consistently over the period.

nominal revenues, but it was located in one of the poorest areas, and had a limited commitment to fees as a means of raising additional resources. In real terms, however, the National Laboratory, Contreras Hospital, and Juan Pablo Pina Hospital experienced a reduction in annual revenues because growth in earnings lagged behind inflation.

Reduced utilization was largely attributed to deterioration in service quality. Lack of drugs, broken machinery, and lack of supplies limited the extent and quality of out-and inpatient services. A 1985 PAHO-supported study of public hospitals found that 90 per cent of incubators, three-quarters of X-ray and laboratory equipment, and almost half the sterilizers were non-functional (SESPAS/PAHO 1985).

While rising fees may be thought to have discouraged use, in practice fee increases were modest, and all patients had the opportunity to have their charges waived (see below). Hospital social workers felt that fee increases had generally not resulted in increased patient requests for waivers. The fact that Aybar Hospital had the highest fee increases and one of the largest rises in outpatients reinforces the view that rising fees did not discourage use. La Forgia (1989) has shown that patient volume rose at the National Laboratory despite frequent adjustments to fees.

The limited growth in government monies and increasingly successful efforts to raise funds through fees and charitable contributions shifted hospital dependence away from government budget allocations. Table 5.6 shows revenue relative to outpatient volume, and operating budget support per outpatient during the years 1984 to 1986. The former measure is an important indicator of cost-recovery performance. The reduction in the number of outpatients during this period prevented a decline in per capita operating budgets, although in real terms their value fell by about 30 per cent. Only Aybar and Carl George Hospitals experienced a per capita reduction, resulting from an increase in outpatients of 13.3 and 12.2 per cent respectively (see Table 5.5). Per capita outpatient revenues rose in nominal terms during this period, and in percentage terms improved at a faster rate than per capita budget levels. Aybar Hospital had the biggest increase in per capita revenues (155 per cent), although from a modest base. Cabral y Báez Hospital's per capita revenues rose by 139 per cent, or over 100 per cent in real terms.

Rising costs and budgetary stringencies appear to have made

Table 5.6 *Government budget and fee revenues in relation to outpatient volume, 1984–1986 (Dominican pesos)*

Facility	1984		1985		1986	
	Revenue/ out-patient	Operating budget/ out-patient	Revenue/ out-patient	Operating budget/ out-patient	Revenues/ out-patient	Operating budget out-patient
Carl George	0.82	6.45	0.78	7.71	1.29	5.75
Dr Dario Contreras	2.97	17.00	3.88	20.39	3.60	19.41
Jaime Mota	0.25	4.90	0.31	5.33	0.20	5.66
José Maria Cabral y Báez	0.90	13.22	1.72	16.63	2.15	18.30
Juan Pablo Pina	0.65	5.85	0.85	6.96	0.84	6.02
N.S. de la Altagracia	0.75	9.10	0.71	10.83	1.08	10.60
Dr Luis E. Aybar	0.20	13.06	0.47	14.78	0.51	12.97
Robert Reid Cabral	0.19	6.90	0.17	8.26	0.22	7.49

facilities more cognizant of the need to raise funds from patients who could pay. The experience over time indicated in Table 5.6 points to the relative commitment of hospitals to share costs with users.

The data presented here suggest that user fees were an important source of funding for public hospitals, that some facilities were much more successful than others at raising funds, and therefore that there remained considerable scope for raising additional funds through a more aggressive stance. The more successful fee systems in the Dominican Republic, from the point of view of per capita outpatient revenues, debt history, and trends in revenue levels, were characterized by: fees that reflected actual resource use; fees for most if not all services, even if they were only token charges; and charges for high-volume services. These conform to efficiency principles, as charges should be a function of costs, and charging something is better than nothing, assuming a basic ability to pay for some services.

Those hospitals that made a commitment to cover some portion of costs through raising funds from patients who could pay raised a good deal of revenue, covering as much as 30 per cent of hospital operating costs, and 66 per cent of the National Laboratory costs. The experience of the latter suggested that raising laboratory charges in other hospitals could increase revenues, and the experience at the Cabral y Báez Hospital reinforced this conclusion. Robert Reid Cabral Hospital, a paediatric hospital, successfully raised resources from its 'Patronato', an option that, while feasible, was probably not as attractive to hospitals with a more general mission.

Thus fees appear to have been the marginal additional resource that kept some hospitals operating. These resources allowed the purchase of basic inputs to medical care, without which the labour component (for example physicians and nurses) could neither function nor be effective. The alternatives to fees were rising supplier credits, fewer patients, or lower quality. Although user fees typically did not entirely substitute for these alternatives they mitigated their effects. Fees were clearly crucial to some hospitals' continued operation, and a key to maintaining quantity and quality of services.

Use of revenues

The use of discretionary resources was determined by the hospital director, and occasionally by department heads. Table 5.7 provides data for nine of the ten facilities, including information on total expenditures of discretionary revenues in 1986, and the distribution of those monies across expenditure categories. Where possible, the value of donated time and materials was imputed and included in the total.

In 1986, drugs were the most frequently purchased item; only the National Laboratory did not buy pharmaceuticals. Such purchases supplemented SESPAS's allocation and paid for costly drugs. Personnel was a priority for a number of facilities, while others believed that funding personnel, especially technical personnel, was an unacceptable use for hospital revenues: government policy was vague on this point. A number of hospitals paid for additional technical and unskilled staff, and some money was used to top-up salaries to attract and keep better technical staff. Hospitals complained about excessive numbers of physicians and inappropriate

Table 5.7 *Expenditures of discretionary revenues for selected hospitals, 1986*

Hospitals*	Total (pesos)	% to drugs	% to personnel	% to maint.	% to equip.	% to supplies	% to food	% to other
Carl George	36221.56	55.9	0.1	15.2	3.5	0.0	5.9	19.4
Dr Dario Contreras	181256.62	29.8	4.1	8.1	0.0	25.7	30.9	1.6
Jaime Mota	6118.19	81.5	5.7	3.5	1.8	0.0	4.9	2.4
José Maria Cabral y Báez	244395.63	13.4	—	37.3	—	29.7	8.3	11.4
Juan Pablo Pina Maternidad, Nuestra	48665.54	53.2	24.3	8.8	2.1	0.0	0.7	10.8
Señora de la Altagracia	119770.04	11.5	14.0	34.1	9.3	18.7	5.2	7.1
Dr Luis E. Aybar	28306.05	19.4	2.4	8.2	0.0	0.0	0.7	69.3†
National Laboratory	488916.05	0.0	23.8	2.5	1.1	69.7‡	0.0	2.9
Robert Reid Cabral	25042.63	8.9	57.1§	2.7	0.0	13.6	12.1	5.6

* Data not available for Dr Padre Billini Hospital. † 87.7% was allocated to the gastroenterology department. ‡ 79.9% for purchase of reagents. § All allocated to administrative and unskilled workers.

staff mixes, and these discretionary resources compensated for the central government's staff allocations, over which hospitals had minimal control.

Most facilities spent something on maintenance; but surprisingly, equipment was rarely purchased. Additional food expenditure was required in a number of facilities, despite the heavy allocation from the SESPAS budget. Supplies were either quite important or facilities spent nothing on them at all. Poor record-keeping systems, which lumped a wide variety of purchases together with little or no explanation, made it difficult to identify other expenditures. Only Aybar Hospital allocated a significant chunk of its earnings to a single department: over 69 per cent of its discretionary funds went to the gastroenterology department.

Trends over time suggested that revenues and other sources of funds only allowed facilities to continue their expenditures; however, the debt levels at most of the hospitals also indicated that they had used supplier credits to cover expenses in the recent past. Even if hospitals' overall financial resources from budgets, revenues, and charity remained the same, debt repayments would claim a certain portion of those resources, and thus constrain their ability to increase expenditures.

The shifts in allocation of discretionary revenue were modest over time. Figure 5.1 summarizes the aggregate changes across hospitals between 1984 and 1986. The National Laboratory was excluded because its much larger earnings skewed the distribution to the 'other' category. Personnel (i.e. additional staff and salary supplements) and maintenance decreased somewhat, and 'other' rose between 1984 and 1986, because of Aybar Hospital's new policy of allocations to gastroenterology as well as increases in expenditures on food and supplies at some hospitals.

The discretionary hospital revenues raised from fees and charitable efforts provided the marginal resources to help keep facilities operating at a minimally acceptable level. Basic inputs such as personnel, drugs, supplies, and maintenance received the bulk of these funds at most facilities, and represented essential elements of proper operation. The National Laboratory raised quality dramatically in terms of the speed and accuracy of tests, and increasingly attracted private patients. Fee revenues ensured availability of supplies and functioning infrastructure, and provided the director with the resources both to hire needed staff and to reward the performance of government personnel.

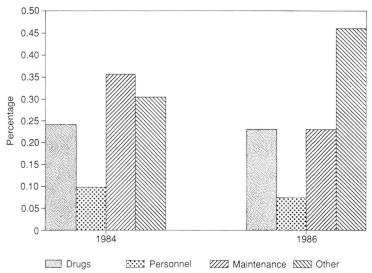

Fig. 5.1   Percentage allocation of resources by function (all hospitals excluding National Laboratory) 1984 to 1986.

Means testing

Every health facility in the sample had a method for waiving fees for those unable to pay even modest charges. Patients who felt they could not pay were interviewed by a social worker who decided, on the basis of a socio-economic assessment, family size, home address, and various qualitative factors, whether full or partial payment was warranted. Some facilities kept detailed accounts of these efforts and the final decision on each patient; and others had no idea of the volume.

Table 5.8 summarizes the information on patients excused payment in five facilities between 1984 and 1986. NS de la Altagracia estimated that less than 1 per cent were fully exempted from fees, and even fewer partially exempt. The National Laboratory required all patients to pay something; and the social worker estimated that about half the patients received a discount. At Dario Contreras Hospital, where data-registration was the most complete and accurate, between a quarter and a third of patients did not pay the full charge, and between 26 and 30 per cent were exempted, so fewer than half paid the full price. Robert

Reid Cabral Hospital's X-ray department had a larger proportion of patients fully exempted, but a smaller proportion partially exempted. Carl George Hospital, with only general estimates about payment waivers, had about 30 per cent of its patients paying full prices. This small sample suggests that hospitals waived payment for around half their patients, and reduced the fee for about another 20 per cent.

Thus a significant portion of patients who used public hospitals were exempted from charges, although little information was available on the characteristics of those who were exempt or those who received discounts. The effectiveness of the system of administering means tests was therefore unknown. All that can be concluded is that there was a system for addressing the government's equity concerns; criteria for determining ability to pay were established; and some patients' fees were waived or partially waived, although it cannot be said that it was only those who could not pay who were exempted. It is reasonable to conclude that the means test was functioning, if imperfectly.

Table 5.8 *Proportion of patients excused from fee payment at selected hospitals, 1984–1986*

Hospital	1984		1985		1986	
	Paid less than fee	Did not pay	Paid less than fee	Did not pay	Paid less than fee	Did not pay
Carl George*	20.0	50.0	20.0	50.0	20.0	50.0
Dr Dario Contreras	25.8	27.3	32.9	30.0	34.1	26.5
Maternidad, Muestra Señora de la Altagracia	0.04	0.09	0.06	1.0	0.02	1.0
National Laboratory*	50.0	0.0	50.0	0.0	50.0	0.0
Robert Reid Cabral†	10.8	37.8	8.1	58.5	9.3	36.1

* Estimates from social worker and director.
† X-rays only. Other services would have fewer patients who made full or partial payment, because the screening practices were less effective.

Conclusions

The Dominican Republic experienced an economic downturn resulting in declining government budgetary allocations to public health during a period of increasing inflation and substantial population growth. The result was pressures on hospitals to raise funds from other sources. User fees were the single biggest source of supplementary funds for all but the national children's hospital, Robert Reid Cabral, which relied more heavily on its 'Patronato'. Charity and supplier credits were also used to help meet recurrent costs.

Each hospital's management team developed and implemented its own schemes to cover rising operating costs, without guidelines or regulation, and without the benefit of knowledge of successful experiences elsewhere. Wide variations in fee structures and revenues resulted. While the autonomy of the facilities may have provided an incentive to raise resources, the lack of regulation and especially of financial oversight left the system open to abuse.

The experience demonstrated which approaches are particularly effective in raising revenues. User fees were primarily charged for outpatient curative care, and were priced well below comparable services in the private sector. Pricing decisions varied, and some appeared better than others. Charging something for every service is important, since revenues are related to service volume. Nominal consultation fees can raise considerable revenue because they are assessed on almost every outpatient. The National Laboratory levied charges for all services and waived fees for no one, although discounts were provided to almost half their patients. Thus mimimum exemptions as well as charges on high-volume services are important to maximizing fee revenue.

Relating prices to cost satisfies an efficiency criterion, contributes to higher revenues, and allows facilities to meet a specific proportion of their operating requirements consistently. Since the system studied generally resulted in modestly priced services subsidizing more costly ones (even aside from outpatients subsidizing inpatients), a more efficient system where costs of service are the basis for fee levels would allow resource-uses to reflect their real value and contribute to cost-recovery. The use of a waiver system can separately address equity considerations. In the Dominican

Republic, the two objectives efficiency and equity were addressed simultaneously.

Public systems implicitly value all inputs equally, since inputs are centrally provided and patients are so rarely expected to pay anything. For example, costly imported equipment has equal value to domestically produced materials, because no prices are attached. Fees based on cost deter overutilization of those services that are most costly, and encourage greater use of less expensive alternatives, because revenues are limited and their expenditure fungible across activities. Where public health resources are as scarce as they were in the Dominican Republic, such a policy may be critical to continuing the supply of basic services.

The issue of ability to pay and the need to take equity considerations into account was addressed in every facility. All had a screening system that waived payment or reduced fees. In the few facilities for which data were available, at least 30 per cent of patients paid the full fee, and typically a much larger proportion did so. If nothing else, this experience suggests that an established system existed to ensure that those who could not pay still received health care, though data were unavailable on whose charges were waived.

The user fee system studied subsidized inpatient care, thereby providing strong incentives to patients to use emergency services or to seek admittance to the hospital to avoid charges. Given the high costs of inpatient care, the deteriorating real value of government transfers, and the shortage of resources in public hospitals, some system of inpatient fees was warranted. If outpatients are expected to help facilities cover costs, then inpatients could and should do the same. The method for ensuring that all citizens had access to care regardless of their ability to pay in theory provided a built-in safeguard to minimize abuse.

The revenues raised from user fees and charitable efforts were allocated to basic inputs of health care, including drugs, equipment, supplies, personnel, and maintenance. Without these complementary inputs, effectiveness, productivity, and staff morale would have been much lower, and at the margin such funds are the key to making public facilities function better. User fees helped to improve health care in public facilities, and at the same time hospitals attempted to meet the government's commitment to equity. The lack of oversight from the centre was on balance beneficial, allowing facilities a free hand to experiment. Continued

latitude would be beneficial to most hospitals, although open
discussion of the scope for alternative revenue-raising options,
and perhaps provision of general incentives such as a requirement
to meet a certain proportion of the operating budget, could spur
on those facilities that were less successful or less interested in
raising their own funds. Clearly, the most important next step was
to recognize the need to expand charges to inpatients who could
pay for services.

References

Ainsworth, M. (1984). User charges for social sector finance: policy and
practice in developing countries, World Bank CDP Discussion Paper
No. 1984–6, March. The Bank, Washington, DC.
Bartlett, L. (undated). Health systems management project financial
analysis. USAID/Santo Domingo [Mimeo].
Bekele, A. and Lewis, M. A. (1986). Financing health care in the Sudan:
some recent experiments in the Central Region. *International Journal
of Health Planning and Management*, **1**, 111–27.
Ceara-Hatton, M. (1987). Hacia una nueva dinamica de la economia
Dominicana. GIE-INTEC, Santo Domingo [Mimeo].
de Ferranti, D. (1985). *Paying for health services in developing countries*,
World Bank Staff Working Paper No 721. World Bank, Washington,
DC.
Dunlop, D. and Donaldson, D. (1987). *Sector review, Ethiopia: a study of
health financing. Issues and options*, Report No 6624-ET. World Bank,
Department of Population, Health, and Nutrition, Washington DC.
Griffin, C. (1987). *User charges for health care in principle and practice*,
Population, Health and Nutrition Technical Note 87–16. World Bank,
Washington, DC.
La Forgia, G. M. (1989). User fees, quality of care and the poor:
lessons from the Dominican Republic. Report to the Inter-American
Foundation, Santo Domingo [Mimeo].
Lewis, M. A. and Parker, C. (1991). Policy and implementation of user
fees in Jamaican public hospitals. *Health Policy*, **18**, 57–85.
Lewis, M. A., Sulvetta, M. B. and La Forgia, G. M. (1990). *Measuring
costs, efficiency and quality in public hospitals: a Dominican case*. Latin
America and the Caribbean Region Internal Discussion Paper, Report
IDP-090. The World Bank, Washington, DC.
Lindsay, C. M. (1975). *Veterans administration hospitals, an economic
analysis of government enterprise*. American Enterprise Institute,
Washington DC.
Overholt, C. (1987). User fee experience in public, acute care hospitals
in Honduras, JSI Reach Project, Washington, DC [Mimeo].

PPSS (President's Private Sector Survey on Cost Control) (1984). *Report on privatisation.* Government Printing Office, Washington, DC.

Ramírez, N., Duarte, I., and Gómez, C. (1986). *Población y Salud en la Republica Dominicana.* Instituto de Estudios de Población y Desarollo de Profamilia, Santo Domingo.

Roth, G. (1987). *The private provision of public services.* Oxford University Press, New York for the World Bank, Washington DC.

SESPAS / PAHO (1985). *Mantenimiento y conservación de infrastructura física de salud.* Estudios de la Primera Etapa Proyecto SESPAS BID-OPS/OMS, Area de Mantenimiento. SESPAS, Santo Domingo.

Shepard, D. S., Carrin, G., and Nyandagazi, P. (1987). *Self-financing of health care at government Health Centres in Rwanda.* Harvard Institute for International Development under AID Contract No. DPE-5927-C-00–5068–00., Cambridge, Mass.

Waddington, C. J. and Enyimayew, K. A. (1989). A price to pay: the impact of user charges in Ashanti-Akim District, Ghana. *International Journal of Health Planning and Management,* **4**, 17–47.

Author's note

I would like to thank the AID-funded REACH project for support in preparing this study; the many officials of the Dominican government who assisted in defining the project; and the hospital managers who facilitated the data-collection. I am also indebted to Charles Griffin and Philip Musgrove for providing useful comments, and to Ranjit Dighe for research assistance.

6

Household participation in financing of health care at government health centres in Rwanda

Donald S. Shepard, Guy Carrin, and Prosper Nyandagazi

Introduction

Rwanda's health financing situation

Rwanda is a small landlocked country in Eastern Africa with an area of approximately 26000 sq.km. and an estimated population of 6.9 million persons in 1989. With a 1989 per capita Gross National Product (GNP) of US$320, Rwanda is classified amongst the poorest countries in the world. Like many developing countries, it faces a serious and growing problem in the financing of its government health services, as new initiatives have outstripped resources. Declining prices for coffee – Rwanda's main export – have meant that the country's revenue, unadjusted for inflation, has barely been maintained since 1981.

During this same period, the Ministry of Public Health and Social Affairs (MINISAPASO) gradually expanded both the number and the quality of its facilities, its goal being to have at least three hospitals per prefecture and one health centre per commune. Fortunately, MINISAPASO enjoyed a relatively high priority within the central government ministries. Yet despite a 7.2 per cent share of the Central Government budget in 1985, or US$13.7 million, finances failed to keep pace with the proliferation in facilities. As a result, pharmaceutical budgets were cut, and the implementation of some preventive programmes was threatened. Throughout this chapter, Rwandan francs (FRW) have been converted to US dollars at the May 1986 rate of 87 FRW equals US$1.00.

This study on alternative financing mechanisms originated in the Programme for Combatting Childhood Communicable Diseases (CCCD) funded by the US Agency for International Development. The CCCD programme emphasizes vaccinations, oral rehydration therapy for diarrhoea, and malaria prophylaxis and treatment. To increase the likelihood that these activities could be sustained after the completion of the five-year CCCD project, Rwanda agreed to support an increasing share of the operating costs of these activities locally. As it was extremely difficult for the Rwandan central government to finance these costs, other revenues – including private sources – had to be found. We examined this question through a combination of facility and household data. Drug fees, as our study shows, appeared to be a very promising approach in Rwanda's search for alternative financing mechanisms.

The remainder of this section further outlines Rwanda's approach to health financing, and reviews the role for user fees generally. Later sections review data from four paired facilities to describe the source and magnitude of revenues and to determine the additional revenue needed for them to operate as intended; present the findings of a household survey of the catchment area of these facilities to assess whether utilization would be maintained despite higher fees; and offer short-run policy recommendations for charging users for drugs.

Financing medical care in Rwanda

Rwanda's health expenditures (from all sources) amounted to about 3.5 per cent of GNP in 1984, or US$5 per capita. External (i.e. foreign) sources financed 49.8 per cent of these expenditures as follows: non-governmental organizations, including missions: 18.4 per cent of total health expenditures; bilateral aid: 21.9 per cent; and multilateral aid: 9.5 per cent. Domestic sources financed the remaining 50.2 per cent, and were made up of: government; 38.6 per cent of total expenditures; individual sources: 8.5 per cent; and insurance institutions: 3.1 per cent (MINISAPASO 1985). External donors financed more than 80 per cent of capital investments in the health sector (MINISAPASO, unpublished data, 1986). Clearly, as in other sub-Saharan African countries, foreign resources played a prominent role in Rwanda.

In 1984, the Rwanda central government sharply curtailed all public-sector outlays in an attempt to halt the country's three-year financial deterioration. Government expenditures were reduced to 12.9 per cent of GNP from 14.6 per cent in 1983. In consequence, public-sector health expenditures per capita were only $2.25 (196

FRW) in 1985, a sum inadequate to meet Rwanda's basic health needs or to maintain its essential infrastructure. In short, Rwanda's public sector could not commit sufficient resources to current health-care demands, and foreign resources were limited to other purposes. Hence alternative sources had to be found so that public health facilities could operate fully.

Role of user fees in Rwanda and other developing countries

Direct financing methods are increasingly advocated as a source of additional resources for health (Shepard and Benjamin 1987; de Ferranti 1985). Such methods include user fees for health services or drugs, and prepayment schemes for health care. The former method requires payment at the time health care is received; the latter, a payment in advance for the right to receive care if and when it is needed. User fees and drug sales are the methods most frequently used (Stinson 1982), because of their greater administrative simplicity, and because the close link between revenues and services makes monitoring cash-flow and book-keeping fairly straightforward. In contrast, prepayment schemes require greater financial management expertise and involve complex administrative duties. Problems arise in applying actuarial principles to set a prepayment level for the prepayment scheme to at least break even; in managing a large amount of working capital (for example, up to a year's prepayment for all members); and in maintaining administrative or enforcement mechanisms to address non-compliance with the prepayment arrangements.

Typically, the revenues generated by user fees in the public sector in developing economies are rather modest. De Ferranti (1985) has estimated user-fee revenues as a percentage of the recurrent expenditures of government health services for 34 countries. The average – and the figure for Rwanda – was only 7 per cent; half the countries surveyed had shares below 2 per cent. In Rwanda's case, modest revenues from user fees were partly due to the fact that the fees for health-care services were relatively low. At the time of this study (April and May, 1986) the fee for an outpatient treatment in a government health centre (GHC) was US$0.23 (20 FRW), while for a hospital bed-day it was US$0.11 (10 FRW). Such fees represented only one-fifth and one-tenth of the minimum daily wage, respectively. Even by Rwandan standards, they were modest.

And yet even these modest revenues were not earmarked for the financing of health services, but instead went into the general fund of the commune. Even if user fees were to be increased, additional funds would not necessarily have become available to improve drug supplies.

The situation in mission health centres (MHCs) was different. Consultation fees were higher – usually more than double those charged in GHCs – and drugs were subject to separate fees. Quality of care and amenities in MHCs were better, with provision of food for hospitalized patients; availability of laundry services; cleaner wards; more frequent nursing care for hospitalized patients; and reliable supplies of needed drugs. However, financial aid from the mission organizations overseas contributed significantly to the care provided at the MHCs.

On the basis of arguments developed in this chapter, we recommended that government health centres in Rwanda should set up a revolving drug fund initially for CCCD drugs, and subsequently for all drugs. A revolving drug fund is a system whereby an initial inventory of drugs is purchased through a donation or levy, and subsequent revenues finance replenishment.

Paired health facilities and their catchment areas

To see whether higher charges to users (such as drug sales) were feasible in Rwanda, three key conditions had to be met: fees should generate enough money to help assure the sustainability of quality services in government facilities; the population should be able to afford and be willing to pay higher fees; and the fees should not substantially deter people from using services. To see whether these conditions were met, the authors conducted an empirical study in rural sections of two of Rwanda's prefectures (provinces) – Gikongoro and Kigali. These two provinces were selected to span a broad range in terms of infrastructure, resources, and availability of medical services, so that it might be possible to generalize the results.

Areas studied and their characteristics

Two health-care facilities were selected for study in each of the two selected provinces. The province of Kigali contained the national capital (Kigali), and was more densely populated than Gikongoro:

the population per sq. km. of agricultural land averaged 443 in Kigali and 395 in Gikongoro. Kigali's population had been growing at a faster rate (5.8 per cent per year from 1978 to 1982) than Gikongoro's (only 1.3 per cent). The higher population-density in Kigali was sustained by good soil and adequate infrastructure. In contrast, Gikongoro was one of the country's poorer regions, where low crop-yields due to acidic soil and a poor road infrastructure hampered improvements in the population's standard of living (Ministère de l'Agriculture, de l'Elevage, et des Forêts 1985).

To assess the population's ability to pay higher fees, we determined the economic resources of some 100 randomly chosen households from each of the four areas. These areas were communes each containing a health centre (one government and one mission health centre in each of the two provinces). A commune was the administrative area below the sub-prefecture, containing about 35000 inhabitants. The health centres, henceforth termed the reference health centres, were those of Musha (GHC) and Rwankuba (MHC) in Kigali, and Ngara (GHC) and Kaduha (MHC) in Gikongoro. A summary of selected indicators of wealth and income is given in Table 6.1.

Surveyed households were asked to describe the size of their holdings of agricultural land as 'very small' (approximately 1/4 ha or below); 'small' (1/2 ha); 'medium' (1 ha); 'large' (2 ha); or 'very large' (4 ha). The responses indicated that Musha and Rwankuba had somewhat larger farms than Ngara and Kaduha, and that a greater percentage of families had small or very small farms in Gikongoro province than in Kigali.

Cash income from the sale of agricultural products (mainly bananas, coffee, sorghum, and tea) and from salaried employment were both higher for households in the Kigali region than for those in Gikongoro (see Table 6.1). The data also confirm that the standard of living (after taking account of household size) in Musha and Rwankuba exceeded that of Ngara and Kaduha. The percentage of households with a per capita cash income at or below 1000 FRW (US$11.50) – a kind of poverty line – was higher in Gikongoro, especially around Kaduha, than it was in Kigali province.

Costs of services and fees at the four facilities

Table 6.2 presents salient data on the costs and financing of the four centres. Government health centres were supported primarily by

Table 6.1 *Economic resources of households in the catchment areas of the health centres*

| Indicator | Kigali Province | | Gikongoro Province | |
	Musha	Rwankuba	Ngara	Kaduha
Household Wealth				
Mean farm size in hectares*	0.8	0.7	0.6	0.5
Households with farms of 0.5 ha or less	49%	53%	62%	73%
Mean value of livestock†	$133.79	$145.31	$129.14	$103.62
Cash Income				
Mean household income from sales of agricultural products	$123.41	$108.75	$68.51	$39.43
From employment	$99.82	$88.79	$21.84	$85.53§
Total cash income	$223.23	$197.54	$90.35	$124.96
Mean cash income per capita§	$40.05	$36.23	$15.99	$22.79
Households with annual cash income per capita of $11.50 (1000 FRW) or less	35%	43%	59%	82%

Notes: * Derived from responses to a 5-category description of farm size: 'very small' (0.25 ha), 'small' (0.5 ha), 'medium' (1.0 ha), 'large' (2.0 ha), and 'very large' (4.0 ha).
    † Amounts converted to dollars at 87 FRW = US$1.
    ‡ From sales of agricultural products and employment.
    § Dominated by large observations.

Table 6.2 *Costs and financing at four health centres in Rwanda, 1985*

| | Kigali Province | | Gikongoro Province | |
	Musha (Gov't)	Rwankuba (Mission)	Ngara (Gov't)	Kaduha (Mission)
Operating expenses				
FRW (000)	1871	1092	2369	4661
US dollars*	21500	12600	27200	53600
Distribution of expenses (%)				
Salaries	68%	62%	48%	49%
Medications	6%	15%	31%	32%
Other expenses	26%	22%	21%	19%
Sources of revenues (%)				
User fees	28%	59%	14%	26%
Government	72%	25%	86%	13%
Mission	0%	16%	0%	61%
Outpatient episodes	30000	10000	10833	24495
Cost/episode				
FRW	44	47	109	142
US dollars	0.51	0.54	1.25	1.63
Basic fee/episode†				
FRW	20	40	20	50
US dollars	0.23	0.46	0.23	0.57
Ratio of basic fee to cost (%)	39%	85%	18%	35%
Inpatient days	5056	1287	1650	9890
Cost/day				
FRW	110	153	316	76
US dollars	1.26	1.76	3.67	0.88

Table 6.2 *(cont.)*

	Kigali Province		Gikongoro Province	
	Musha (Gov't)	Rwankuba (Mission)	Ngara (Gov't)	Kaduha (Mission)
Basic fee/day				
FRW	10	10	10	20
US dollars	0.11	0.11	0.11	0.23
Ratio of basic fee to cost (%)	9%	10%	3%	26%
Overall cost recovery (%)‡	28%	59%	14%	26%

* FRW=Rwandan franc. US$1.00=87 FRW (1986).
† Basic fee included consultations in all facilities and medications in government facilities. Laboratory examinations cost from 5 FRW for malaria slides to 40 FRW for some stool examinations in most facilities. All medications except antibiotics were free in Rwankuba.
‡ User fees from inpatient and outpatient care, medications, laboratory examinations, and ambulance as a percentage of total cost.

the national government, which paid staff salaries and provided drugs and supplies, although local government – the commune – contributed to the maintenance of buildings and vehicles. User fees, collected according to a schedule unchanged since 1975, had formerly reverted to the Treasury, but at the time of the study were remitted to the commune. As noted earlier, the standard fee for a new outpatient episode at a GHC was US$0.23 (20 FRW), while inpatient care cost US$0.11 per day. Medications, when available, were included in the consultation fee. Laboratory examinations, such as a blood smear or stool examination, generally cost US$0.11 each. Persons certified as indigent by their commune, along with schoolchildren and civil servants, were exempted from these fees.

One of the mission facilities, Rwankuba, was remarkably self-sufficient in its financing, generating 59 per cent of its overall operating costs and 85 per cent of its outpatient costs from user charges. While the other mission facility, Kaduha, actually generated greater revenues per visit, its staffing and drug costs were much higher, so the share of self-financing there was smaller. Both facilities demonstrated that user fees could finance an important

Table 6.3 *Availability of drugs at Musha Health Centre by source and recall period (per cent)*

	Sources							
	Today		Last month		Last year		Overall[†]	
Drug	From HC only	From HC & sales woman	From HC only	From HC & sales woman	From HC only	From HC & sales woman	From HC only	From HC & sales woman
Antimalarials								
Chloroquine*	0	100	48	100	50	100	33	100
Fansidar	0	100	0	100	0	100	0	100
Quinimax	0	100	0	100	5	100	2	100
Antiparasitics								
Mebendazole	100	100	50	100	40	100	63	100
Metronidazole	100	100	0	100	0	100	33	100
Piperazine*	100	100	100	100	100	100	100	100
Thiabendazole*	100	100	100	100	60	60	87	87
Antibiotics								
Penicillin*	0	100	60	100	50	100	37	100
Tetracycline	0	100	0	100	0	60	0	87

Other drugs

Aluminium*	100	100	90	90	100	100	97	97
Anti-cough syrup*	100	100	100	100	100	100	100	100
Aspirin*	100	100	45	45	60	60	68	68
Belladonna	100	100	100	100	80	100	93	100
Ear-drops	100	100	100	100	100	100	100	100
Eye-drops	100	100	100	100	100	100	100	100
Iron fortification*	100	100	100	100	100	100	100	100
Noscapine*	100	100	0	100	20	30	40	77
Nose drops	100	100	100	100	100	100	100	100
Niclosamide	100	100	100	100	40	100	80	100
Polyvitamins*	100	100	100	100	100	100	100	100
Means								
All drugs	75	100	65	97	60	86	67	94
10 leading drugs	80	100	80	99	76	89	79	96

Note: The ten most important drugs are those marked with an asterisk.
† Overall average is the unweighted average of the availabilities in the three reference periods.

part, or even a majority, of health expenditures. Observed fee levels supported costs of outpatient care to a greater extent than those of inpatient care.

Quality of services

Rwanda health-providers believed, as empirical research elsewhere (Akin *et al.* 1986) has shown, that higher-quality health services will be more heavily used, controlling for other variables. While, conceptually, quality can be measured in terms of the structure (types of facilities and services), process, and outcome of care, only structure can be assessed without an extraordinarily large and complex study. Since structure captures those characteristics most noticed by patients, the availability of drugs – a salient and readily observable structural indicator – was used as our primary indicator of quality.

All four facilities received allocations of drugs from government, although these were often inadequate, with some needed drugs frequently unavailable. Since the two MHCs were able to use their fee revenues to purchase additional drugs, they did not experience shortages. In contrast, the fees charged by the GHCs were given to the commune, and the law did not allow the heads of GHCs to charge supplementary fees, nor to earmark them for drug purchases.

Instead, the directors of GHCs sought alternative ways to provide patients with drugs. In Ngara, patients were sometimes advised to purchase needed drugs at the private pharmacy in the provincial seat of Gikongoro, about 25 km from Ngara, or to travel to a MHC. In Musha, a young woman under the auspices of a nearby mission was allowed to sell both oral and injectable drugs on the premises of the health centre, and these were then administered by health-centre personnel.

Tables 6.3 and 6.4 attempt to quantify drug availability at government health centres, including the retail sales in Musha. The directors of the two health centres were asked to estimate the availability (in percentage terms) of some 20 drugs at three different time-periods; the same day as the interview, during the last month, and during the last year. Availability on the day of the interview was answered by yes (100 per cent), or no (0 per cent). Supplies during the last month and the last year were reported as the percentage of weeks or months of

Table 6.4 *Availability of drugs at Ngara health centre by recall period (per cent)*

Drug	Today	Last month	Last year	Overall[†]
Antimalarials				
Chloroquine*	100	100	80	93
Fansidar	0	0	0	0
Quinimax	100	100	50	83
Antiparastic drugs				
Mebendazole	100	50	40	63
Metronidazole ᵥ	100	100	100	100
Piperazine*	0	50	80	43
Thiabendazole*	100	100	100	100
Antibiotics				
Penicillin*	100	100	100	100
Tetracycline	0	0	40	13
Other drugs				
Aluminium*	100	0	75	58
Anti-cough syrup	0	0	85	28
Aspirin*	0	0	75	25
Belladonna	100	100	75	92
Ear drops	0	0	0	0
Eye drops	0	0	25	8
Iron fortification*	0	0	0	0
Noscapine*	0	0	25	8
Nose drops	0	50	90	47
Niclosamide	100	100	25	75
Polyvitamins*	0	0	25	8
Means				
All drugs	45	43	55	52
Ten leading drugs	50	45	64	53

Notes: see Table 6.3.

the reference period that drugs were available. The data showed that drug availability varied both within each health centre over time and between health centres. To facilitate the interpretation of the data, we computed an availability index for all drugs as well as for the ten most important ones. We also computed an overall index, averaging the three reference periods. This overall index combined the better recall of the more recent periods with the opportunity to get more representative data over a longer period.

Four findings emerged from this analysis. First, overall drug availability at the Musha health centre was higher than that in Ngara (for example, 79 per cent versus 53 per cent for the 10 leading drugs). Second, the saleswoman in Musha did much to alleviate shortages, raising the overall availability of basic drugs to 96 per cent. The success of this arrangement indicated a clear willingness to pay for essential drugs, even when those same drugs were dispensed free at other times. Third, drug availability differed through the year. For example, in Musha, the availability during 'last month' (April, 1986) exceeded that of 'last year' (1985–6). In Ngara, the pattern was reversed. Fourth, drug availability in both of these centres was much lower than in mission health centres, where it was always 100 per cent for regularly used drugs.

In effect, the MHCs and the saleswoman in Musha operated successful revolving drug funds. Drug availability was adequate under both these systems, and inadequate elsewhere. Their smooth and competent administration by local personnel suggested that such systems would be feasible elsewhere. As salaries and other expenses were, in general, adequately covered, a revolving drug fund would suffice to cover the drug expenses. More importantly, such a scheme would provide the financial autonomy essential to ensure that additional revenues were available to the health centre and were used for health. On the basis of these considerations we concluded that a revolving drug fund could resolve the present financing and administrative problems of government health centres.

Population-based utilization, expenditures, and willingness to pay

Survey methods

The necessary random sample of households was obtained by using the technique of cluster sampling, adapted to Rwanda's administrative structure. Each administrative unit or commune is divided into approximately 8 sectors, and each sector has approximately 7 cells of approximately 100 households. Geographically, each cell is one of the thousands of hills that lace Rwanda's countryside, and is headed by a chairman who knows well, and is known by, these households.

A sample size of 100 households for each health centre's catchment area was planned, to ensure a sampling error below 5 per cent for any estimated proportions under simple random sampling. The sample was composed of 25 clusters of 4 households per cluster. To select the clusters, we adapted the sampling methods used for coverage surveys, and developed a cumulative list of the population of each area by sector. Within each sector, we knew only the number of cells, and assigned the average population to each. We chose a random starting number and added the sampling interval (one-twelfth of the cumulative population) 12 times. The cells in which these cumulative populations fell constituted a systematic sample of 12 cells. We chose one cell at random (based on cumulative populations) for over-sampling, as described below. For each systematically selected cell, one of the survey organizers visited the chairman and asked him to prepare a numbered list of the households in his cell. We selected two households (but three in oversampled cells) in each cell by systematic sampling by computing a sampling interval, randomly selecting a starting household number, and adding the sampling interval to obtain subsequent systematically chosen households. At each systematically chosen household, we obtained data from that household and from the three households closest to it.

Description of health expenditures

Table 6.5 shows out-of-pocket per capita health expenditures which were extrapolated from survey responses. These expenditures included services from the reference health centre, other health centres, and hospitals within and outside the commune, other service-providers, and private pharmacies. Annual expenditures ranged from US\$3.01 to US\$4.52 per capita, equivalent to US\$17 to US\$24 per household, or an average 2.4 per cent of household income.

Table 6.6 shows the types of services for which expenditures were incurred. Modern primary health care was predominant,

Table 6.5 *Per capita health expenditures in four areas in Rwanda*

	Kigali Province		Gikongoro Province		Average
	Musha (Gov't)	Rwankuba (Mission)	Ngara (Gov't)	Kaduha (Mission)	
Sample size (no. of):					
Households	101	102	100	100	101
Persons	572	556	565	535	557
Persons per household	5.66	5.45	5.63	5.35	5.52
Number of completed illnesses in sample (4 weeks' recall)					
Total	68	57	48	56	57
Percentage with any treatment	87%	86%	92%	89%	86%
Mean health expenditure per episode ($)*	1.95	2.48	2.90	3.32	2.66
Mean value per person per year:					
Number of illness episodes	1.55	1.33	1.10	1.36	1.34
Health expenditure ($)	3.01	3.31	3.20	4.52	3.51
Cash income (from employment and cash crops) ($)	41.04	36.24	15.99	22.80	29.02
Total income (incl. value of subsistence farming) ($)	186.53	115.23	117.16	113.30	133.06
Health expenditure as percentage of:					
Cash income	4.7%	11.3%	13.3%	15.2%	11.1%
Total income	1.0%	3.6%	1.8%	3.1%	2.4%

* FRW = Rwandan franc. US$1.00 = 87 FRW (1986).

Table 6.6 *Health expenditures per episodes of illness by type of expenditure (US dollars) (1US$ = 87 Rwandan francs)*

Type of expenditure	Kigali Musha	Rwankuba	Gikongoro Ngara	Kaduha	Average
	(68)*	(57)*	(48)*	(56)*	
Modern primary care:					
Government HC	$0.18	$0.04	$0.11	$0.05	$0.10
Mission HC	$0.09	$0.50	$0.49	$0.90	$0.50
Doctor or nurse	$0.02	$0.01	$0.00	$0.00	$0.01
Drugs at pharmacy	$0.33	$0.22	$0.45	$0.78	$0.44
Total primary care	$0.62	$0.77	$1.05	$1.73	$1.04
Other care:					
Traditional medicine	$0.44	$0.11	$0.35	$0.06	$0.24
Government hospital	$0.19	$1.01	$0.06	$0.00	$0.32
Mission hospital	$0.00	$1.18	$0.45	$0.75	$0.60
Grand total	$1.25	$3.07	$1.92	$2.54	$2.20

* Number of illness episodes.

with drugs constituting about half of the primary health-care expenditures. Hospital care was more heavily subsidized, and figured less prominently as an out-of-pocket expenditure. Overall, 76 per cent of reported episodes received some form of modern treatment (such as consultation, hospital care, or medications), indicating that respondents had a high regard for such medical care. While many minor problems may not have been identified as illnesses, once individuals defined themselves as ill, they almost always sought treatment.

The self-reported incidence of illness was strikingly low. The 229 episodes were derived from a population surveyed of 2228 persons with a four-week recall period. This is equivalent to 1.34 episodes per person per year. If there were errors in recall, they should not affect this rate substantially. While some illnesses may not have been reported, others that occurred more than four weeks ago may have been reported within the recall period. Influenza, malaria, and worms accounted for almost 60 per cent of the episodes of illness.

Effects of fees on utilization

The possible effect of higher user charges on utilization has important policy implications. If higher prices substantially reduce demand, then the social benefit of promoting access to health care would be considerably reduced. The health benefits of each service would have to be carefully assessed, or a policy of higher user fees would have to be implemented selectively. If, conversely, demand is little affected or not at all, then a more broad-based policy of higher user fees can be recommended.

From our household survey, we ascertained the mean and median prices shown in Table 6.7. As the data were skewed, median prices tended to be somewhat lower than means. This table shows how total prices paid by users exceeded the official prices for consultations alone. In all GHCs, the official price for the consultation and drugs was US$0.23 (20 FRW), except for persons entitled to free care. Actual mean consultation fees in GHCs were consistent with official policy, except in Musha, where several respondents reported paying more. Exemptions explain why mean consultation fees in GHCs were below US$0.23 in the other areas. In Kaduha mission health centre, the fee for an episode was US$1.15 (100 FRW) to register for the first time and US$0.57 (50 FRW) for subsequent episodes. Drugs in MHCs were sometimes subject to additional charges. Although the prices per episode for care by a trained provider (doctor or nurse), for traditional medicine, for drugs in a pharmacy, and for government or mission hospital care, were relatively high, the low mean expenditures on these services (in Table 6.6) show that these services were infrequently used.

The difference in prices between mission and government centres is striking, with overall prices in mission health centres about four times as high as those in government centres. The higher total prices at mission facilities were the result of higher standard consultation fees (about twice as high); fewer exemptions for free care; and higher and separate charges for drugs. Note that the price at Kaduha was eight times as high as the mean fee for government facilities around Rwankuba.

Table 6.8 shows that substantially higher fees were associated with some reduction in utilization of services. Within Kigali prefecture, the mission facility had fees that were 2.3 times as high as the government facility, and the rate at which the local population used the reference health facility was 42 per cent lower $(57-33)/57 = 42$

per cent). In Gikongoro province, the total price in the mission facility was almost five times that in the government facility, and utilization was 19 per cent lower.

Higher fees did not affect the overall probability of receipt of modern treatment for an illness episode. Patients who were able to walk had several health centres, hospitals, pharmacies, or other sources of care to choose from. The results show that higher fees in Kigali prefecture (at Rwankuba) were associated with higher overall utilization of modern care. In Kaduha, higher fees were associated with slightly lower utilization, though the effect was small. These findings are consistent with earlier results (Heller 1982), which suggest that fees affect the choice of provider more than the decision to seek care.

Table 6.7 *Total prices by treatment type paid by users of that treatment (US$)*

Type of treatment	Kigali Musha	Rwankuba	Gikongoro Ngara	Kaduha	All areas
	(68)*	(57)*	(48)*	(56)*	
Government health centre					
Consultations	$0.30	$0.19	$0.19	$0.19	$0.22
Laboratory exams and drugs	$0.26	$0.07	$0.23	$0.14	$0.18
Subtotal	$0.56	$0.26	$0.42	$0.31	$0.39
Median	$0.23	$0.23	$0.23	$0.23	$0.23
Mission health centre					
Consultations	$1.12	$0.48	$0.53	$0.63	$0.69
Laboratory exams and drugs	$0.40	$0.82	$1.27	$1.56	$1.01
Subtotal	$1.52	$1.30	$1.80	$2.19	$1.70
Median	$1.26	$1.21	$1.84	$1.12	$1.36
Trained provider	$0.57	$0.57	$0.00	$0.00	$0.29
Drugs at pharmacy	$1.47	$1.37	$6.21	$1.67	$2.68
Trad. medicine	$4.26	$1.59	$0.60	$4.23	$2.67
Government hospital	$6.55	$57.47	$0.00	$1.55	$16.39
Mission hospital	$0.00	$7.49	$8.37	$5.40	$5.32
All users	$1.44	$3.57	$2.09	$2.85	$2.49

* Number of illness episodes.

Table 6.8 *Percentage of ill persons receiving treatment at various facilities*

Source of Treatment	Kigali		Gikongoro	
	Musha	Rwankuba	Ngara	Kaduha
	(68)*	(57)*	(48)*	(56)*
Reference health centre†	57	33	48	39
Other type of health centre	6	19	27	20
Other modern care‡	6	36	8	16
All modern care	69	88	83	75

* Number of illness episodes.
† The reference health centres are those for which the service areas were defined (Musha, Rwankuba, Ngara, and Kaduha). Musha and Ngara are government health centres, while Rwankuba and Kaduha are mission centres. 'Other type of health centre' means mission centres around Musha and Ngara, where the reference centres are government-owned, and government centres around Rwankuba and Kaduha, where the reference centres are mission-owned.
‡ Other types of modern care were treatment by an individual trained provider, purchase of 'modern' pharmaceuticals, and inpatient care in a health centre or hospital.

To understand better how higher fees might affect utilization, we needed to control simultaneously for all important influences. When ill, individuals face a series of choices regarding their use of medical services. First, and most importantly, they must decide whether to seek care at the reference facility. Once there, they may be told that their condition requires a laboratory test, a drug, a follow-up visit, or inpatient hospitalization. Some of these services require an additional payment. Whether these services are obtained undoubtedly depends on a number of factors: on how strongly the need for them is presented; whether the patient actually has the required cash at the time; and whether they would have to wait or to return to the facility to receive the service.

Multivariate logistic regression analysis was used to analyse the initial decision of whether or not to seek care at the reference facility. The explanatory variables that proved statistically significant were the price of that medical care, the patient's sex, and the duration of their illness (a proxy for the severity of illness). Median total payments to a facility as reported by the patient for an episode of illness were taken as the 'price': these comprised the sum of fees for registration and consultations, laboratory examinations, and drugs, adjusted for exemptions due to indigence or other reasons. Since this price was derived from information reported by the patients (or their households), it was based on their understanding of the fee schedule. That understanding is what influences the patient's decision to seek care.

The statistical results, reported fully elsewhere (Shepard *et al.* 1987), indicated that females were more likely to receive care at the reference facility, and that longer illnesses were also more likely to receive treatment than shorter ones. The price variable is, of course, of the greatest policy interest in this analysis. We estimated that a doubling of the price would reduce the rate at which people sought care at the reference government health centre from 53 per cent to 50 per cent of episodes. This effect, while statistically significant, is not large enough to be of great concern. At the mean price across all health centres, the price elasticity of demand was −0.25. Hence fees for medications should substantially increase revenues, without imposing a substantial deterrent on utilization.

Furthermore, Table 6.8 showed that the proportion of episodes treated with 'modern' care from all sources was not substantially affected by higher fees in the reference health centre. Our data did not allow us to estimate the effect of prices in all health facilities on total utilization. Yet the rather low price elasticity of −0.25 suggests that higher fees at all facilities would have only a modest effect on total utilization of all modern care.

Willingness to pay more for health care

Two survey questions examined whether households would be willing to pay more for health care. Table 6.9 presents responses to the following question: 'Suppose that the government found that it needed to raise medical fees to assure the availability of medications. Which do you prefer, the current situation or the proposed modification?' It is striking that the preference for the higher fees was overwhelming (88–93 per cent) in all four areas. Furthermore, the preference was just as strong in low-income households as amongst normal-income households.

Table 6.9 *Percentage of households willing to accept higher fees to improve drug availability, by income level*

Income category	Kigali province		Gikongoro province	
	Musha	Rwankuba	Ngara	Kaduha
All households	80	88	93	89
(No. of households in group)	(100)	(101)	(99)	(100)
Low income	81	95	96	86
(No. of households in group)	(31)	(41)	(48)	(80)
Normal income	91	83	90	100
(No. of households in group)	(69)	(60)	(51)	(20)

Table 6.10 reports the percentage of households in each area reporting difficulties in paying for medical care. As would be expected, difficulties were somewhat more frequent amongst low-income households than amongst normal-income ones. The difference was greatest in Kaduha, the poorest area. Nevertheless, 70 per cent of low-income households still did not experience payment difficulties.

Furthermore, Table 6.10 shows that differences in fee levels had a minor effect compared to the influence of other factors.

Table 6.10 *Percentage of households reporting difficulties in paying for medical care (by income level)**

Cash income per capita	Kigali		Gikongoro		All areas
	Musha (96)†	Rwankuba (102)†	Ngara (100)†	Kaduha (100)†	
$11.50 or below	25	28	30	36	30
Above $11.50	16	20	22	14	18
All	19	24	27	32	26

* Based on index. Households reporting 'never' counted as 0 per cent, those reporting 'always' counted as 100 per cent, and those reporting 'sometimes' as 50 per cent.
† Number of households.

Although mission fees were triple those of the government, only 5 per cent more households in areas served by MHCs reported payment difficulties. Relative incomes would appear to be important determinants of utilization, with households in the poorer province (Gikongoro) reporting 8 per cent more payment difficulties than those in similar areas in Kigali province. This contrast between lower and normal income was associated with a 12 per cent increase in payment problems.

In summary, if fees in GHCs were to be raised to the levels in mission facilities, it could be argued that about 5 per cent more households would experience payment difficulties. However, provided higher fees led to improved drug availability, 90 per cent of households would applaud the change!

To determine whether the proposed drug charges would be affordable, we estimated the resulting increase in consumer health expenditures. Suppose that a revolving fund in GHCs covered all the costs of drugs currently incurred in those health centres, and that medications absorbed 18 per cent of total costs (the average of their share) in the two government health centres. Cost recovery averaged 21 per cent of total costs in these same health centres. Thus, the proposed drug fees would be 86 per cent as large as observed user fees. As Table 6.6 showed, on a population basis, observed user fees at GHCs constituted US $0.10 out of US $2.20 spent for the treatment of an average episode of illness. The proposed drug fees would add only US $0.09 to these costs (86 per cent of $0.10). This represents a 4 percent addition to the average expenditure per illness episode. Thus, on average, there should be no problem with the affordability of higher drug fees. Problems might arise in individual cases, but an exemption mechanism will be proposed to address them.

Establishing fees for drugs at government health centres

As the first step in financing CCCD services from internal sources within Rwanda, we recommended that a revolving drug fund should first be established for chloroquine and oral rehydration solution under the CCCD programme. Fees should be based on the total cost of these drugs, including raw materials, distribution costs, and losses due to damage, expiry, or theft. We recommended this initially narrow focus for several administrative reasons. First, the distribution system was partly under the control of the CCCD programme, so the problems of coordination were minimized. Second, the distribution of drugs and collection of revenues could be handled by existing personnel (head nurses and regional coordinators). Third, this step moved closer to implementing a policy to which the Government of Rwanda agreed when it requested the CCCD project to examine and implement options to improve the self-financing of CCCD services.

This analysis of household expenditures suggested that higher fees were affordable by almost all households. The overall proportions of ill persons who sought modern care was 76 per cent across all four areas studied. The multivariate analysis indicated that higher fees, combined with higher quality, deterred utilization at the reference health centre by only 3 percentage points (i.e. from 53–50 per cent of episodes). However, in order to ensure that truly indigent patients were not denied essential drugs, we recommended for them a system that waives drug fees. This mechanism must limit waivers to a small number of needy persons, so that the financial integrity of the system is not undermined. The lost revenue should be recovered through a surcharge on the price charged to paying patients. It was recommended that the waivers should be monitored and controlled through a special free drug register, containing the dates, names, and locations of patients given free drugs, and the value of the free drugs. The locations would allow the head of the health centre to verify the patient's need with administrative personnel, such as the chairman of the cell in which the patient lives. If patients misrepresented their financial status to obtain an exemption improperly, they and others in their household could be denied care at the centre in the future.

Drug fees should be administratively and politically feasible in Rwanda, since the fee schedule had been in place for at least ten years, and the principle of user fees in government facilities was already long established. Many other developing countries lack this history; their national governments have officially maintained a policy of 'free' care, though in practice user fees may be levied by local governments, the facilities themselves, or health workers.

We considered raising the consultation fee as an alternative to selling drugs, but we did not recommend this approach for several reasons. First, our household survey showed the acceptability of raising user fees to ensure availability of drugs. Second, a consultation fee would have to be paid regardless of whether facilities had the required drugs available, which seemed unfair. Third, tying fees to drugs should facilitate retaining the revenues locally and earmarking their use for drug resupply. Fourth, it may be possible to institute user fees for drugs without awaiting the legislative approval that would be required for a change in the long-established consultation fee.

As a further step in improving the financing of government health centres, we recommended that the revolving drug fund should be broadened to include all drugs. The additional revenue would almost double the collections from users in the two government health centres, and should eliminate the 30–50 per cent of regularly used medicines that were often out of stock. Although transportation and inventory-control may contribute to exhaustion of stocks in some countries, in Rwanda the problem seemed to be primarily lack of money.

Conclusion

The present study was sufficiently modest in its requirements that it could readily be replicated in other settings. Fieldwork (planning, visiting health centres, organizing interviews) took about 45 person-days of professional effort, with about 108 person-days for interviewers and the survey co-ordinator, and about 10 days' use of three vehicles with drivers. After excellent planning by the CCCD programme, fieldwork was completed in 21 calendar days.

The methodology of household surveys on the utilization of health services and attitudes also generalizes readily to other countries. The methods outlined above were subsequently used in a study of health-care financing in West Mali (Carrin *et al*. 1987). Some adaptations of the questionnaire were necessary to account for a more complex family structure, in which women played a more significant role in the generation of household revenues. Overall, the results in that study are quite consistent with those obtained in the present chapter: they do confirm a capacity and willingness to pay on the part of a rural population for low-cost primary health care.

References

Akin, J. S., Guilkey, D., and Popkin, B. (1986). The demand for adult outpatient services in the Bicol Region of the Philippines. *Social Science and Medicine*, **22** (3), 321–28.

Carrin, G., Kegels, G., and Reveillon, M. (1987). *Evaluation économique du système de recouvrement des coûts des soins de santé dans le cercle de Kita (Mali)*. Medicus Mundi Belgium and PDS Bamako, Mali.

De Ferranti, D. (1985). *Paying for health services in developing countries: an overview*, World Bank Staff Working Paper, No.721. World Bank, Washington, DC.

Heller, P. (1982). A model of the demand for medical and health services in peninsular Malaysia. *Social Science and Medicine*, **16**, 267–84.

Ministère de l'Agriculture, de l'Elevage, et des Forêts (1985). *Resultats de l'Enquête Nationale Agricole 1984*, Vol.1, Rapport 1. Kigali, Rwanda.

Ministère de la Santé Publique et des Affaires Sociales (MINISAPASO) (1983–1986). *Annual reports*. Kigali, Rwanda.

Shepard, D. S. and Benjamin, E. (1987). User fees and health financing in developing countries: mobilizing financial resources for health. In *Health, nutrition and economic crises: approaches to policy in the Third World* (ed. D. E. Bell and M. R. Reich), pp. 401–24. Oelgeschlager, Gunn & Hain, Boston, Mass.

Shepard, D. S., Carrin, G., and Nyandagazi, P. (1987). *Self-financing of health care at government health centres in Rwanda* [Mimeo]. Harvard Institute for International Development, Cambridge, Mass.

Stinson, W. (1982). *Community financing of primary health care*, American Public Health Association, PHC Issues Series, No.4. The Association, Washington, DC.

Authors' note

We are grateful to the staff of the health centres we visited and to the mayors, cell chairmen, and regional officials whose generosity in making their time available made this study possible. We thank the interviewers and personnel of the CCCD project for their thorough work in limited time. We thank Andrew Agle, John Akin, Jacques Baudouy, Roger Bernier, Michael Deming, Alan Fairbank, Stanley Foster, Stephen Tores, Wendy Roseberry, and especially Maryanne Neill for support and comments on the report from which this chapter derives. Naturally, views expressed are those of the authors alone.

7

Economic determinants of demand for modern infant-delivery in low-income countries: the case of the Philippines

J. Brad Schwartz, John S. Akin, and Barry M. Popkin

Introduction

A majority of births in the Philippines take place at home, and a significant proportion are either attended by a traditional midwife or friends and relatives of the mother. Women continue to choose this pattern of delivery despite large investments by the health sector in modern prenatal and obstetrical health services. Even though a large majority of the pregnant women have direct contact with modern delivery services, there still appears to be a preference for traditional home deliveries. It turns out that this choice can to a large extent be explained by the characteristics of the modern and the traditional delivery systems, and by the socio-economic characteristics of the households.

Health-policy decisions on how to provide and finance modern delivery care in low-income countries require that important questions should be answered, especially where traditional and modern health-providers co-exist. The factors that affect mothers' choices of types of health care are ultimately those same choices that determine how many infants live or die, are healthy, or are chronically ill. We examine the determinants of the choice of type of delivery care, including economic factors, health facility characteristics, and delivery-practitioner characteristics for both traditional and modern delivery providers in one region of the Philippines. The sensitivity of the choice of birth-delivery method to factors such as these has important implications for the location, organization, and financing of modern delivery services.

The data come from a survey of health facilities and delivery practitioners combined with a survey of over 3000 women who delivered babies during 1983–4 in the Cebu region of the Philippines. In subsequent sections, we describe the traditional and modern delivery sectors in low-income countries; present an overview of the economic model that guides the analysis; discuss the data and provide descriptive statistics; discuss the estimation technique and the results of the multivariate analysis; and finally, discuss the policy implications and our conclusions.

Background

The traditional sector

Over two-thirds of the babies born in low-income countries are delivered by traditional birth attendants, who are often poorly educated and have no formal medical training. A national survey of traditional midwives conducted in 1974 in the Philippines found that over 50 per cent had only elementary school training, and most had either learned midwifery on their own or from relatives (Mangay-Maglacas 1981; Akin *et al.* 1984). It is this lack of formal medical training which differentiates traditional midwives from modern medical professionals. The modern health sector consists mainly of physicians and nurses with university education and licensed midwives with some formal medical training.

The heavy reliance on traditional birth attendants in developing countries may be related to the heavy concentration of modern practitioners in urban areas and of traditional practitioners in rural areas. While typically some 60–80 per cent of the population live in rural areas, some 70–90 per cent of the doctors are located in urban areas (Akin *et al.* 1984). The urban facilities at which these doctors work are often inaccessible (either for geographical or economic reasons) to the lower-income and rural populations.

The traditional sector ·generally provides greater coverage of the rural population than does the modern sector. While in Asia and Africa the modern sector may be physically accessible to only 10–30 per cent of the population, in many countries 100 per cent of the population is within walking distance of a traditional midwife. It is not unusual, therefore, for the population per practitioner ratio for traditional midwives to be only one-fifth to one-half that of modern practitioners.

The work of the typical traditional midwife is diverse. She not only delivers babies, but also assists women during the prenatal and postnatal periods, and is involved in a number of important aspects of maternal and child health care. During prenatal care, they often:

. . . Use massage to relax muscles, relieve discomfort, and estimate the progress of pregnancy. As delivery approaches, massage is used to position the fetus . . . During labor, the traditional midwife may massage the woman and administer herbal beverages . . . At delivery, many midwives help to extract the baby and the placenta (Simpson-Hebert *et al.* 1980, pp. J-444–5).

It is generally believed that some of the practices of the traditional birth attendants are harmful, and that many others, while probably harmless, are of uncertain effect. Harmful practices, or those which can be potentially harmful, include dietary restrictions, mishandling the umbilical cord (associated with neonatal tetanus), misuse of drugs (for example, heavy use of inappropriate antibiotics), postpartum feeding practices which exclude the feeding of colostrum, and incorrect responses to complications of pregnancy (Popkin 1984). Both surveys of modern medical personnel and data from hospital records repeatedly identify neonatal tetanus as the major infant-mortality risk associated with deliveries attended by untrained midwives (Mangay-Maglacas 1981).

Modern obstetrical care and primary health care

In the last decade there has been a major effort to expand modern health services in Third World countries. One major goal of this expansion has been the provision of inexpensive modern prenatal and delivery services. Usually, when planning the allocation of these services, planners have concentrated on simple formulae related to the geographical distribution of health services rather than on how best to provide services, given the available resources and the benefits of alternative approaches. Few studies have documented the impact of changes in health facilities and practitioners on the proportion of deliveries attended by modern practitioners, and even fewer have evaluated the health effects of such changes. An exception is a project in the province of Bohol, Philippines, which implemented and evaluated a maternal and child health and family-planning project. Over the period of the project, the availability of low-cost modern care led to a reduction from 67 per cent to 1 per cent in the proportion of births attended by untrained midwives. Concurrent declines in the number of cases of neonatal tetanus and in the prevalence of many inappropriate delivery practices (for example, the use of bamboo slivers to cut the umbilical cord) were observed (Williamson 1982; Parado 1979). Another study found that the introduction of modern care to the area led to a reduction in fetal deaths (Akin *et al.* 1984).

The realignment of delivery patterns

For government investments in improved delivery services to achieve their objectives, it is essential that the determinants of the type of infant delivery should be considered. Surprisingly, few systematic studies have considered the factors associated with the choice of delivery services – be it for modern or traditional, public or private care. Elsewhere, the authors have reviewed the existing studies and presented the results of a small case study of the factors associated with the choice of modern or traditional delivery services (Akin *et al.* 1984, 1986). That earlier research, based on an analysis of about 500 births from the Bicol region of the Philippines, concluded that the choice between a modern or a traditional birth attendant was made mainly on non-economic grounds. The important explanatory variables were found to be mother's education and urban residence.

Previous studies, including the earlier work of these authors, of choice of infant-delivery method have been based on small samples, and, more importantly, have failed to control for some important economic and quality-of-service characteristics of the available delivery-service options. In this study, we expand on previous work by analysing a large data set, which includes information not only on the socio-economic characteristics of the demanders of delivery services, but also on the economic cost and service-quality characteristics of all suppliers of delivery services in the community analysed. Moreover, because the data were collected on a prospective basis, they represent a significant improvement over those for other studies based on retrospective recall data.

Economic demand model

In this section, we briefly outline a delivery-service demand model which is detailed elsewhere (Akin *et al.* 1984, 1986). We assume that a model for analysis of delivery services must take into account the facts that delivery services can be provided either publicly or privately, either by untrained or trained practitioners, and either at home or away from home. In the model, each type of delivery has an associated set of characteristics, including time and money prices, availability, and service quality. We assume that a woman maximizes her own well-being, which is a function of the health of her infant. The outcomes predicted as a result of this maximization process are that a woman's choice of type of delivery service will be determined by the prices, availability, and quality of the services, plus a set of socio-economic, demographic, and community factors. In general terms, the relationship between type of delivery used and the exogenous factors is as follows:

$$Y_i = f(P_i, T_i, H_i, Q_i; Z)$$

where Y_i = the ith delivery type;

i = at home by relatives, at home by traditional practitioners, at home by modern public practitioners, at home by modern private practitioners, away from home (at clinics or hospitals) by modern public practitioners, or away from home by modern private practitioners (6 possible choices);

P_i = cash price paid to delivery-service provider of type i;

T_i = time price of travelling between the delivery-provider of type i and the woman's residence;

H_i = the hours of availability for delivery service of type i;

Q_i = the perceived quality of delivery service of type i; and

Z = the set of household and community characteristics (such as income, assets, education, insurance coverage, residence, season, and household composition) affecting the income available to, the time constraints of, and the knowledge and preferences of, the mother.

Survey background

The study site is Metropolitan Cebu, an area embracing both the City of Cebu and rural areas of the Island of Cebu in the Central Philippines. Metropolitan Cebu is located on the eastern coast of Cebu Island, and includes, besides Cebu City, coastal towns and a number of mountain villages. While basically of Malayan stock, the Metropolitan Cebu population (particularly in the urbanized areas) also contains people who are of Spanish and Chinese ancestry.

Metropolitan Cebu is composed of three administratively distinct cities (among them Cebu City, the second largest city of the country) and six other municipalities. At the time of the 1980 census the administrative entities contained 243 barangays, with 171702 households and slightly more than one million inhabitants. (The barangay is the smallest administrative unit in the Philippines, and in the rural areas is usually identical with a village). The barangay was the initial sampling unit for the survey from which the data are derived. Separate random samples taken from the universes of urban and rural metropolitan Cebu barangays resulted in a sample of 17 urban and 16 rural barangays.

All households in the 33 barangays were surveyed to collect data on all women who had births between 1 May 1983, and 30 April 1984. Baseline surveys were obtained during the sixth month of pregnancy for the 3327 pregnant women who gave birth during the twelve-month period. For the analysis of delivery patterns, the sample consists of 3075 women for whom both baseline and birth information were collected, and who delivered non-twin births. Of the 3327 baseline women, 38 (1.1 per cent) had stillbirths, 13 (0.4 per cent) had miscarriages, 26 (0.8 per cent) had twin births, 135 (4.1 per cent) outmigrated between the baseline and birth interviews, and 17 (0.5 per cent) refused birth interviews. An additional 57 women in the sample communities who gave birth during the twelve-month period but either did not live in the communities during their pregnancy or were missed in the screening for pregnant women are omitted from this analysis.

The public and private health facilities serving the 33 sample barangays were also surveyed. Included in the sample were all facilities and personnel within each barangay, plus those personnel and facilities located outside the barangays but identified by proximity to the barangay, by legal jurisdiction over the community (for public clinics and hospitals), or by barangay informants (on questions asked during the baseline) as servicing the sample households. In total, data from 48 modern public and modern private hospitals, clinics, and health centre facilities and 88 private modern and traditional health practitioners were used in this analysis. In addition, data were collected from part-time government health facilities (Barangay Health Stations (BHSs)) located in 23 of the 33 barangays.

Variables

The pattern of delivery choice across the six methods represented in the dependent variable is presented in Table 7.1. Table 7.2 describes each independent variable used, and Table 7.3 shows the mean values and standard deviations of the independent variables. All variables are presented separately for urban and rural samples for reasons discussed below.

The data shown in Table 7.1 indicate that over one-third of the sample women delivered their babies at home either with relatives or with traditional practitioners. In the rural areas, the proportion in these categories was significantly larger (72 per cent) than for

Table 7.1 *Pattern of delivery*

Category and delivery type	Urban No.	%	Rural No.	%	Total No.	%
1. Relatives and friends, at home	130	5.45	64	8.84	194	6.25
2. Traditional practitioner, at home	511	21.77	460	63.54	971	31.62
3. Public practitioner, at home	405	17.26	112	15.47	517	16.83
4. Private practitioner, at home	200	8.48	14	1.93	214	6.94
5. Public practitioner, away from home	508	21.64	35	4.83	543	17.68
6. Private practitioner, away from home	597	25.40	39	5.39	636	20.68
Total	2351	100.00	724	100.00	3075	100.00

the urban areas (27 per cent). There was also a large urban – rural difference in the delivery pattern for home deliveries (categories 1, 2, 3, and 4) and delivery away-from-home (categories 5 and 6). While only slightly over 10 per cent of the rural sample delivered away from home at public or private facilities, approximately 47 per cent of the urban sample delivered away from home. The difference between the urban and rural samples in the use of modern trained practitioners for home deliveries (categories 3 and 4) was relatively small. About 17 per cent of the rural women and about 26 per cent of the urban sample chose this option.

As is shown in Table 7.3, there was a fairly wide variation in the money prices paid for the different types of delivery. In general, the price differences were notably large between delivery at home and delivery away from home, as well as between public and private away-from-home delivery. Interestingly, in the Philippines there is a cultural norm which dictates payment for delivery in the form of a gratuity even where there is no explicit market price. Thus even relatives were paid a 'fee for service', and this is included in our empirical specification as an expected price, to control for differences in money prices across all delivery choice options. The average delivery-price did not differ markedly by location. The urban sample paid an average of Pesos (P) 136.61, and the rural sample slightly less, at P120.27. Slightly larger prices were charged to the urban sample for each type of delivery choice.

The travel time between the household and the delivery practitioner was significantly greater for the rural women than for their urban counterparts for each type of delivery service. The average travel time for the rural sample was approximately 25 minutes; but the average urban dweller was located only 6.41 minutes away from a general practitioner.

Private facilities for deliveries away from home were open for more hours per week (approximately 32 hours more) than were public facilities. In rural barangays, the difference was about 68 hours, and in urban areas about 21 hours. Drugs were available at public and private facilities in about the same proportions for the urban and rural samples. There were more hospitals (both public and private) which were open 24 hours a day in the urban than in the rural areas.

Individual and household characteristics varied between urban and rural samples. On average, the urban sample had larger

Table 7.2 *Variable descriptions*

Delivery–specific variables:

Price — The average price, in pesos, for each delivery type in each barangay are used as the prices facing women in each barangay.

Travel time — The time, in minutes, between the household and the delivery-practitioner.

Hours available — The number of hours per week that the practitioner and/or facility is available.

Drugs available — Whether drugs are available at the public or private facility (yes = 1; no = 0).

Untrained practitioner — Whether the delivery-practitioner has had formal medical training (yes = 0; no = 1).

Trained midwife — Whether the usual delivery-practitioner at the public and private facility was a trained midwife (yes = 1; doctors, nurses, or combinations of doctors, nurses and midwives = 0).

Individual and household characteristics:

Household income — Annual household income, in thousands of pesos.

Household assets — Total value of assets, in thousands of pesos, owned by the household, including land, housing, consumer goods, vehicles, etc.

Mother's education — Years of formal schooling.

Father's education — Years of formal school interacted with whether the father was present.

Father present — Whether the father is present in the household (yes = 1; no = 0).

Mother's age — Age in years.

Children under age 6 — Number of children aged 0–6 years.

Females over age 13 — Number of females in the household aged 13 and older.

Cebuano — Ethnic origin indicated by language spoken in the household (Cebuano spoken by both husband and wife = 1; otherwise = 0).

Table 7.2 (*cont.*)

Individual and household characteristics (*cont.*)	
Electricity	Whether the household has electricity (yes = 1; no = 0).
Insurance coverage	Whether the woman is covered by health insurance (yes = 1; no = 0).
Wet season	Whether the childbirth occurred during the rainy season (June–October = 1; otherwise = 0).
Dry season	Whether the childbirth occurred during dry months (February–April = 1; otherwise = 0).
Private prenatal visit	Whether a prenatal visit was made to a private practitioner (yes = 1; no = 0).
Public prenatal visit	Whether a prenatal visit was made to a public practitioner (yes = 1; no = 0).
Traditional prenatal visit	Whether a prenatal visit was made to a traditional practitioner (yes = 1; no = 0).

incomes and assets, were better educated, were slightly younger, had fewer children under the age of six, and had more insured mothers.

Estimation method and results

The dependent variable in the delivery model is in the form of a set of unordered, mutually exclusive categories. An appropriate statistical method for estimating the relationships is the mixed multinomial logit technique. This estimation procedure allows two types of independent (explanatory) variables to be used – *conditional* variables, such as the price of delivery, which differ in value for any given mother on the basis of choice made; and *unconditional* variables, such as mother's age, which do not change as a result of the choice.

If we let X_{ij} represent a vector of values for a set of independent variables (for example, the set of prices in Table 7.3) that vary by choice ($j = 1, 2, \ldots, N$) and by woman ($i = 1, 2, \ldots, M$), and Z_i

Table 7.3 *Sample means and standard deviations of independent variables*

Variables	Urban		Rural		All	
	Mean	SD	Mean	SD	Mean	SD
Delivery–specific variables:						
Prices (in pesos)						
Relatives	48.66	(20.14)	27.36	(8.47)	43.64	(20.22)
Traditional	56.96	(15.85)	48.33	(17.09)	54.92	(16.56)
Public, home	51.27	(14.74)	41.17	(6.62)	48.89	(13.96)
Private, home	66.98	(16.11)	66.37	(39.92)	66.83	(23.94)
Public, away	169.80	(48.75)	162.13	(70.33)	167.99	(54.69)
Private, away	426.81	(104.70)	378.04	(102.93)	391.94	(121.84)
All	136.61	(28.28)	120.27	(13.80)	128.95	(25.40)
*Travel time (in minutes)**						
Traditional	7.27	(4.73)	24.15	(21.13)	11.25	(13.16)
Public	11.23	(5.66)	32.51	(24.67)	16.24	(15.79)
Private	4.39	(2.91)	30.15	(25.16)	10.46	(16.57)
All	6.41	(2.44)	24.99	(15.21)	10.78	(11.04)
Hours available (per week)†						
Public, away	127.77	(58.06)	58.74	(42.25)	111.49	(62.09)
Private, away	148.95	(36.16)	127.94	(42.76)	143.99	(38.85)
Drugs available						
Public, away	0.51	(0.50)	0.53	(0.26)	0.51	(0.49)
Private, away	0.45	(0.49)	0.36	(0.42)	0.43	(0.49)
Untrained						
practitioners‡	0.33	(0.06)	0.33	(0.06)	0.33	(0.06)
Trained midwives						
Public, home	0.41	(0.49)	0.59	(0.49)	0.44	(0.50)
Private, home	0.45	(0.50)	0.43	(0.48)	0.45	(0.47)
Public, away	0.32	(0.47)	0.95	(0.21)	0.47	(0.50)
Private, away	0.00		0.00		0.00	
Individual and household characteristics:						
Household income	0.30	(0.47)	0.19	(0.27)	0.28	(0.44)
Household assets	14.25	(54.42)	5.76	(19.35)	12.25	(48.63)
Mother's education	7.62	(3.29)	5.46	(2.29)	7.11	(3.31)
Father's education	7.49	(3.41)	5.09	(3.01)	6.93	(3.51)
Father present	0.94	(0.24)	0.95	(0.21)	0.94	(0.23)
Mother's age	25.88	(5.84)	26.70	(6.46)	26.07	(6.00)
Children under 6	1.49	(1.14)	1.67	(1.12)	1.53	(1.14)
Females over 13	0.51	(0.90)	0.36	(0.76)	0.47	(0.87)
Cebuano	0.91	(0.29)	0.95	(0.21)	0.92	(0.27)

Table 7.3 (*cont.*)

Variables	Urban		Rural		All	
	Mean	SD	Mean	SD	Mean	SD
Individual and household characteristics (*cont.*)						
Electricity	0.60	(0.49)	0.18	(0.38)	0.50	(0.50)
Insurance	0.12	(0.32)	0.05	(0.21)	0.10	(0.30)
Wet season	0.50	(0.50)	0.47	(0.50)	0.49	(0.50)
Dry season	0.18	(0.38)	0.20	(0.40)	0.19	(0.39)
Private prenatal visit	0.24	(0.43)	0.07	(0.26)	0.20	(0.40)
Public prenatal visit	0.53	(0.50)	0.47	(0.50)	0.52	(0.50)
Traditional prenatal visit	0.47	(0.50)	0.58	(0.50)	0.49	(0.50)
n	2351		724		3075	

* Travel time for relatives assumed equal to zero.
† Hours available per week for at-home deliveries equals 168.
‡ Sample average across all choices.

represent a vector of independent variables that vary only by woman, then the log of the odds of any particular choice being made is

$$\log \left[\frac{P(Y_i=j)}{P(Y_i=1)} \right] = \gamma(X_{ij} - X_{i1}) + \beta_j Z_{ij} \quad (j = 2, ..., N)$$

where the γ's represent coefficients associated with the choice-varying (conditional) independent variables. A positive value for a particular coefficient implies that the corresponding independent variable has positive weight in the individual's indirect utility function (i.e. that an increase in the value of that variable is considered to be a favourable change by the individual), and that an increase in the value of that variable for a particular choice will make that choice more likely. If, for example, the coefficient on the quality of delivery is positive, this indicates that adding to the service quality at any type of provider will tend to increase the individual's likelihood of choosing to use that type of delivery service, and that because of this service-quality increase, the individual is able to obtain a higher level of welfare.

The β_j coefficients vary by choice, and a positive value for a particular coefficient implies that as the corresponding inde-pendent variable increases, the probability that choice j will be chosen increases *relative* to other choices. The use of choice 1 in the denominator of the equation, as the basis for comparison of other choices defining the log odds, is arbitary. All odds ratios can be computed, and we present all comparisons in the results.

The estimation of this model entails solving the above equations for probabilities and setting up a likelihood function. Details of the procedure can be found in Maddala (1983).

Model-specification issues

Urban/rural residence. Because urban and rural residents could reasonably have behaved differently in seeking delivery services, we test for such differences. A likelihood-ratio test of the null hypothesis 'no behavioural difference between urban and rural residents' is rejected at the 1 per cent level of significance, indicating that the two samples do behave differently. Because of this structural difference, we stratify the sample into urban and rural sub-samples, and all results are presented for both urban and rural groups.

Distance to facilities. In the model, the travel time between the mother and the practitioner represents the proximity of each delivery option, and whether the mother chooses to travel to the practitioner or to have the practitioner travel to her home for delivery. The quantification of this variable is complex. From the mother, we determined the specific facility of each type she would use, and from the facilities we determined the populations they served. We carried out an analysis of transportation patterns, topography, and distance to estimate the travel time of each household to the relevant public, private, or traditional facility.

Choice of prenatal care. The type of prenatal care chosen by the mother (traditional, public, or private practitioner) may be an important factor in the choice of delivery-practitioner. However, it is possible that the choices of prenatal care and delivery-practitioner are jointly determined, and that the choice of prenatal care is therefore endogenous to the delivery model. A statistical procedure to correct for such endogeneity is to estimate the probability that each type of prenatal care is chosen by the mother and then enter these probabilities in the delivery model as lagged (pre-delivery) endogenous variables. Unfortunately, this procedure is impossible in the multinomial logit model because the error term assumptions for the instrumental variables violate the necessary logit model error assumptions. Because no perfect answer to the endogeneity problem in the logit model exists, we carry out two alternative estimation procedures, each of which is consistent with a specific set of assumptions about the true model. We estimate a reduced-form model, in which prenatal care-type is excluded as an explanatory factor, and assume the results and simulations to be appropriate if the choice of prenatal care actually is endogenous to the model. As an alternative, we present estimation and simulation results for a model in which the prenatal care choice is included as an exogenous explanatory variable, a model which is appropriate if in reality the choice of prenatal care-type is exogenous to the choice of type of delivery service.

Qualifications of delivery-practitioner. In order to tak e into account the differences in quality of the delivery-practitioners providing the actual delivery services under the alternative choices of delivery type, we include two binary variables that indicate whether the actual practitioner has received little or no formal medical training (i.e. relatives and traditional practitioners), or conversely, whether the practitioner who normally makes the delivery is a certified trained midwife. For infant-deliveries performed at public and private facilities, and for deliveries performed at home by practitioners from public and private facilities, we thereby capture the effects both of having a practitioner with or without formal medical training, and of the practitioner providing the delivery services being or not being a trained midwife. The omitted dichotomous variable is defined as the practitioner performing the delivery being a doctor, a nurse, or a combination of doctors, nurses, and midwives. In the sample, the second most common provider of a modern delivery after a trained midwife was a combination of practitioners.

Lack of data on some spouses. There were nearly 200 households without a spouse for whom information for the spouse's education was unavailable. In order to control for the presence of the spouse, we have included a binary variable to indicate whether the father was present. As an additional variable, we also have interacted this binary variable with father's education.

Multivariate results

Tables 7.4 and 7.5 present the results from estimation of the mixed multinomial logit model for both the urban and rural samples. The

Table 7.4 Multinomial logit results ■ urban sample (T-stats)

Unconditional variables

	Log REL/APUB	Log TRAD/APUB	Log HPUB/APUB	Log HPRIV/APUB	Log APRIV/APUB	Log REL/HPUB	Log TRAD/HPUB	Log HPRIV/HPUB	Log APRIV/HPUB	Log REL/HPRIV	Log TRAD/HPRIV
Household income	-0.6367 (-1.065)	-0.1153 (-0.396)	0.2725 (1.189)	-0.1299 (-0.341)	0.3624 (1.790)*	-0.9092 (-1.529)	-0.3878 (-1.387)	-0.4024 (-1.075)	0.0899 (0.447)	-0.5068 (-0.768)	0.0146 (0.036)
Household assets	-0.0655 (-0.863)	-0.0035 (-1.272)	-0.0025 (-1.078)	-0.0029 (-0.818)	0.0007 (0.519)	-0.0030 (-0.454)	-0.0010 (-0.306)	-0.0004 (-0.099)	0.0032 (1.405)	-0.0026 (-0.368)	-0.0006 (-0.143)
Mother's education	-0.1283 (-3.132)***	-0.1154 (-4.335)***	-0.0810 (-3.060)***	-0.1452 (-4.355)***	0.1126 (4.570)***	-0.0473 (-1.139)	-0.0344 (-1.253)	-0.0643 (-1.880)*	0.1936 (7.098)***	0.0170 (0.368)	0.0298 (0.875)
Father's education	-0.0527 (-1.316)	-0.0682 (-2.618)***	-0.0572 (-2.117)**	-0.0603 (-1.801)*	0.1325 (5.118)***	0.0045 (0.111)	-0.0110 (-0.414)	-0.0031 (-0.092)	0.1897 (6.678)***	0.0076 (0.170)	-0.0079 (-0.237)
Father present	0.0307 (0.064)	0.3656 (1.078)	0.4238 (1.285)	0.3512 (0.865)	-1.8167 (-5.645)***	-0.3931 (-0.806)	-0.0582 (-0.167)	-0.0726 (-0.176)	-2.2404 (-6.409)***	-0.3205 (-0.592)	0.0144 (0.034)
Mother's age	-0.0148 (0.879)	0.059 (0.529)	0.0007 (-0.064)	0.0053 (0.395)	0.0143 (1.321)	0.0141 (-0.837)	0.0066 (0.592)	0.0060 (0.442)	0.0150 (1.283)	-0.0200 (-1.082)	0.0007 (0.048)
Children under 6	0.1541 (1.665)*	0.1155 (1.912)*	0.0469 (0.741)	0.0895 (1.160)	-0.1615 (-2.616)***	0.1072 (1.149)	0.0686 (1.114)	0.0426 (0.540)	-0.2084 (-3.106)***	0.0646 (0.625)	0.0260 (0.342)
Females over 13	-0.1648 (-1.112)	-0.1150 (-1.348)	0.0166 (0.203)	-0.1921 (-1.664)*	0.0345 (0.473)	-0.1813 (-1.212)	-0.1316 (-1.497)	-0.2086 (-1.766)*	0.0179 (0.218)	0.0273 (0.160)	0.0770 (0.643)
Cebuano	-0.9046 (-2.663)***	-0.5014 (-1.933)*	-0.3840 (-1.546)	-0.7133 (-2.480)**	-0.8900 (-4.159)***	-0.5207 (-1.544)	-0.1175 (-0.459)	-0.3293 (-1.141)	-0.5060 (-2.199)**	-0.1914 (-0.525)	0.2118 (0.727)
Electricity	-0.4383 (-1.992)**	-0.4612 (-3.214)***	-0.2459 (-1.637)	0.2761 (1.481)	0.6858 (4.207)***	-0.1924 (-0.868)	-0.2154 (-1.477)	0.5220 (2.771)***	0.9317 (5.470)***	-0.7144 (-2.892)**	-0.7374 (-4.044)***
Insurance	0.3579 (1.012)	0.2943 (1.264)	0.2792 (1.151)	0.1312 (0.418)	0.4623 (2.278)**	0.0788 (0.221)	0.0151 (0.063)	-0.1480 (-0.462)	0.1831 (0.805)	0.2267 (0.555)	0.1631 (0.525)
Wet season	-0.1650 (-0.742)	0.0365 (0.244)	0.0791 (0.512)	-0.3880 (-2.014)**	0.1968 (1.350)	-0.2441 (-1.080)	-0.0427 (-0.274)	-0.4672 (-2.344)**	0.1177 (0.721)	0.2231 (0.878)	0.4245 (2.184)**
Dry season	0.0335 (0.112)	0.5099 (2.638)***	0.3152 (1.540)	0.3916 (1.689)*	-0.0318 (-0.154)	-0.2816 (-0.945)	0.1948 (1.014)	0.0764 (0.328)	-0.3469 (-1.589)	-0.3580 (-1.128)	0.1184 (0.534)

*** Significant at α = 0.01. ** Significant at α = 0.05. * Significant at α = 0.10.

where REL = probability of home delivery with relatives
where TRAD = probability of home delivery with traditional practitioner
where HPUB = probability of home delivery with public practitioner
where HPRIV = probability of home delivery with private practitioner
where APUB = probability of away-from-home delivery with public practitioner
where APRIV = probability of away-from-home delivery with private practitioner

Table 7.4 (cont.) *Multinomial logit results – urban sample (t-stats)*

Unconditional variables (cont.)

	Log $\frac{\text{APRIV}}{\text{HPRIV}}$	Log $\frac{\text{REL}}{\text{APRIV}}$	Log $\frac{\text{TRAD}}{\text{APRIV}}$	Log $\frac{\text{TRAD}}{\text{REL}}$
Household income	0.4923	-0.9990	-0.4777	0.5213
	(1.332)	(-1.687)*	(-1.726)*	(0.859)
Household assets	0.0036	-0.0062	-0.0041	0.0020
	(1.020)	(-0.970)	(-1.542)	(0.303)
Mother's education	0.2579	-0.2409	-0.2280	0.0129
	(7.556)***	(-5.786)***	(-8.244)***	(0.324)
Father's education	0.1928	-0.1852	-0.2007	-0.0155
	(5.565)***	(-4.497)***	(-7.210)***	(-0.395)
Father present	-2.1679	1.8474	2.1822	0.3349
	(-5.148)***	(3.733)***	(6.078)***	(0.740)
Mother's age	0.0091	-0.0291	-0.0084	0.0207
	(0.649)	(-1.675)*	(-0.696)	(1.324)
Children under 6	-0.2510	0.3156	0.2770	-0.0386
	(-3.119)***	(3.296)***	(4.248)***	(-0.426)
Females over 13	0.2265	-0.1992	-0.1495	0.0497
	(1.944)*	(-1.333)	(-1.706)*	(0.331)
Cebuano	-0.1767	-0.0147	0.3885	0.4032
	(-0.653)	(-0.045)	(1.643)	(1.297)
Electricity	0.4097	-1.1241	-1.1471	-0.0230
	(2.006)**	(-4.792)***	(-6.932)***	(-0.106)
Insurance	0.3311	-0.1044	-0.1680	-0.0636
	(1.092)	(-0.302)	(-0.762)	(-0.184)
Wet season	0.5848	-0.3618	-0.1603	0.2014
	(2.928)***	(-1.575)	(-0.997)	(0.921)
Dry season	-0.4233	0.0653	0.5417	0.4764
	(-1.734)*	(0.211)	(2.575)**	(1.666)*

Conditional variables

Price	-0.0016
	(-3.380)***
Travel time	-0.0088
	(-1.283)
Hours available	0.0149
	(12.386)***
Drugs available	0.2621
	(3.174)***
Untrained midwife	0.8457
	(2.088)**
Trained midwife	0.5035
	(5.631)***

*** Significant at α = 0.01. ** Significant at α = 0.05. * Significant at α = 0.10.
where REL   = probability of home delivery with relatives
where TRAD   = probability of home delivery with traditional practitioner
where HPUB   = probability of home delivery with public practitioner
where HPRIV   = probability of home delivery with private practitioner
where APUB   = probability of away-from-home delivery with public practitioner
where APRIV   = probability of away-from home delivery with private practitioner

Table 7.5 *Multinomial logit results – rural sample (t-stats)*
Unconditional variables

	Log REL/APUB	Log TRAD/APUB	Log HPUB/APUB	Log HPRIV/APUB	Log APRIV/APUB	Log REL/HPUB	Log TRAD/HPUB	Log HPRIV/HPUB	Log APRIV/HPUB	Log REL/HPRIV	Log TRAD/HPRIV
Household income	-4.0438	-0.3176	-0.3655	-1.8023	-0.1903	-3.6782	0.0480	-1.4368	0.1752	-2.2414	1.4848
	(-2.512)**	(-0.495)	(-0.510)	(-0.723)	(-0.282)	(-2.315)**	(0.077)	(-0.579)	(0.238)	(-0.788)	(0.605)
Household assets	-0.0011	-0.0085	-0.0046	0.0065	0.0100	0.0034	-0.0039	0.0110	0.0145	-0.0076	-0.0150
	(-0.060)	(-0.820)	(-0.401)	(0.290)	(1.344)	(0.183)	(-0.351)	(0.480)	(1.367)	(-0.281)	(-0.668)
Mother's education	-0.3032	-0.1374	-0.0396	0.1202	-0.1716	-0.2636	-0.0978	0.1598	-0.1321	-0.4234	-0.2576
	(-3.195)***	(-1.795)*	(-0.508)	(0.881)	(-1.863)*	(-3.459)***	(-1.854)*	(1.282)	(-1.792)*	(-3.130)***	(-2.098)**
Father's education	0.0112	-0.1290	-0.0583	-0.0756	0.0193	0.0695	-0.0706	-0.0173	0.0776	0.0868	-0.0534
	(0.118)	(-1.680)*	(-0.718)	(-0.558)	(0.202)	(0.933)	(-1.372)	(-0.141)	(0.997)	(0.658)	(-0.445)
Father present	1.4149	2.3200	1.3530	2.7420	-0.3155	0.0619	0.9670	1.3890	-1.6685	-1.3270	-0.4220
	(1.388)	(2.770)***	(1.592)	(1.602)	(-0.313)	(0.072)	(1.504)	(0.865)	(-1.965)**	(-0.770)	(-0.260)
Mother's age	-0.0578	0.0180	0.0010	-0.1568	0.0480	-0.0589	-0.01904	-0.1579	0.0469	0.0990	0.1388
	(-1.509)	(-0.567)	(0.032)	(-2.133)**	(1.321)	(0.072)	(-0.904)	(-2.271)**	(1.366)	(1.366)	(2.002)**
Children under 6	0.1260	-0.0243	0.0052	0.2701	-0.4792	0.1207	-0.0296	0.2649	-0.4845	-0.1442	-0.2944
	(0.575)	(-0.130)	(0.027)	(0.759)	(-1.950)*	(0.741)	(-0.249)	(0.816)	(-2.410)**	(-0.426)	(-0.923)**
Females over 13	0.3774	0.1659	0.0264	-0.5463	-0.3715	0.3510	0.1395	-0.5728	-0.3979	0.9237	0.7123
	(1.288)	(0.679)	(0.105)	(-0.915)	(-1.094)	(1.384)	(0.804)	(-1.004)	(-1.315)	(1.548)	(1.253)
Cebuano	-0.2292	0.4230	0.0986	-0.7159	0.0382	-0.3278	0.3244	-0.8145	-0.0604	0.4867	1.1389
	(-0.301)	(0.634)	(0.156)	(-0.754)	(0.050)	(-0.546)	(0.669)	(-0.980)	(-0.096)	(0.529)	(1.356)
Electricity	0.4184	-0.1674	0.0851	0.2279	0.4726	0.3333	-0.2524	0.1429	0.3876	0.1904	-0.3953
	(0.730)	(-0.349)	(0.172)	(0.290)	(0.817)	(0.752)	(-0.786)	(0.204)	(0.841)	(0.252)	(-0.576)
Insurance	-0.3974	-0.5009	-0.2716	0.9548	0.3098	-0.1258	-0.2298	1.2264	0.5814	-1.3521	-1.4556
	(0.702)	(-1.125)	(-0.584)	(1.290)	(0.574)	(-0.276)	(-0.764)	(1.860)*	(1.339)	(-1.844)*	(-2.256)**
Wet season	0.0115	-0.0503	-0.2023	-1.1097	-0.0391	0.2138	0.1520	-0.9074	0.1632	1.1212	1.0594
	(0.023)	(-0.1179)	(-0.450)	(-1.479)	(-0.072)	(0.563)	(0.551)	(-1.344)	(0.372)	(1.577)	(1.604)
Dry season	-0.3519	0.2733	-0.1991	-0.8203	0.0218	-0.1528	0.4723	-0.6212	0.2209	0.4684	1.0935
	(-0.510)	(0.481)	(-0.334)	(-0.835)	(0.031)	(-0.292)	(1.348)	(-0.711)	(0.403)	(0.497)	(1.276)

*** Significant at $\alpha = 0.01$. ** Significant at $\alpha = 0.05$. * Significant at $\alpha = 0.10$.

where REL = probability of home delivery with relatives
TRAD = probability of home delivery with traditional practitioner
HPUB = probability of home delivery with public practitioner
HPRIV = probability of home delivery with private practitioner
APUB = probability of away-from-home delivery with public practitioner
APRIV = probability of away-from-home delivery with private practitioner

Table 7.5 (cont.) *Multinomial logit results – rural sample (t–stats)*

Unconditional variables (cont.)

	Log APRIV/HPRIV	Log REL/APRIV	Log TRAD/APRIV	Log TRAD/REL
Household income	1.6120 (0.647)	-3.8534 (-2.391)**	-0.1272 (-0.196)	3.7262 (2.469)**
Household assets	0.0035 (0.159)	-0.0111 (-0.619)	-0.0185 (-1.960)**	-0.0074 (-0.439)
Mother's education	-0.2918 (-2.180)**	-0.1316 (-1.454)	0.0343 (0.486)	0.1659 (2.589)***
Father's education	0.0948 (0.711)	-0.0081 (-0.090)	-0.1482 (-2.103)**	-0.1401 (-2.179)**
Father present	-3.0575 (-1.790)*	1.7304 (1.724)*	2.6355 (3.284)***	0.9051 (1.240)
Mother's age	0.2048 (2.860)***	-0.1058 (-3.099)***	-0.0660 (-2.531)**	0.0398 (1.616)
Children under 6	-0.7494 (-2.093)**	0.6052 (2.760)***	0.4549 (2.448)**	-0.1503 (-1.091)
Females over 13	0.1749 (0.282)	0.7489 (2.165)**	0.5374 (1.870)*	-0.2115 (-0.965)
Cebuano	0.7541 (0.797)	-0.2674 (-0.354)	0.3849 (0.595)	0.6522 (1.183)
Electricity	0.2447 (0.321)	-0.0543 (-0.101)	-0.6400 (-1.498)	-0.5858 (-1.454)
Insurance	-0.6450 (-0.893)	-0.7071 (-1.329)	-0.8106 (-2.041)**	-0.1035 (-0.249)
Wet season	1.0706 (1.444)	0.0506 (0.104)	-0.0112 (-0.028)	-0.0618 (-0.193)
Dry season	0.8421 (0.882)	-0.3737 (-0.580)	0.2514 (0.500)	0.6251 (1.358)

Conditional variables

	Price
Price	-0.0002 (-0.148)
Travel time	-0.0312 (-8.639)***
Hours available	0.0073 (2.048)**
Drugs available	0.3889 (0.963)
Untrained midwife	1.3886 (1.693)*
Trained midwife	0.4924 (1.841)*

*** Significant at $\alpha = 0.01$. ** Significant at $\alpha = 0.05$. * Significant at $\alpha = 0.10$.

where REL   = probability of home delivery with relatives
TRAD = probability of home delivery with traditional practitioner
HPUB = probability of home delivery with public practitioner
HPRIV = probability of home delivery with private practitioner
APUB = probability of away-from-home delivery with public practitioner
APRIV = probability of away-from-home delivery with private practitioner

coefficients for the conditional variables indicate how changes in each of the variables affect the household's utility (welfare), and represent the effect of these factors irrespective of the delivery choice actually made. For example, because the coefficient on price is negative for both the urban and rural samples, it follows that increasing the price of any of the delivery choices will decrease the utility of the household, and will decrease the probability of choosing that option for which price was increased, relative to the other delivery options. The coefficients on the unconditional variables, however, are allowed to differ for each delivery-method choice, with the data being allowed to indicate how a change in each of these variables affects the probability of choosing each specific type of delivery.

For the urban households, an increase in the money price of delivery services is both a statistically significant and a negative factor in the choice of delivery. For rural mothers, price is found to have a negative influence on the choice, but is not statistically significant. The negative coefficient findings suggest that an increase in the money price for any type of delivery will tend to reduce the likelihood of choosing that type of delivery. The relationship between travel time from the household to the delivery-practitioner and the type of delivery chosen is also found to be negative for both samples, but is statistically significant only for the rural sample. This finding suggests that increased distance to a facility will reduce its usage only in the rural areas.

The lack of statistical significance for time (distance) prices in the urban areas can be explained by the fact that the urban sample was relatively close to all delivery options (6.41 minutes, on average) and that there was little variation in travel time between options (2.44 minutes). It appears that, in these urban situations, the time spent to reach a practitioner, though negatively related to delivery choice, was not an important factor in the choice. The opposite was true for the rural households, who lived much farther away from all types of delivery care (24.99 minutes, on average) and for whom the variation in travel time to the choices could be great. For this rural sample, time is negatively related to delivery choice, and the statistical tests suggest that it is an important factor in the choice.

The hours per week that each delivery choice was available is a positive and statistically significant factor for both the urban and the rural samples, indicating that an increase in hours of availability will increase the probability that any delivery option will be chosen. Whether or not drugs were available at the public and private facilities is entered as a quality-of-service variable, and, as expected, is positively related to delivery choice. The availability of drugs is statistically significant for the urban sample; but we have less confidence in the finding for the rural households.

For the delivery-practitioner either to be a midwife with no formal training or a formally trained midwife is found to be positively associated with the choice of delivery service with which that practitioner was associated. This type of practitioner variable (midwife) is statistically significant for both the urban and rural samples. The results suggest that households preferred delivery services from midwives, whether or not they were formally trained, to deliveries performed by combinations of doctors, nurses, and midwives (the excluded category).

The results found for the unconditional variables (factors which do not change according to the delivery method chosen) may be interpreted as the influence of these factors on each delivery option relative to each other option. In most cases, household income and household assets are found not to be statistically significant factors in delivery-method choice in either the urban or rural samples, although, in the one exception, having greater income or assets does appear to increase the probability that deliveries away from home (at both public and private facilities) will be chosen. As the mother's education level increases, she is more inclined to choose a delivery away from home if she lives in an urban area, and to choose modern delivery if she is a rural resident. Having insurance coverage appears to increase the probability that modern private-practitioner deliveries will be chosen, but to have little effect on other delivery choices.

The wet season and dry season dummy variables, along with the omitted class (other seasons), are included in the estimations to control for such seasonal factors as cash availability and workload, such as crop planting or harvesting. During the wet season, it appears that urban households are more likely to choose options other than home private deliveries. During the dry season, it seems that these households are more likely to prefer traditional and home private deliveries to both public and private away-from-home deliveries. Seasons do not appear to be statistically significant factors of the choice of delivery type for rural households.

Simulation results

The interpretation of the meaning of the magnitude of the coefficients in a multinomial logit model is difficult because the estimated parameters are the logarithm of the ratio of two probabilities. Table 7.6 presents simulations performed using the logit estimates to obtain predicted probabilities. Probabilities of choices are estimated for hypothetical households having the sample means for all independent variables, and then changes in these probabilities are determined which result from changes in the specific conditional and unconditional variables. The simulation results are revealing because the statistical significance of a relationship does not necessarily indicate whether the effect of that independent variable on the dependent variable will be large. An effect could be strongly significant but almost infinitely small, and therefore not 'significant' in the non-statistical sense of the word. The simulations present the effects of changes in the characteristics of public delivery services on the choice of home and away-from-home delivery in order to examine the policy implication of such changes. The changes examined are in travel time, money price, hours of operation, and drug availability – the factors most likely to be affected by government service-provision and financing decisions. To complete the picture, the effects of changes in factors less amenable to government policy manipulation, such as household income, assets, insurance coverage, mothers' education, and choice of prenatal care are also examined.

From the information presented in Table 7.6, we see that if each woman in the sample had a value for each independent variable set at its sample mean (see Table 7.3), approximately 27 per cent of the urban sample and 73 per cent of the rural sample would choose to deliver at home, with either a traditional practitioner or a relative attending; about 26 per cent of the urban and 17 per cent of the rural sample would choose delivery at home with a modern public or private practitioner; and 47 per cent of the urban and 10 per cent of the rural sample would choose away-from-home delivery with a modern public or private practitioner.

The simulation results, indicating the expected changes in these average probabilities that result from changes in the explanatory variables, show that changes in money and time prices for public delivery services have differential impacts on women in the urban and the rural samples. When the money prices of public deliveries,

Table 7.6 *Predicted probabilities and changes in probabilities of delivery choice by residence*

	Urban						Rural					
	REL	TRAD	HPUB	HPRIV	APUB	APRIV	REL	TRAD	HPUB	HPRIV	APUB	APRIV
Probabilities at mean values of independent variables	0.0553	0.2130	0.1717	0.0930	0.2124	0.2546	0.0828	0.6455	0.1573	0.0166	0.0445	0.0533
Changes in probability for:												
Price increased by one standard deviation												
Public, home (51 to 66 for urban; 41 to 48 for rural)	0.0003	0.0010	−0.0037	0.0004	0.0011	0.0009	0.0	0.0002	−0.0002	0.0	0.0	0.0
Public, away (170 to 218 for urban; 162 to 232 for rural)	0.0010	0.0042	0.0037	0.0017	−0.0142	0.0036	0.0001	0.0007	0.0002	0.0	−0.0010	0.0
Travel time increased by one standard deviation (11 to 16 for urban; 33 to 57 for rural)												
Public, home	0.0005	0.0022	−0.0078	0.0009	0.0024	0.0018	0.0071	0.0694	−0.0889	0.0008	0.0079	0.0037
Public, away	0.0004	0.0027	0.0024	0.0011	−0.0090	0.0024	0.0027	0.0259	0.0074	0.0003	−0.0377	0.0014
Hours available increased by one standard deviation Public, away (128 to 168 hrs/wk for urban; 60 to 100 hrs/wk for rural)	−0.0081	−0.0343	−0.0304	−0.0141	0.1161	−0.0292	−0.0016	−0.0159	−0.0045	−0.0002	0.0231	−0.0008

Drugs available changed *(from 0 to 1)*											
Public, away	−0.0034	−0.0142	−0.0126	−0.0059	0.0482	−0.0121	−0.0016	−0.0155	−0.0045	−0.0002	0.0226	−0.0008
Trained midwife changed *(from 0 to 1)*											
Public, home	−0.0054	−0.0229	0.0821	−0.0094	−0.0249	−0.0195	−0.0057	−0.0538	0.0716	−0.0007	−0.0064	−0.0030
away	−0.0068	−0.0286	−0.0253	−0.0117	0.0967	−0.0243	−0.0019	−0.0189	−0.0054	−0.0002	0.0274	−0.0010
Household income increased by one standard deviation *(from 0.30 to 0.77 urban; from 0.19 to 0.46 rural)*	−0.0147	−0.0181	0.0199	−0.0080	−0.0073	0.0282	−0.0041	−0.0260	−0.0050	0.0025	0.0098	0.0228
Household assets increased by one standard deviation *(from 14 to 69 urban; from 6 to 25 rural)*	−0.0101	−0.0216	−0.0095	−0.0062	0.0223	0.0251	0.0006	−0.236	0.0004	0.0021	0.0085	0.0120
Insurance coverage changed *(from 0 to 1)*	−0.0053	−0.0281	−0.0134	0.0094	0.0528	0.0153	−0.0025	−0.0869	0.0162	0.0166	0.0290	0.0278
Mother's education increased by one standard deviation *(from 8 to 11 for urban; from 5 to 8 for rural)*	−0.0150	−0.0564	−0.0322	−0.0296	0.0225	0.1107	−0.0330	−0.0438	0.0337	0.0057	0.0116	0.0258
Prenatal care changed *(from 0 to 1)†*											
Public	−0.0102	−0.0045	−0.0099	−0.0282	0.1023	−0.0495	−0.0469	−0.0988	0.1077	0.0035	0.0241	0.0104

* For key to abbreviations in headings see note to Table 7.5. † Note that simulations of the effects of public prenatal care are from a separately estimated model where prenatal care is assumed not to be jointly determined with the choice of delivery.

either at home or away, are increased by one standard deviation, the results indicate that there will be little or no change in the choices of delivery care made by the rural sample. The women in the urban sample also appear to be relatively insensitive to moderate changes in money prices, although the urban women are more responsive than rural women to changes in public delivery prices.

The simulation results for changes in the time prices of public practitioners indicate only a limited responsiveness for the urban sample, while the rural sample appears to be more sensitive. When the travel time between the mother and a public practitioner for home delivery is increased by one standard deviation, the model predicts a decrease of about 0.09 in the probability that the mother will choose to use the 'public practitioner at home' option. The results also indicate that women would be likely to switch to a traditional practitioner ($+0.07$) when faced with such a distance increase. Increasing the travel time to public facilities for deliveries away from home also appears to decrease greatly the probability of a rural woman's choosing this option (-0.0377). (Note that the probability of this choice at the means is only 0.0445.)

The number of hours per week that public facilities are available is increased by 40 hours for the purpose of the simulation exercise. For the urban sample, this change represents an increase to 168 hours per week (i.e. 24-hours-a-day availability), and significantly increases the odds that public delivery away from home will be chosen. The predicted 0.116 increase represents an increase of over 50 per cent in the probability that a woman in the urban sample with mean characteristics would choose this option. The rural sample also appears to be very responsive to increases in the hours of availability of public facilities. When hours of operation are increased from 60 to 100 hours per week, women are 0.0231 more likely to choose this modern away-from-home option, an increase of over 50 per cent of the probability predicted at mean values.

A dummy variable for whether drugs are available at the public facility is entered in the model as a proxy for the quality and range of services offered there. The simulation results indicate that adding drug availability at a public facility where drugs are not available will cause a relatively large increase in the probability that the public delivery option will be chosen. The likelihood that this modern away-from-home option will be chosen is increased by 0.0482 for the urban sample, representing an increase of about 25 per cent of the predicted probability when all variables are at their mean values. For the rural sample, the increase is 0.0226, and represents a change of over 50 per cent of the probability predicted at the mean values.

In general, both the urban and rural samples are highly responsive to having trained midwives perform deliveries either at home or at public facilities away from home. For the urban sample, having trained public midwives as the only practitioners to perform at-home deliveries would increase the probability of this option's choice by 0.0821. For away-from-home deliveries at public facilities, the result of having trained midwives as the practitioners is similar, a 0.0967 increase. For the rural sample, at-home public trained midwives are predicted to increase the probability of the choice of at-home public delivery by 0.0716, and for away-from-home public delivery by 0.0274. In each of these four cases, the increase in the probability of choosing the delivery option represents over 49 per cent of the predicted probability at sample mean values. Also, in each case, large reductions in the likelihood of selecting traditional delivery occurs. It is obvious that, for the Cebu samples, trained midwives are highly regarded as birth attendants.

If household income is increased by one standard deviation, the model predicts that urban mothers will be more likely to choose both home deliveries by public practitioners and away-from-home deliveries at private facilities, although the magnitudes of these predicted changes are relatively small. For the rural sample, an increase in household income increases the likelihood of both public and private away-from-home deliveries, as well as that of home deliveries by private practitioners. Increases in household assets appear to increase the probability of choice of the modern away-from-home option for the urban sample, and to shift the pattern of delivery away from the traditional types of delivery for the rural sample. In general, however, the magnitudes of the simulation results suggest that changes in household wealth do not markedly affect the pattern of delivery.

The results for mother's insurance coverage indicate that insurance increases the likelihood of choosing home private, away public, and away private deliveries for members of both the urban and the rural samples. In the urban sample, the largest response to insurance coverage is an increase of 0.0528 in the probability of the choice of public away-from-home deliveries, a change which represents about 25 per cent of the predicted probability of choosing that option at mean values for all variables. For the rural sample, insurance coverage greatly increases the probability of choosing public home, and both public and private away-from-home delivery. With coverage, the predicted probability of public away-from-home deliveries is increased by 0.0290, roughly 65 per cent of the expected probability at the means. The increase in private away-from-home deliveries (0.0278) represents more than 52 per cent of the mean expected probability of choosing this option.

Simulations to test the effect of increases in the mother's education (increasing the number of years of education by one standard deviation) indicate that urban mothers who are more highly educated will be more likely to choose modern public and private away-from-home deliveries than will those with less education. In the rural sample, more highly educated mothers are more likely to choose modern practitioners, both at home and away-from-home, rather than relatives and traditional practitioners.

Using the coefficient results from the alternative estimation, which included dummy variables for whether the woman had received prenatal care from a traditional, public, or private practitioner, simulations were performed to test the effect of the woman's choosing public prenatal care. The use of this model implies that choice of type of prenatal care is exogenous to the choice of delivery service-type. For the urban sample, the effect of using public prenatal care is seen to be a 0.1023 increase in the likelihood that a modern public away-from-home delivery is chosen, representing nearly a 50 per cent increase over the probability of this choice when all variables are at their mean values. For the rural sample, choosing public prenatal care increases the probability that a modern delivery, either away from home, at home, or from public or private practitioners will be chosen. The largest increase (0.1077) is for the probability of a home delivery with a public practitioner, an increase of 68.5 per cent over the probability at the means. The increase in the probability of choosing delivery at a public facility for those who use public prenatal care is also relatively large (0.0241), representing a 54 per cent increase over the probability at the means. The likelihood of choosing a traditional delivery is reduced by 0.0988, a decrease of 15.3 per cent of the probability at the mean values. For the urban sample, the largest effects of using public prenatal care are reductions in the probabilities of choosing both at-home (-0.028) and away-from-home (-0.05) private-practitioner delivery.

Summary and policy implications

This study examined the determinants of the choice of infant-delivery in the Cebu region of the Philippines. The study focused on the effects of certain characteristics of delivery services and socio-economic characteristics of the households on the choice of different types of delivery-care, especially modern delivery-care. A unique data set, with choice-specific measures, designed expressly for this analysis, was used in combination with prospective information for over 3000 mother – infant pairs. The estimation technique allowed us to examine the effect of delivery choice-specific factors as well as unconditional household-specific factors.

The results suggested that the choice of delivery service-type was relatively insensitive to changes in money prices. Consequently, a policy designed to increase the use of modern publicly-provided delivery services by decreasing money prices would be expected to do little to increase demand for these services. The results found for the travel-time price of infant-delivery suggested that in urban areas decreasing the travel time between expectant mothers and modern public delivery services also would have a minor effect on the use of these services. In rural areas, however, decreasing the travel time between expectant mothers and modern public delivery services by locating practitioners and facilities nearby would increase use. In another paper, we further investigate the degree of sensitivity of the choice of delivery type to changes in prices and income (Schwartz *et al.* 1987).

In addition to increasing the accessibility of public delivery practitioners and facilities in urban areas, other public policy changes, such as increasing the hours of operation, increasing the availability of drugs, and providing trained midwives at public facilities would be likely to increase the use of modern delivery services.

The provision of such health services has been a major concern in many low-income countries. In particular, the provision of modern infant-delivery services is especially important because the type of delivery chosen is likely to influence infant mortality and morbidity in these countries. As resources for modern health systems are becoming more scarce and many developing countries are seeking alternative approaches to financing health care, this study provides a method to examine the feasibility of an alternative financing approach which would partially reduce government responsibility for paying for modern health care. For infant-delivery in the Philippines, the results suggest that increasing the money price charged for modern publicly-provided delivery services would decrease usage very little. Similar research to examine the price-sensitivity of various publicly-provided health services in other developing countries is needed to determine the effect of increasing user charges on the demand for modern care.

References

Akin, J.S., Griffin, C., Guilkey, D. K., and Popkin, B. M. (1984). *The demand for primary health care in the Third World*. Littlefield, Adams, and Company, Totowa, NJ.

Akin, J.S., Griffin, C., Guilkey, D. K., and Popkin, B. M. (1986). The demand for primary health services in the Bicol region of the Philippines. *Economic Development and Cultural Change*, **34**(4), 755–82.

Maddala, G. S. (1983). *Limited dependent and qualitative variables: econometrics*. Cambridge University Press.

Mangay-Maglacas, A. (1981). Philippines: the development and use of the National Registry of Traditional Birth Attendants. In *The traditional birth attendant in seven countries: case studies in utilization and training*, World Health Organization Public Health Papers No. 75 (ed. A. Mangay-Maglacas and H. Pizurki), pp. 37–70. WHO, Geneva.

Parado, J. P. (1979). Experiences in the Bohol MCH/FP Project. In *Maternal and Child Health Family Planning Program: technical workshop proceedings*, pp. 86–99. October 31 – November 2, 1979, New York City. International Programs, The Population Council, New York.

Popkin, B. M., Yamamoto, M. E., and Griffin, C. C. (1984). Traditional and modern health professionals and breast-feeding in the Philippines. *Journal of Pediatric Gastroenterology and Nutrition*, **3**, 765–76.

Schwartz, J. B., Akin, J. A., and Popkin, B. M. (1987). Price and income elasticities of demand for modern health care: the case of infant delivery in the Philippines, [Mimeo]. Carolina Population Center, University of North Carolina at Chapel Hill, Chapel Hill, NC.

Simpson-Hebert, M., Piotrow, P. T., Christie, L. J., and Streigh, J. (1980). Traditional midwives and family planning. *Population Reports*, Vol. VIII, No. 22, Series J, pp. J-437–8.

Williamson, N. E. (1982). An attempt to reduce infant and child mortality in Bohol, Philippines. *Studies in Family Planning*, **13**, 106–17.

8

Quantity rationing and the demand of adults for medical care in rural Côte D'Ivoire

Avi Dor and Jacques van der Gaag

Introduction

The principal providers of health care in many developing countries are ministries of health and other public-sector institutions. Slow economic growth and record budget deficits in the 1980s have forced reductions in public spending. This has placed severe pressures on public health-care systems, unable to meet growing needs even during the economic growth periods of the 1960s and 1970s. Whereas funds for capital investment are often funded by international donors, recurrent costs are typically financed by the public treasury. Revenues from user charges usually contribute only about 10 per cent of recurrent expenditures (Ainsworth 1983; de Ferranti 1985). Consequently, little attention has been paid to market forces.

Public health-care systems have been widely criticized. While a large share – if not the majority – of the population resides in rural areas, a disproportionate share of resources has been allocated to health-care in urban centres. Moreover, although infections and parasitic diseases continue to be the leading causes of death and morbidity, there has been an emphasis on technology-intensive care at the hospital level that is more suited to the treatment of chronic diseases.

In these respects Côte d'Ivoire is typical of many developing countries, particularly those in Africa. The Ministry of Public Health and Population (MOPHP) is the principal provider of health-care in Côte d'Ivoire. The private sector, which consists primarily of a number of clinics, is concentrated in the Abidjan area.

In 1984 recurrent expenditures accounted for 90 per cent of the MOPHP budget. Although primary health-care services were available free of charge, hospital-based care and urban centres received a disproportionate share of the government budget. Urban areas, with populations constituting less than 50 per cent of the population, received nearly 89 per cent of the recurrent health budget, while two university hospitals in Abidjan alone accounted for 22 per cent of the total budget. Such imbalances in the health-care system were also apparent in the distribution of medical personnel. About 36 per cent of doctors and 22 per cent of dentists worked at the two university hospitals. A further 34 per cent of doctors and 32 per cent of dentists worked in other hospitals. Similarly, nearly 70 per cent of nurses were assigned to public hospitals and other urban facilities, while only 13 per cent worked in rural areas. The remainder worked in autonomous health institutions.

The strongest argument in favour of the policy of providing medical care free of charge or at very low cost is that it promotes equal access by eliminating financial barriers. However, given the distorted regional distribution of facilities, the policy has not resulted in an equitable health-care delivery system. In fact, the policy has tended to be regressive, with most beneficiaries living in the higher-income urban areas. Furthermore, given the limited supply of health-care services, prospective patients in rural areas may incur considerable access costs associated with queuing, lengthy travel times, and transportation. This suggests that a policy that combines an expansion of health infrastructure with an effective system of user charges could enable the public health-care sector to recover at least part of its recurrent costs, while holding consumers' other out-of-pocket expenditures constant. Using a mixed discrete choice/continuous demand analytical framework, we show here that the absence of user fees *per se* does not guarantee equal access to all adult consumers. Private costs, represented by travel time, result in non-price rationing similar to the conventional money price mechanism. Our results strongly suggest that if revenues obtained from user fees are used to improve the regional distribution of services, the resulting system may improve equity over the long run.

Analytical framework

To date there have been relatively few studies of household demand for health-care in developing countries. Most have focused on the discrete choice problem of selecting amongst alternative providers. These include Dor *et al.* (1987), Gertler *et al.* (1987), Birdsall and Chuhan (1986), Akin *et al.* (1986), and Heller (1982). Conventional analyses of the amount of care demanded, as measured by medical expenditures or numbers of consultations, are found in Musgrove (1983) and Heller (1982). In general, the literature has not been able to establish an unambiguous relationship between money prices and utilization. However, using a model in which price effects depend on income, Gertler *et al.* (1987) showed that health-care demand is highly elastic with respect to prices for low-income groups, but that the price effect diminishes as income increases.

As was mentioned earlier, travel time may be expected to be a particularly powerful rationing device in poor countries, where the majority of the population inhabit rural areas, and health infrastructures are concentrated in the cities. It has been shown (Acton 1975, 1976) that, when money prices are low, time becomes the dominant rationing mechanism. Past studies in developing countries have not been able to confirm this, primarily because of data limitations. The main purpose of this chapter is to identify the impact of travel time and other economic variables on health-care utilization by adults in rural Côte d'Ivoire, where medical services are rendered free of charge. In order to address this issue we define a general health-care demand function:

$$M = M (P, Y, H, Z)$$

with M the demand for medical care;
P a vector of prices, including time prices;
Y a measure of income;
H a measure of health capital; and
Z a vector of socioeconomic variables.

Looking first at the determinants of market entry, we analyse the question of who obtains medical care in case of an illness or injury. M, the demand for medical care, is thus defined as a zero-one dummy variable. We adapted the standard logit model for this part of the analyses. We then estimate a provider-choice model that gives the probabilities of seeking care from a doctor or a nurse, relative to not seeking care at all. We use the multinomial logit model for this step of the analyses. Finally, we analyse the determinants of the number of consultations with each provider.

A more complete presentation of the theoretical model, with a discussion of sample-selection bias issues, is found in Dor and Van der Gaag (1986).

Data and summary statistics

The Ivorian living standards survey

The data used in this study are drawn from the Côte d'Ivoire Living Standards Survey (CILSS), a multi-purpose household survey which was started in February 1985. During the first 12-month period, 1588 households were interviewed, of whom 950 were located in rural areas. Approximately 93 per cent of these households were farming households. Detailed information on health-care utilization was obtained from all household members who reported an illness or injury during the four weeks prior to the interview. Information on medical consumption included the number of visits to each type of provider, expenditures on consultations (if any), and expenditures on drugs. The CILSS also contains extensive information on many socio-economic aspects relevant to the demand for medical care.

In addition to household data, the CILSS collected community-level information in rural areas. Most relevant to the current study are data on the availability of various types of health-care facilities and travel time to the nearest health-care provider (for example, a hospital, clinic, or maternity centre or some type of health worker).

In the rural areas 38 per cent of all adults (those aged 16 or above) reported an illness in the last 28 days, of whom about 49 per cent obtained some form of formal or traditional health-care. While over half those who obtained medical care in Abidjan consulted a doctor, only 17 per cent of those in the villages did so. Still fewer rural dwellers consulted a traditional healer (10 per cent), the majority choosing to consult a nurse (69 per cent).

The rural sample and variables

Persons interviewed in CILSS belonged to 665 households in 56 statistical clusters (i.e. villages). The corresponding community survey provided information on travel time to the nearest sources of care in only 49 villages. Summary statistics in Table 8.1 refer to the reduced sample of individuals with complete information. The overwhelming majority of households, some 637, were headed by males, whose mean age was 48.87 years (s.d. = 13.96), and whose mean years of schooling were only 1.05 years (s.d. = 2.50).

Household consumption or income was used as a measure of the household's economic well-being. Demographic variables such as age, education, sex, and the composition of the household (number of adults and number of children) enter the model in a simple linear fashion. Non-linearities in age were accounted for by dividing the sample into age-groups. The education variable was years of schooling: educational attainment was typically low, and there was little variation in schooling. Approximately 83 per cent of the adults had no education, with the remainder ranging from 1 to 12 years of schooling.

The choice of health-provider is held to depend on certain preconceptions or cultural biases of the decision-maker, although these are not thought to affect the amount of health-care obtained once a provider has been selected. Such biases in favour of one type of health-provider rather than another may be expressed as a function of a person's nationality, ethnic group, religion, or tribal affiliation. Since our sample was almost wholly Ivorian, and because the remaining variables were not available (future CILSS surveys incorporate such variables), we opted for a regional dummy variable (Savannah) as a proxy for these cultural differences. This variable enters only the discrete-choice models.

Health status was measured by the number of days during the past four weeks that individuals were *not* restricted in their normal activities. This variable is expected to reduce the probability of seeking medical care. Since elderly persons typically have more sick time than prime-age adults, they can expect a higher number of restricted-activity days to be their normal state. This implies that an elderly person may require a relatively large number of restricted-activity days in order to motivate an initial visit to a health practitioner, so that the anticipated positive effect of restricted activity days on the probability of seeking medical care would decrease with age. Conversely, the positive effect of unrestricted days on the probability of seeking medical care is likely to increase with age (i.e. to become less negative). For this reason we include an interaction term between our health measure and age in the adult discrete-choice models.

Table 8.1 *Summary statistics: rural adults with illness or injury*

Sample Number of persons with positive sick time	Ages 16–49		Age 50+	
	702		492	
Variables	Mean	Standard deviation	Mean	Standard deviation
Endogenous				
Probability of obtaining formal medical care	0.43	0.50	0.32	0.47
Probability of seeing a doctor	0.10	0.31	0.08	0.27
Probability of seeing a nurse	0.32	0.48	0.25	0.43
Number of doctor consultations	0.31	1.46	0.31	1.88
Number of nurse consultations	0.92	1.98	0.95	2.34
Exogenous				
Travel time to doctor (in hours)	0.86	0.70	0.92	0.95
Travel time to nurse (in hours)	0.56	0.62	0.56	0.63
Income, annual household consumption (in millions of CFAF)	1.32	1.21	1.09	0.96
Years of age	32.82	10.00	61.56	9.78
Sex (male=1, female=0)	0.37	0.48	0.51	0.50
Years of education	1.46	2.82	0.12	0.72
Number of adults in the household (age 16+)	5.61	4.93	5.17	3.84
Number of children in the household (age <16)	5.66	5.71	4.36	4.39
Number of unrestricted activity days (maximum = 28)	20.60	8.56	16.06	11.05
Savannah resident (= 1 answer is yes; = 0 otherwise)	0.29	0.45	0.32	0.46

Once a person selects a health-care provider, healthiness is likely to affect the number of medical consultations in opposite directions. On the one hand, the healthier the person the fewer the consultations needed. On the other hand, relatively healthier patients are better equipped to undertake trips to their preferred provider. In order to see which of the two effects prevails, the unrestricted days variable enters the quantity demand regressions in a quadratic fashion.

Travel time to a doctor or to a nurse is given in hours. At the time of the survey 12 villages had a nurse on location, while none had a doctor. All the individuals in the sample obtained health-care from providers in the public-sector, where services were available at no charge. In the following sections we test whether, in the absence of money prices, travel time replaces the conventional price mechanism in the health-care market.

Estimation of demand for health-care

Entry to the health-care market

In order to measure the effect of travel time and other exogenous variables on the probability of adults seeking medical care, we estimated a market-entry equation in logit form. For those adults reporting illness (i.e. those with a positive sick-time) the dependent dummy variable takes a value of 1 if the person consulted a medical practitioner. In Table 8.2 we present the estimation results for prime-age adults (those between the ages of 16 and 49 years), for elderly persons (aged 50 years or above), and finally for all adults taken together (i.e. the pooled adult sample). The coefficients (the β's) are reported, together with asymptotic t-values. Throughout this paper, the marginal effects are also reported for all dichotomous regressions.

In all the regressions in Table 8.2 the age variable had the expected negative effect on demand; and it is statistically significant in the elderly and pooled samples. We also ran the pooled regression with quadratic and splined age terms, but this did not improve the results.

Healthiness – measured as the number of unrestricted activity days – has a significantly negative impact on overall utilization, although, as anticipated, this effect is dampened somewhat at old age. The positive sign of the healthiness and age interaction

Table 8.2 Determinants of decision to seek medical care in case of illness (logit model)

	Prime-age Adults (age 16–49)			Elderly (ages 50+)			All adults		
	β	t	Marginal effect	β	t	Marginal effect	β	t	Marginal effect
Constant	2.76	(3.36)	0.676	3.69	(2.99)	0.792	2.59	(5.50)	0.610
Average travel time	0.38	(2.37)	-0.090	-0.36	(2.06)	-0.076	-0.36	(3.03)	-0.081
Income	0.24	(2.86)	0.059	0.13	(0.93)	0.027	0.20	(2.69)	0.048
Age	-0.05	(2.60)	-0.013	-0.07	(3.61)	-0.015	-0.05	(5.79)	-0.011
Male	0.00	(0.02)	0.001	0.15	(0.73)	0.032	0.04	(0.29)	0.011
Education	-0.01	(0.30)	-0.003	-0.03	(0.18)	-0.006	-0.02	(0.61)	0.009
Adults	-0.08	(2.04)	-0.020	-0.01	(0.19)	-0.002	-0.06	(2.30)	-0.014
Children	0.03	(1.46)	0.008	0.07	(1.79)	0.016	0.04	(2.01)	0.010
Unrestricted days	-0.15	(3.33)	-0.035	-0.20	(2.03)	-0.043	-0.11	(5.36)	-0.026
Unrestricted days × Age	0.002	(1.97)	0.0005	0.003	(2.79)	0.001	0.002	(4.00)	0.0004
Savannah	-0.15	(0.72)	0.036	0.42	(1.65)	-0.090	-0.25	(1.60)	-0.058
Log likelihood	-444.65			-286.64			-737.76		
χ^2	70.16			48.81			119.04		
Income elasticity	0.183			0.095			0.156		
Travel time elasticity	-0.149			-0.181			-0.154		

variable suggests that, *ceteris paribus*, an older person requires relatively fewer healthy days (i.e. requires more sick days) in order to have the same probability of seeking health-care as a younger person.

Home care may be viewed as a substitute for formal medical care. Since home care is normally provided by adults, the number of adults in the household is expected to reduce the probability of seeking formal care. However, since adults in the extended households must also devote a certain portion of their time to child-care, the number of children in the household is likely to increase the probability of seeking care. Estimation results confirm our expectations. The household-size variables always have the anticipated sign, and are usually significant.

The resulting demographic variables appear to be less important determinants of market entry. Living in savannah areas has a negative impact on market entry in all age categories, but is significant at a 10 per cent level only in the elderly category. Sex and education variables do not have any effect on the decision to seek health-care.

With the exception of health status itself, economic variables are the most important determinants of health-care utilization. Individuals living in households with a relatively high income show, *ceteris paribus*, a significantly greater propensity to seek care than their poorer counterparts. The income elasticity of the pooled sample, at the sample means, is 0.16, which is comparable to the results usually obtained for industrialized countries.

Travel-time differences prove to have a most important influence on utilization. The travel time variable was obtained by averaging travel time to the nearest doctor and travel time to the nearest nurse. The estimation result (Table 8.2) shows a time-price elasticity ranging from −0.15 to −0.18, and supports the proposition that, in the absence of money prices, other private costs of obtaining medical care play the role of the conventional price mechanism.

Even though actual fees for medical care were zero, total out-of-pocket expenditures are likely to have been positive on account of transportation costs. Unfortunately, information on the money cost of travel associated with the consumption of medical care was not available in the survey.

The goodness of fit criterion χ^2 (chi-square), which is given in Table 8.2, is based on the general log likelihood ratio of the form

$$LR = L(\hat{\beta})/L'(0)$$

$L(\hat{\beta})$ is the value of the maximized log likelihood using the estimated parameters and $L'(0)$ is the maximized log likelihood function under the null hypothesis that all β are equal to zero. It can be shown that $-2 \times \ln (LR)$ is approximately distributed as a χ_k^2 (chi-squared), where k degrees of freedom are equal to the number of zero restrictions (Wilks 1962). Throughout this study, χ^2 statistics are sufficiently large to reject the null hypothesis that the estimated β are equal to zero.

Finally we tested the validity of pooling across age-groups. To do this we used another aproximation of the χ^2 test, also known as the Wald test.

$$\chi^2 \simeq [\beta_1 - \beta_2] [V_1 + V_2]^{-1} [\beta_1 - \beta_2]'$$

where β_1 is the parameter vector belonging to prime age adults, β_2 is the parameter vector from the elderly regression, and V_1, V_2 are the respective variance matrices. The result was 15.4, well below the 95 per cent critical level of 19.7. Consequently we cannot reject the null hypothesis that $\beta_1 = \beta_2$ and hence pooling is appropriate.

Before showing how the above results hold up when other models of demand for health-care are estimated, concerns about selectivity bias should be mentioned. Although data were available for all persons who completed the interview, the estimating sample excludes all healthy people. To see whether this severely biases the sampled data, the Probit demand equation was estimated conditional upon the probability of being ill or injured. The procedure (from Van der Ven and Van der Praag 1981) yielded small change in the coefficients and virtually no change in the slopes. Therefore it was concluded that no severe selection bias arose because of the exclusion of healthy persons.

Provider choice, a multinomial logit model

In the previous section we analysed the decision of whether or not to seek medical care in case of an illness or injury. In this section we analyse the choice of alternative health-care providers (i.e. a visit to a doctor or a nurse, relative to not obtaining medical care at all). In a later section we discuss the choice of how much care to consume (i.e the number of consultations with each provider).

The multinomial logit model is specified in the following form:

$$\ln (P_j/P_0) = \sum_{k=1}^{2} \beta_{jk} T_{jk} + \gamma_j Z$$

with

P_j	the probability of choosing provider j;
$j = 1$	doctor;
$j = 2$	nurse;
T_{jk}	travel time to a given provider;
Z	composite of socio-economic variables; and
β_{jk}, γ_j	the corresponding coefficients for choice j.

P_0 is the default option, the probability of not seeking care when ill, with coefficients normalized to zero. Thus, $\ln (P_j P_0)$ is the logarithm of the probability of consulting provider j, relative to the probability of not seeking care at all. The composite Z contain the same exogenous variables as in the previous section. The T_k variables denote travel time, and may be interpreted as choice-related price variables. Note that travel time for the 'don't go' option is equal to zero.

The elasticity of P_j with respect to X_k where X_k represents any of the exogenous variables, is given by

$$E_{jk} = \left(\beta_{jk} - \sum_{j=1}^{2} P_{jk} \beta_{jk} \right) X_k$$

From the above, one may calculate own time elasticities ($j = k$), cross time elasticities ($j \neq k$), or elasticities with respect to a trait of a decision-maker (replace β by γ).

Estimation results are given in Table 8.3. Time prices are represented by the time needed to travel to the nearest doctor and travel time to the nearest nurse. All own time-price effects have the expected negative sign. In the doctor alternative the coefficient is -1.95, with a t-value of 4.03. In the nurse alternative there is a highly significant negative own time-price effect of -0.89.

In both alternatives cross time effects are positive and significant at the 0.99 significance level. These results suggest that in Côte d'Ivoire the services of nurses and doctors are substitutes, rather than complements. The income effects in both alternatives are positive and significant. Income and travel time elasticities are given in Table 8.4.

The multinomial logit model strongly confirms and augments the results obtained from the simpler bivariate model: own time price effects are negative, cross time-price effects are generally positive. The magnitude of these effects is substantially greater than those found by Akin *et al.* (1986) in the Philippines.

We finally note that the impact of socio-economic variables is generally stable across the entry-to-the-market and provider-choice models. In particular, the coefficient of age is negative and highly significant. The effect of gender (i.e. of being male) is negative and insignificant in the nurse alternative, but positive and significant in the case of doctor visits. This indicates that

Table 8.3 *Determinants of choice between doctor, nurse, and home care (multinomial logit model, all adults)*

	Nurse alternative β	t	Doctor alternative β	t
Constant	2.125	(4.23)	2.135	(3.39)
Doctor travel time	0.325	(3.38)	−1.953	(4.03)
Nurse travel time	−0.887	(5.57)	1.028	(2.31)
Income	0.234	(2.84)	0.259	(2.86)
Age	−0.048	(5.46)	−0.050	(4.54)
Male	−0.043	(0.29)	0.439	(1.95)
Education	−0.042	(1.54)	0.010	(0.21)
Adults	−0.054	(1.99)	−0.080	(1.99)
Children	0.039	(1.73)	0.053	(1.49)
Unrestricted days	−0.106	(4.81)	−0.130	(4.46)
Unrestricted days × Age	0.002	(3.86)	0.001	(2.52)
Savannah	0.093	(0.53)	0.407	(1.31)
Log likelihood			−967.49	
χ^2			198.66	

males are more likely to obtain higher-quality health-care. These results are not compatible with the notion drawn from the standard utility model framework such as Acton's, that individuals with higher opportunity cost of time, for example working-age males, demand less medical care. Furthermore, negative age effects are not predicted by Grossman's household production model (1972). The results of this study suggest that individuals who are relatively more productive obtain the largest share of medical care in the household.

An implicit assumption in our model is that the probability choice set of an individual includes all prices, and is therefore analogous to the conventional demand function. While our specification is convenient it is not consistent with the random utility maximization framework developed by McFadden (1981, 1982). In this framework each alternative may be chosen only on the basis of alternative specific variables. Thus deciding whether to visit a doctor depends on travel time to that doctor, not on travel time to the nurse. Similarly, the choice of a nurse depends on travel time to that nurse. Strict adherence to the random utility maximization framework would require the exclusion of socio-economic variables that do not vary across alternatives. However, Gertler *et al.* (1987) show that under certain behavioural assumptions, socioeconomic variables may affect each alternative differently. This leads us to the following specification of the multinomial logit model.

$$\ln(P_j/P_0) = \beta_j T_j + \gamma_j Z$$

This model is identical to the previous model, except for imposing the restriction that the coefficients of the cross time variables are

Table 8.4 *Income and travel time elasticities of the probability of choosing a doctor or nurse (multinomial logit model)*

	Nurse alternative	Doctor alternative
Income elasticity	0.183	0.214
Travel time elasticities		
Nurse	−0.385	1.082
Doctor	0.310	−1.075

equal to zero. Henceforth we will refer to it as the restricted multinomial logit model.

The own-time elasticity becomes:

$$E_j^{P_j} = \beta_j T_j (1 - P_j)$$

As in the case of binary logit, the cross elasticity of the probability of alternative j with respect to travel time to alternative m is:

$$E_m^{P_j} = - \beta_m T_m P_m$$

In practice, the restricted version of the multinomial logit model is not expected to yield significant changes in the coefficients of the socio-economic variables. This is not the case with the travel time variable, where actual and spurious correlations (the correlation between the nurse and doctor travel time was 0.61) may have biased the estimates in the unrestricted model.

Results of the unrestricted version of the multinomial logit model are given in Table 8.5. As anticipated, the coefficients of the various socio-economic variables remain fairly stable compared with the previous multinomial logit model. There is no significant change in the own-time effect in the nurse alternative. In the doctor alternative, the coefficient of travel time was reduced by nearly one half.

Elasticities obtained from the restricted model are presented in Table 8.6. Although all own-time and cross-time elasticities are lower in absolute values than the corresponding elasticities in Table 8.4, the basic results of both models are the same. The t-values tend to be slightly higher in the restricted model. However, the unrestricted model does better in term of goodness-of-fit criteria. Since both models were estimated on the same sample and with the same set of alternatives, their likelihood ratios are directly comparable. We can thus construct a likelihood ratio test for the null hypothesis that cross-time coefficients are zero:

$$\chi^2 \simeq -2 \ln \left[\frac{L(\hat{\beta}_2)}{L(\hat{\beta}_1)} \right]$$

Table 8.5 *Determinants of choice between doctor, nurse, and home care (restricted multinomial logit model, all adults)*

	Nurse alternative β	Nurse alternative t	Doctor alternative β	Doctor alternative t
Constant	2.28	(4.46)	2.180	(3.44)
Doctor travel time			−1.160	(4.35)
Nurse travel time	−0.658	(4.89)		
Income	0.202	(2.48)	0.255	(2.32)
Age	−0.047	(5.31)	−0.032	(4.68)
Male	-0.061	(0.42)	0.046	(2.07)
Education	−0.073	(1.54)	−0.002	(0.30)
Adults	−0.053	(1.95)	−0.077	(1.79)
Children	0.038	(1.71)	0.039	(1.11)
Unrestricted days	−0.102	(4.67)	−0.129	(4.44)
Unrestricted days × Age	0.002	(3.69)	0.001	(2.49)
Savannah	0.035	(0.20)	−0.280	(0.93)
Log likelihood		−966.73		
χ^2		180.18		

Table 8.6 *Income and travel time elasticities (restricted multinomial logit model)*

	Nurse alternative	Doctor alternative
Income elasticity	0.154	0.219
Travel time elasticity		
Nurse	−0.261	0.107
Doctor	0.072	−0.953

$\hat{\beta}_1$ denotes the coefficients from the unrestricted model, while $\hat{\beta}_2$ denotes the coefficients from the restricted model. The test yielded a χ^2 value of 1.4, compared with $\chi^2_{22,.010} = 42.0$. Consequently the null hypothesis of zero cross-time effects cannot be rejected.

Number of consultations with doctors and nurses

In this section we turn to the actual 'quantity' of care demanded, as measured by the number of visits to each type of provider. Demand is estimated conditional on first entering the health-care market (i.e. for all individuals who visit). Owing to the small size of the conditional sample, the quantity-demand equations were estimated from the pooled sample.

Tables 8.7 and 8.8 show results obtained from ordinary least-squares regressions. The coefficients of each of the demographic and health variables display the same signs for both the doctor and

Table 8.7 *Demand for medical consultations (ordinary least squares, all adults)*

	Nurse alternative		Doctor alternative	
	β	t	β	t
Constant	2.275	(5.62)	2.010	(3.06)
Doctor travel time	0.149	(1.10)	−0.737	(1.01)
Nurse travel time	−0.267	(1.67)	0.550	(0.84)
Income	0.141	(1.66)	0.150	(0.97)
Age	0.007	(1.17)	0.002	(0.25)
Male	0.095	(0.68)	0.501	(1.68)
Education	−0.033	(0.83)	−0.092	(1.50)
Adults	−0.039	(1.19)	−0.164	(2.36)
Children	0.059	(2.34)	0.130	(2.44)
Unrestricted days	0.021	(0.66)	0.083	(1.64)
(Unrestricted days)^2	−0.002	(1.64)	−0.003	(1.58)
R^2	0.102		0.103	
F value	3.600		1.250	
Sample size*	330		109	

* Excluding observations with more than 7 consultations.

Table 8.8 *Elasticities of quantity demand (adults, conditional upon market entry)*

	Nurse consultations	Doctor consultations
Income elasticity	0.075	0.098
Travel-time elasticity		
Nurse	–0.043	0.066
Doctor	0.051	–0.155

Note: These estimates apply strictly to the conditional sample of entrants to the health-care market, and not to the whole population.

nurse alternatives, although they are more significant and larger in magnitude in the doctor alternative. The demographic variables with the greatest impact on doctor consultations are the number of adults and the number of children in the household. There is a negative association between the number of adults and utilization, and a positive association between the number of children and utilization. Since the interpretation is the same as in the preceding provider-choice models, we need not discuss it here.

While the education variable had no effect on the decision of whether or not to choose a doctor, it had a significantly negative effect on the number of doctor consultations. This result is compatible with the notion that more education makes people more efficient at the 'home production' of health, and may therefore reduce the amount of medical care required (Grossman 1972).

It is also interesting to note that being male has a significantly positive and large effect on the number of doctor consultations, and a negligible effect on nurse consultations. The provider-choice model indicated that males are more likely to obtain health-care provided by doctors and less likely to obtain care provided by nurses. Assuming that doctors provide higher-quality health-care, these results imply that households bias their use of health-care in favour of males.

Although the economic variables travel time and income fail to attain critical t-values (with the exception of the own-time parameter in the nurse alternative), the results do confirm and augment conclusions drawn from the provider-choice model. Negative own-time effects and positive cross-time effects indicate that travel time may replace the conventional monetary price mechanism, and that the medical care provided by nurses and by doctors are indeed substitutes for each other.

Summary and conclusion

Total utilization response

In this chapter we have estimated various health-care demand models in order to assess the extent of quantity rationing in the health-care system in Côte d'Ivoire. Quantity rationing is defined as the effect of travel time to the nearest provider on the decision to seek medical care, on the choice of the health-care provider, and on the total number of consultations with each provider.

We summarize our main results in Table 8.9. Note that total demand, M_j, for services of provider j is given by

$$M_j = P_j (N_j \mid N_j > 0),$$

where P_j is the probability of choosing j, and N_j is the number of consultations with j, only observed if j is chosen. Thus:

$$\frac{\partial M_j}{\partial X} = P_j \frac{\partial N_j}{\partial X} + N_j \frac{\partial P_j}{\partial X}$$

for any exogenous variable X. The total elasticity of demand for provider j is given by

$$E_j = \epsilon_j + n_j$$

i.e., the sum of the probability elasticity of demand and the conditional elasticity of demand for consultation (in Tables 8.6 and 8.8).

The results in Table 8.9 demonstrate that, in the absence of user fees, travel time acts as a rationing mechanism in the health-care market. It also seems appropriate to state that access to higher-quality care, i.e. doctors, is always completely restricted by long travel times. On the other hand, because medical care

Table 8.9 *Total demand elasticities*

	Nurse alternative	Doctor alternative
Income elasticity	0.229	0.317
Travel time elasticities		
Nurse	−0.304	0.173
Doctor	0.123	−1.108

is free, income elasticities in the Ivorian health-care market are relatively low, much like they are in the developed countries, in which the market for medical care is generally characterized by a high level of insurance coverage.

Policy implications

The case against user fees in the health-care market stems from the desire to allow free access to medical care to everyone who needs it. However, while money prices may be zero, as they are in rural Côte d'Ivoire, private costs to the patients may still be considerable. As we have shown in this paper, the absence of user fees *per se* does not guarantee equal access for all. In fact, the private costs (here represented by travel time), much like a money price, serve as a rationing mechanism, with those living further from health-care facilities being most restricted. Thus the case against user fees cannot be based on some *a priori* notion of an otherwise existing equity.

The results of this study imply that the demand for medical care in rural areas can be significantly increased if the regional distribution of health-care providers is improved. This improvement, which could be funded by user fees, may offset the expected negative impact on the demand for medical care that is likely to result from the introduction of fees. The resulting system may turn out to be more equitable, rather than less equitable, as is usually feared. The net outcome depends on many issues: which medical services are charged for; whether the fees result in sufficiently high revenues to improve the system; whether fees have the same impact on poor and rich households; and whether fees are to be income-dependent.

Answers to such questions depend on the money price elasticity of demand, the willingness-to-pay for medical care, and the cost structure of health-care facilities. In order to help policy-makers make the difficult decisions necessary to solve the severe financial problems that are prevalent in the health-care delivery systems of many developing countries, more research is needed.

References

Acton, J. P. (1975). Nonmonetary factors in the demand for medical services: some empirical evidence. *Journal of Political Economy*, 83, 595–614.

Acton, J. P. (1976). Demand for health-care among the rural poor, with special emphasis on the role of time. In *The role of health insurance in the health services sector* (ed. Richard N. Rosett). National Bureau of Economic Research, New York.

Ainsworth, M. (1983). User charges for cost recovery in the social sectors: current practices [Mimeo]. World Bank, Washington, DC.

Akin, J., Griffin, C. C., Guilkey, D. K., and Popkin, B. M. (1986). The demand for primary health services in the Bicol Region of the Philippines. *Economic Development and Cultural Change*, 34(4), 755–82.

Birdsall, N. and Chuhan, P. (1986). Client choice of health-care treatment in rural Mali. [Mimeo]. The World Bank, Washington, DC.

de Ferranti, D. (1985). *Paying for health services in developing countries: an overview*. World Bank Staff Working Papers No. 721. World Bank, Washington, DC.

Dor, A. and van der Gaag, J. (1986). *The demand for medical care in developing countries: quantity rationing in rural Côte d'Ivoire*, LSMS Working Paper no.35. World Bank, Washington, DC.

Dor, A., Gertler, P., and van der Gaag, J. (1987). Non-price rationing and the choice of medical care provided in rural Côte d'Ivoire. *Journal of Health Economics*, 6, 291–304.

Gertler, P., Locay, L., and Sanderson, W. (1987). Are user fees regressive? The welfare implications of health-care financing proposals in Peru. *Journal of Econometrics*, 36, 67–88.

Grossman, M. (1972). On the concept of health capital and the demand for health. *Journal of Political Economy*, 80, 233–55.

Heller, P. S. (1982). A model of the demand for medical and health services in peninsular Malaysia. *Social Science and Medicine*, 16, 267–84.

McFadden, D. (1981). Econometric models of probabilistic choice. In *Structural analysis of discrete data with econometric applications* (ed.) C. Manski and D. McFadden), pp. 198–272. MIT Press, Cambridge, Mass.

McFadden, D. (1982). Qualitative response models. In *Advances in Econometrics:* invited papers for the Fourth World Congress of the

Quantity rationing and the demand of adults for medical care 213

Econometric Society (ed. W. Hildenbrand), pp. 1–38. Cambridge University Press.

Musgrove, P. (1983). Family health-care spending in Latin America. *Journal of Health Economics*, 2(3), 245–58.

Van der Ven, W. and Van der Praag, B. M. S. (1982). The demand for deductibles in private health insurance: a probit model with sample selection. *Journal of Econometrics*, 17(2), 229–52.

Wilks, S. S. (1962). *Mathematical statistics*. Wiley, New York.

9

Setting global priorities for strategies to control diarrhoeal disease: the contribution of cost-effectiveness analysis

Margaret Phillips

Introduction

Agencies involved in health-programme policy, planning, and implementation continually face the problem of choosing between alternative approaches to improve the health of their populations. In the context of increasingly severe financial constraints, 'value for money' is recognized as an important criterion for choice, and countries are now paying more attention to the cost-effectiveness of their health programmes. However, it is difficult, time-consuming, and costly to evaluate all alternative investments each time a decision on programme development has to be made. There are clearly advantages in being able to identify health strategies which can be widely recommended even if their detailed implementation needs to be adapted to local circumstances. Such was the thinking behind, for example, the advocacy of selective primary health care (Walsh and Warren 1979), and UNICEF's promotion of GOBI-FFF – growth monitoring, oral rehydration therapy, breast-feeding, immunization, family planning, female education, and food supplementation. These were also the kind of considerations which led the World Health Organization, an organization with a special responsibility to guide countries in their decision-making about health, to support research to identify diarrhoea-control strategies that could be promoted internationally.

Diarrhoea is estimated to be responsible for the deaths of nearly five million children under five years of age annually (Snyder and Merson 1982). A major breakthrough in the treatment of diarrhoea was achieved in the 1960s with the development of oral rehydration therapy (ORT), which is effective in preventing dehydration and

Table 9.1 *Potential non-clinical interventions for diarrhoea control amongst young children*[1]

Area	Potential intervention	Reference to published effectiveness review	Status[2]
Maternal health	Preventing low-weight babies	Ashworth and Feachem (1985b)	?
	Enhancing lactation	Ashworth and Feachem (1985c)	?
Child health	Promoting breast-feeding	Feachem and Koblinsky (1984)	*
	Improving weaning practices	Ashworth and Feachem (1985a)	*
	Supplementary feeding programmes	Feachem (1983)	—
	Growth monitoring	Ashworth and Feachem (1986)	?
	Increasing child spacing	In preparation	?
	Vitamin A supplementation	Feachem (1987)	?
Immuno- and chemo prophylaxis	Rotavirus vaccination	de Zoysa and Feachem (1985a)	*
	Cholera vaccination	de Zoysa and Feachem (1985a)	*
	Measles vaccination	Feachem and Koblinsky (1983)	*
	Chemoprophylaxis	de Zoysa and Feachem (1985b)	*
Inter- rupting trans- mission	Improving water supply and santitation facilities	Esrey et al. (1985)	*
	Promoting personal and and domestic hygiene	Feachem (1984)	*
	Improving food hygiene	Esrey and Feachem (1989)	?
	Controlling zoonotic reservoirs	No publication	?
	Controlling flies	Esrey (1991)	—
Epidemic control	Epidemic surveillance, investigation, and control	No publication	?

[1] Adapted from Feachem (1986).
[2] Status:
    – interventions which are ineffective and/or of limited feasibility
    * effective interventions
    ? interventions of uncertain effectiveness and/or feasibility.

consequently death, is relatively simple to administer, and is, moreover, inexpensive. However, ORT has little impact on mortality that is due to non-watery diarrhoeas, or on the morbidity rates of any type of diarrhoea.

Fortunately, a number of other potential control strategies for diarrhoea have been identified, ranging from improved water-supplies to fly-control (Feachem *et al.* 1983). WHO, in order to decide which interventions to advocate most strongly, initiated research to study systematically non-clinical interventions that might possibly play a role in diarrhoea control.

After an initial round of analysis which reviewed published studies of effectiveness, several of the proposed interventions were found to be of unknown effectiveness, infeasible, or obviously too costly. Some, however, appeared to be highly effective anti-diarrhoea measures, and of potential interest to both international and national agencies concerned with diarrhoeal diseases control. The list of interventions studied and their potential for diarrhoeal disease control is shown in Table 9.1.

Before wholeheartedly advocating the implementation of these measures or attempting to indicate priorities, the Diarrhoeal Disease Control Programme of WHO felt it desirable to complement the effectiveness analysis with a detailed study of resource requirements for the interventions with the greatest potential to control diarrhoea. The results of that analysis are the subject of this chapter. The principal objective of the research was to derive estimates of cost-effectiveness to guide decision-makers by showing which interventions would have maximum impact on diarrhoea for a given level of investment. A secondary objective was to elaborate on the characteristics of possible interventions as a broad guide to designing intervention strategies. Of the interventions shown in Table 9.1, the following were studied:

- measles, rotavirus and cholera vaccination;
- breast-feeding promotion;
- improved weaning practices; and
- promoting personal hygiene through handwashing.

The next section in this chapter discusses the variety of methodologies applied to data drawn from the literature on diarrhoeal disease control in order to calculate costs and cost-effectiveness.

The results of these calculations are presented briefly in section three. The fourth section discusses the interpretation of the cost-effectiveness results, and the final section the limitations of cost-effectiveness analysis in assisting decision-making, noting in particular the variety of costs and benefits not captured in the summary measures of 'cost per diarrhoea case averted' and 'cost per diarrhoea death averted'.

The methodology used to calculate cost and cost-effectiveness

Since the conclusions of the study were intended to be of relevance to a wide range of countries, and a number of different interventions were being reviewed, field-based research was not considered appropriate until a desk study had been carried out. It is this desk study of published data on real programmes that is the subject of this chapter. Relevant literature on studies reporting effectiveness provided the starting-point for the research. Where cost data on these same projects were available they were extracted, and if necessary adapted to derive cost-effectiveness results for each project. For some interventions, few if any of the projects whose effectiveness was known also had cost data. For these interventions, plausible cost estimates were constructed based on descriptions of resource use and on prices. Only those costs associated with the *provision* of the intervention were estimated. User costs were ignored. Data limitations dictated the choice of 'diarrhoea cases averted' or 'diarrhoea deaths averted' as the summary measures of intervention effectiveness.

Since the methodology used to derive estimates of cost and cost-effectiveness for each intervention differed to some degree depending on data availability, the approach used for each intervention is briefly described below. Further details are provided in Phillips *et al.* (1987).

Vaccination against measles, rotavirus diarrhoea, and cholera

A considerable body of evidence, reviewed by Feachem and Koblinsky (1983), suggests that measles vaccination can have a modest impact on diarrhoea morbidity and a substantial impact on diarrhoea mortality. New oral vaccines against cholera and rotavirus diarrhoea are under field trial. It appears that rotavirus vaccines could play an important role in reducing diarrhoea illness and death in children, while new cholera vaccines may provide an effective intervention in countries, such as Bangladesh, which experience relatively high rates of endemic cholera (de Zoysa and Feachem 1985*a*).

In contrast to other interventions against diarrhoea explored in this chapter, there already exists a substantial literature documenting cost breakdowns for various vaccination programmes in a number of countries. These data provided a useful base from which to derive estimates of the likely costs of vaccinating a child with measles, rotavirus, and cholera vaccines. The method employed was as follows.

Data on 13 vaccination programmes in 9 countries provided estimates of the cost per child fully vaccinated with the vaccines available in that particular programme, as well as breakdown of those costs by major component: central and local staff, transport, materials, vaccines, and capital items (vehicles, buildings, equipment, training). For each of these major cost components, a 'model' of how they were likely to change with the addition of different kinds of new vaccines was developed and applied to the data collected. Three key assumptions underpinned these calculations. The first assumption was that measles, rotavirus, or cholera vaccination programmes would involve the addition of certain inputs to an existing infrastructure (i.e. that the analysis was concerned with the intervention's additional or incremental costs). This seemed appropriate given that most countries already had established vaccination programmes for at least some of the major immunizable childhood diseases.

The second assumption was that vaccination costs vary depending on whether the vaccine is given orally or injected; whether it is administered at the same time as other vaccines or at a separate contact; and whether it is in the same dose as another vaccine or in a separate dose. The third assumption was that the schedule and dosage (i.e. treatment regime) for each of the vaccines would be an injected dose of measles vaccine at about 9 months; oral doses of rotavirus diarrhoea vaccine before 6 months; and oral doses of cholera vaccine in the second year of life.

The extra costs incurred in adding measles (or rotavirus diarrhoea or cholera) vaccination to each programme were calculated (for instance, costs for salaries, transport, and vaccines). These separate cost components were then summed to give estimates of the incremental cost per fully vaccinated child for each vacination programme (i.e. measles, rotavirus diarrhoea, or cholera). Using the data from de Zoysa and Feachem (1985*a*) on the estimated percentage of diarrhoea episodes and deaths averted by each ~prevent from happening~ vaccine and assumptions concerning the pre-intervention incidence of diarrhoea, a range of estimates of cost per episode and death averted was calculated for each vaccine.

The method used for estimating incremental salary costs requires special mention, since salaries are a key input, comprising on average about 60 per cent of the total costs of the vaccination programmes studied. In the absence of time-and-motion studies it is difficult to predict how manpower costs and utilization will respond to the addition of a new vaccine. To overcome this, a hypothetical standardized workload unit – the 'injected-dose-equivalent' (IDE) – was adopted, one unit representing the amount of time required to administer an injectable vaccine to a child that has already come for a vaccination. Based on assumptions about the relationship between the IDE and the amount of staff time required for each of the differently administered vaccines, it was possible to estimate, for each of the 13 programmes analysed, the amount and value of the additional time required by staff to administer each of the new vaccines. Details of this methodology and the assumptions adopted in calculating the value of other inputs required are given in Phillips *et al.* (1987).

Breast-feeding promotion

The association between a failure to breast-feed and diarrhoeal incidence and severity has been convincingly demonstrated. So too has the possibility of influencing breast-feeding rates through various strategies (Feachem and Koblinsky 1984). Five strategies appear to be particularly important: changes in hospital routine in maternity wards; face-to-face education of women; the use of mass media; the discouragement of alternatives to breast-milk; and improvements in conditions for working mothers. Since cost data on these strategies are scarce, it was necessary to develop plausible descriptions of the nature of each strategy in order to be able to derive realistic assessments of the type and quantity of their resource-input requirements. Salary-rates used for manpower (one of the key inputs) were based on the results of a small informal survey conducted at the London School of Hygiene and Tropical

Medicine using a questionnaire addressed to 30 experienced health professionals with detailed knowledge of one or more developing countries.

Changes in hospital routine. One of the strategies most carefully studied for its impact on breast-feeding is changes in hospital routine. This includes keeping neonates in the same room as their mother and encouraging skin-to-skin contact and early breast-feeding after delivery (Winikoff and Baer 1980). No studies were located which provided estimates of the resource costs of such changes, and few studies even describe in any detail the process involved in preparing an institution for a change in routine. Hales (1981) and Durongdej and Israel (1986) are two exceptions. On the basis of their descriptions of an attempt to institutionalize 'rooming-in' in one hospital and the preparation of a one-week national workshop for key hospital staff, probable costs were estimated and expressed in terms of both cost per hospital and cost per delivery for a variety of differently-sized hospitals. Because most of such costs are relatively fixed with respect to the number of deliveries, hospital size is likely to be an important determinant of average incremental costs.

Face-to-face education and support. The provision of information and support to women in hospital for childbirth has been shown to have a positive impact on breast-feeding rates. This strategy may involve seminars for nurses or a discussion with mothers, together with a survey of breast-feeding rates of mothers leaving hospital designed to measure the success of the education interventions. Such surveys are often an important source of motivation for staff – in one example, the only intervention was a survey, and it is to this that the subsequent changes in breast-feeding rates were cautiously attributed (Smart and Bamford 1976). None of the studies located provided data on costs. For this study the resources that these activities might require were estimated on the basis of descriptions of the strategies in the literature. Total costs and costs per delivery were calculated using a range of assumptions concerning the size of classes held and the number of births per hospital per year – both factors which are likely to be important determinants of incremental cost per delivery.

Use of mass media. Although several countries have embarked on national campaigns to promote breast-feeding using mass media, data on their effectiveness and costs are scanty. However, there is some evidence from other educational campaigns that mass media can be successful in changing health-related behaviour. Some data on the costs of these campaigns have been published. The potential range of costs in mounting a breast-feeding promotion campaign using mass media is vast, not only because the choices concerning the intensity and length of the campaign and the variety of ways of packaging the components are essentially limitless, but also because the costs of each of the components can vary substantially.

To develop some rough estimates, a plausible range of possible types of promotional campaign was considered, from a basic campaign restricted to radio and costing $20000 (type A), through to a more comprehensive model involving the intensive use of a wide range of media, including television, and costing over $500000 (type E). The size of the population exposed to mass media is clearly a crucial determinant of cost-effectiveness, since the majority of the costs of mass media are fixed. Costs per child whose mother is exposed to mass media were derived using a variety of assumptions concerning population size (0.5 to 50 million) and media coverage (20 per cent to 80 per cent). The effect of mass media programmes was assumed to last for only one year.

Discouragement of breast-feeding alternatives. Legislation to discourage the use of infant formula has been demonstrated to increase breast-feeding rates (Baer 1981). However, insufficient data are available on the costs of establishing and policing legislation in developing countries to allow any accurate cost estimates to be derived. Such costs are difficult to measure, and may be relatively small in circumstances where efficient legislative and policing machinery exists already. On the assumption that legal services, publicity, and policing costs amount to $50000, the cost per child affected was calculated for different assumptions of population size (again 0.5 to 50 million), and for different assumptions of the length of time for which legislation is effective (1 to 5 years).

Facilities for working women. Maternal employment is widely cited as a major reason for the decline in breast-feeding throughout the world. The provision of maternity leave, nursing breaks during working hours, and crèches at or near a work site are possible strategies for encouraging employed women to breast-feed. The total costs of enacting legislation to support these activities may be similar to the costs of legislation to encourage breast-feeding. However, the average costs (per child affected) are likely to be considerably higher in any given country, because women in the formal sector constitute only a proportion of the total population of mothers of infants. Governments enacting legislation may also need to finance the implementation of some of the changes required under the legislation, either by virtue of being employers themselves or through subsidizing private industry's costs. Using a range of plausible salaries for baby-minders and working women, and assumptions about the changes required based on International Labour Organization recommendations (for example, that women should be given 6 to 12 weeks' maternity leave) and developing-country experience, incremental salary costs for implementing these strategies were calculated.

Package of breast-feeding strategies. As was noted above, there is already a substantial literature documenting the impact on breast-feeding of changes in hospital routine, and to a lesser extent, of the education of mothers whilst in hospital (Winikoff and Baer 1980). Data are more scanty for the other options (i.e. mass media, legislation concerning breast-milk substitutes, and the provision of facilities for working women), and their effectiveness is often measured only in terms of intermediate attitudinal or behavioural variables. For these reasons, no attempt was made to derive cost-effectiveness results for each strategy, and instead a package of strategies was assessed. It was conservatively assumed that the impact of a package of breast-feeding promotional strategies was no more than the average impact on breast-feeding of the selection of individual strategies reviewed by Feachem and Koblinsky (1984). These authors explored the consequences of three hypothetical intensities of intervention and three different pre-intervention patterns of breast-feeding and diarrhoeal morbidity and mortality. The results were combined with the estimated range of costs likely to be required for the package of interventions (excluding the provision of facilities for working women because of the highly speculative nature of the costs) to derive estimates of the incremental cost per diarrhoea episode averted and cost per diarrhoea death averted.

Improved weaning practices for better nutrition

Weaning is a period of high health-risk for children, which can largely be attributed to the contamination of weaning foods (Black *et al.* 1982) and – the cause discussed in this section – inadequate nutrition (Ashworth and Feachem 1985*a*). Strategies to reduce the risk of malnutrition (and the consequent risk of mortality from diarrhoea) can be categorized broadly in terms of increased education, and increased access to food. Food-price subsidies (including the free distribution of food) are one approach employed to help improve nutrition. In practice, however, the results of supplementary feeding schemes have been disappointing (Beaton and Ghassemi 1982), and others have concluded that it is unlikely that these programmes are a cost-effective intervention for national diarrhoeal disease control programmes (Feachem 1983). For these reasons, this section focuses on measures which increase education, reflecting the assertion (admittedly controversial) that 'a major proportion of malnutrition at weaning age has been shown to be caused by ignorance, incorrect food and health beliefs and resultant poor feeding and health practices, rather than lack of basic food resources' (Zeitlin and Formacion 1981).

Although nutrition education programmes are incorporated into many nutrition projects (Austin *et al*. 1978), published evaluations are relatively rare. Evaluations which measure nutritional status as well as knowledge or behavioural changes are rarer still. To estimate the impact of education on diarrhoea mortality, nutritional data of a specific kind are necessary. The association of poor nutritional status with diarrhoea mortality has been demonstrated for moderately and severely malnourished children (i.e. 60–74 per cent weight-for-age and less than 60 per cent weight-for-age respectively) (Black *et al*. 1984; Chen *et al*. 1980). Consequently information is required on the changing proportion of children in these categories resulting from the education programme. Ashworth and Feachem (1985*a*) identify nine projects which provide data on nutritional status that are adequate to estimate the impact on diarrhoea mortality.

Only seven weaning education projects with cost estimates were located, four of them providing data on both costs and nutritional impact. It is these four projects that were studied in some detail, and for which cost-effectiveness estimates were calculated. One, in Morocco, was attached to a supplementary feeding programme (Gilmore *et al*. 1980). The other three were community-based: one in Burkina Faso (Zeitlin 1981), a second in the Philippines (Jones and Munger 1978), and the third in Indonesia (Zeitlin 1984). All four involved the face-to-face education of mothers.

The cost data presented in each of the four studies were used to derive a cost per child whose mother received education from the project. The effectiveness data from the studies (expressed originally in terms of impact on malnutrition) were converted into the expected number of diarrhoeal deaths averted (using data from Black *et al.* 1984 and Chen *et al.* 1980), and then combined with cost data to give estimates of the incremental cost per diarrhoea death averted for each of the four projects. The consequences of varying some of the key assumptions (for example, the proportion of diarrhoea deaths in under-fives benefiting from the intervention, the annual diarrhoea mortality rate per 1000 under-five-year-olds, and the different cost estimates) were explored.

None of the studies with adequate data used mass media as an educational strategy, so it was not possible to derive cost-effectiveness estimates for weaning education involving mass media. Although mass media weaning education has been demonstrated to reach a large audience and to improve knowledge, the scope for exploiting mass media to improve weaning is likely to be limited: the ideal weaning message is quite circumstance-specific (depending on the age of the child, accessible foodstuffs, and the amount of time and money available), and involves conveying skills which are more easily taught through direct face-to-face demonstration.

Handwashing

Studies of the impact of handwashing on bacterial counts (for example, de Wit and Kampelmacher 1982) and on the incidence of diarrhoea (for example, Khan 1982) confirm the potential for a reduction in diarrhoeal disease through improved personal hygiene. To estimate the cost-effectiveness of handwashing promotion, attention was focused on the few projects demonstrated to have had an impact on diarrhoea. The studies analysed consisted of: a hygiene and education programme in Guatemala directed at mothers of young children (Torun 1982); the intensive short-term education of families with an identified case of shigellosis to encourage them to wash their hands after defecation and before taking food (Khan 1982); and a programme of instruction for day-care employees to encourage them to wash their own hands and those of the children after using the toilet and changing nappies, and before handling food (Black *et al.* 1981). These published studies were used in order to develop a plausible picture of procedures and resource use, and hence of costs. These costs were combined with data on the effectiveness of these projects in reducing the incidence of diarrhoea in order to derive individual cost-effectiveness ratios for each project.

Schoolchildren are well documented as a source of diarrhoeal infection for younger siblings (Dingle *et al.* 1964), and schools do appear to be a potentially low-cost and important venue for promoting hygiene messages aimed at reducing diarrhoea in young children (see, for example, Rohde and Sadjimin 1980). While hygiene education is a common component of school syllabuses, there are unfortunately few published papers which describe either the inputs required for these programmes or their impact on knowledge or behaviour. No papers were located which measure the impact on diarrhoea incidence. One study in Colombia (Koopman 1978) provided data showing lower rates of diarrhoea in schoolchildren and their younger siblings with improved levels of hygiene in school. These data, together with estimates of the likely cost in staff time, training, and materials, were used to develop rough estimates of the incremental cost per diarrhoea episode in under-fives averted by a school education programme.

No convincing studies documenting the impact of hygiene education at health centres were located. It seems likely that, with careful planning and execution, health centre-based education could be cost-effective; but practical experience suggests that this potential remains largely untapped.

Promotion of handwashing may be particularly suited to a mass-media approach: the required behaviour is easily defined and universally relevant. Furthermore, soap is already widely advertised in the Third World, and it should be possible to capitalize on this by linking specific hygiene messages to soap promotion. However, no studies were located which describe in sufficient detail any mass-media hygiene campaign and its impact on diarrhoea or on a relevant behavioural variable, such as handwashing.

Inadequate facilities rather than a lack of information appear to be the primary determinant of poor hygiene in several documented cases (Elmendorf and Buckles 1980). If lack of access to soap or the price of soap is an obstacle to improved hygiene, governments could subsidize commercial soap production or encourage small-scale, community-based production by providing information on techniques or by subsidizing ingredients. However, descriptions of efforts to make soap more widely available and of data on the costs or effects of these efforts are absent. There are many communities where soap is available and purchased, but is used for washing clothes and periodic bathing rather than regular handwashing. Reducing the price of soap in these circumstances may simply give rise to cleaner shirts.

Cost and cost-effectiveness results

The sections below report the results of the analysis and comment on the quality of data and thus the reliability of the cost-effectiveness estimates.

Measles, rotavirus, and cholera vaccination

The average incremental costs per child vaccinated with measles, rotavirus or cholera vaccine were as follows (values in $ US):

	median	range
measles vaccine	1.30	(0.60–12.00)
rotavirus vaccine	1.90	(1.20–12.00)
cholera vaccine	3.20	(1.70–26.00)

Combining these results, first with estimates of the impact of each vaccine on diarrhoea morbidity and mortality (Feachem and Koblinsky 1983; de Zoysa and Feachem 1985*a*); and second, with assumptions concerning average diarrhoea morbidity and mortality in developing countries (for rotavirus diarrhoea and measles and, in the specific case of Bangladesh, for cholera), gives estimated effectiveness and costs per episode and per death averted as shown in Tables 9.2 and 9.3. The cost-effectiveness of measles and rotavirus vaccines in terms of diarrhoea control are of a similar order of magnitude, while the cost-effectiveness of cholera vaccine is significantly lower, even for a country such as Bangladesh where cholera rates are relatively high.

All the studies from which the above cost data were gathered employed the WHO guidelines for costing immunization programmes (WHO 1979*a*) or similar approaches which attempt both to take account of *all* the resources used in providing vaccination programmes and to value them in a consistent manner. The vaccination programmes represent a broad range of cost-influencing conditions in low- and middle-income countries: different vaccination schedules, different kinds of strategies (routine, fixed/mobile, mass campaigns), different population densities, levels of existing infrastructure, sizes of output, and cost structures. The method used to derive the incremental average costs of adding new vaccines to existing schedules employed several assumptions designed specifically to provide conservative estimates of costs. To minimize further the possibility of underestimating costs, the costs shown above were rounded up to $2 per child vaccinated with measles or rotavirus vaccine and $4 per child vaccinated against cholera. Sensitivity analysis revealed that cost-effectiveness values (and certainly their ranking) were fairly insensitive to changes in the assumptions adopted for the variables in the model.

Breast-feeding

Considerable variation in cost was found amongst the strategies for increasing breast-feeding, from several hundred dollars to less than 10 cents per mother exposed to breast-feeding promotion. However, with a judicious selection of strategies (excluding, for example, expensive mass-media campaigns in small countries) it

Table 9.2 *Diarrhoea morbidity and mortality averted through vaccinations against measles, rotavirus diarrhoea, and cholera*

Vaccine	The number of diarrhoea episodes and deaths averted per 1000 vaccinated children per year in children under 5 years of age	
	Morbidity (episodes averted)	Mortality (deaths averted)
Measles*	55.0	2.8
Rotavirus diarrhoea†	88.0	1.8
Cholera‡	4.6	0.4

* assuming 85 per cent efficacy of vaccine, and average diarrhoeal incidence found for developing countries.
† assuming 80 per cent efficacy of vaccine, and average diarrhoeal incidence found for developing countries.
‡ assuming 70 per cent efficacy of vaccine, and cholera incidence as in Bangladesh.

should be possible in many circumstances to implement a package of breast-feeding promotional strategies for between about $1.00 and $10.00 per mother exposed (not including the relatively expensive strategy of providing facilities for working women). The size of the population, access to the media, and the size of hospitals are all important factors, and will influence average incremental costs.

Putting estimates of cost per mother exposed to breast-feeding promotion of $1.00, $5.00, and $10.00 together with the effectiveness results (Feachem and Koblinsky 1984) gives the estimated costs per diarrhoea case and diarrhoea death averted shown in Table 9.4. The cost per diarrhoea case averted ranges from between $2.4, with a high-impact promotional programme costing $1.00 per mother exposed in a country with moderate levels of exclusive and partial breast-feeding and moderate rates of diarrhoea, to about $140 for a low-impact programme costing $10.00 per mother exposed in a country with relatively low levels of breast-feeding and low rates of diarrhoea. The cost per diarrhoea death averted ranges between about $100 and $10000. This wide range of potential cost-effectiveness figures is due in roughly equal measure to variations in both costs and effectiveness. Some narrowing of the range of cost-effectiveness results could be achieved by allowing for the fact that costs and effectiveness are not independent: more resources in many circumstances will mean greater effectiveness.

Table 9.3 *Cost per diarrhoea episode and diarrhoea death averted through measles, rotavirus diarrhoea, and cholera vaccinations*

Vaccine	Cost per diarrhoea episode and death averted in children under 5 years of age * ($US 1982)	
	Morbidity ($ per episode averted)	Mortality ($ per death averted)
Measles	7	143
Rotavirus diarrhoea	5	222
Cholera	174	2000

* assuming vaccine effectiveness given in Table 9.2 and costs estimated at $2 per measles and per rotavirus diarrhoea vaccination and $4 per cholera vaccination.

Table 9.4 *Cost per diarrhoea episode and diarrhoea death averted through breast-feeding promotion in children under 5 years*

Pre-intervention breast-feeding levels *	Cost per mother exposed (US$)	Cost per diarrhoea episode and diarrhoea death averted in children under 5 years by effectiveness of breast-feeding promotion †								
		Morbidity					Mortality			
		high impact	medium impact	low impact			high impact	medium impact	low impact	
A	10.00	37.0	73.0	142.9			2500	5376	10753	
	5.00	18.5	36.5	71.4			1250	2688	5376	
	1.00	3.7	7.3	14.3			250	538	1075	
B	10.00	23.6	48.8	96.2			1188	2375	4000	
	5.00	11.8	24.4	48.1			594	1188	2000	
	1.00	2.4	4.8	9.6			119	237	400	
C	10.00	26.4	60.6	106.4			874	1603	2747	
	5.00	13.2	30.3	53.2			437	801	1374	
	1.00	2.6	6.1	10.6			87	160	275	

* Breast-feeding pattern A is one of high rates of partial and no breast-feeding; pattern C has relatively high rates of exclusive breast-feeding; and pattern B is mid-way, with a substantial proportion of children partially breast-fed (see Table 3, Feachem and Koblinsky 1984).

† Using effectiveness results derived from Feachem and Koblinsky (1984).

Although those effectiveness studies with serious methodological flaws were rejected in the analysis of Feachem and Koblinsky, there are some problems with the quality of the data (for example, failure to control for confounding variables and to specify the feeding mode precisely). The almost complete lack of expenditure data or detailed input descriptions makes it difficult to know whether the relevant inputs have been accurately identified for costing purposes.

Weaning

The four weaning education projects for which both cost and suitable nutritional impact data were available were calculated to have cost-effectiveness results in the range $70 to $1700 per diarrhoea death averted (Table 9.5), with considerable potential variation for any one project depending on the assumptions adopted. The studies differed in several important respects: in their country settings (and hence their price structure), and in their scale and approaches to cost measurement (notably whether or not voluntary labour and start-up costs were included). On the effectiveness side, some studies measured impact only in terms of the immediate target group, and neglected consideration of siblings who may also benefit. Others failed to take into account the impact of other interventions which are frequently provided alongside weaning education, and which may have some potential to influence nutritional status (such as the use of growth charts, provision of ORT, and education on breast-feeding). Useful comparisons between different strategies aimed at the face-to-face education of mothers are therefore difficult. In all cases research here considered only the nutritionally-related diarrhoea consequences, and ignored any impact that weaning education might have as a result of reduced contamination of food.

Handwashing

Analysis of the three studies of hygiene education for which data on diarrhoea impact were available gives a range of cost-effectiveness estimates for hygiene education of under $20 per childhood diarrhoea case averted for village-based group education and education of employees of day-care centres; and $300–500 for face-to-face education of *Shigella* index families. Though hard evidence concerning effectiveness is lacking, a school education programme could cost less than $5 per case averted. In some circumstances a quite substantial mass-media campaign could be mounted for less than $0.50 per year per child whose mother is exposed to the mass media. The likely impact on handwashing and diarrhoea incidence of efforts to make soap more accessible is uncertain, and deserves more research: 'It is quite astonishing that so little attention has been paid to soap' (Greenough 1985).

Comparison of interventions

The ranges of cost-effectiveness results for the six interventions discussed in this chapter are presented in Table 9.6. The table also shows the estimated cost per diarrhoea death averted by ORT

Table 9.5 *Summary of cost–effectiveness calculations for four weaning education case studies*

Country	Total number of diarrhoea deaths averted in children under 5 years per 1000 benefiting children per five years * (A)	Total annual cost for nutritional education ($US1982) (B)	Number of benefiting children per year (C)	Number of years each benefiting child participates (D)	Cost per diarrhoea death averted in children under 5 years ($US 1982) (E = $\frac{B}{C} \times \frac{D}{A} \times 1000$)
Morocco	5.64	300000	300000	2.5	443
Burkina Faso	7.16	1880	5400	1.5	73
Philippines	5.63	7890	836	1.0	1676
Indonesia	5.40	63000	12000	1.2	1167

* Assuming that:
   (i) differences between controls and participants represent the impact of the weaning programme;
   (ii) children less than 75% (or 80%) weight-for-age have a two times higher diarrhoea mortality rate than other children (see Ashworth and Feachem 1985c);
   (iii) the impact of the weaning education programme is on 60% of diarrhoea deaths in the first five years of life (the average of the conservative (47%) and optimistic (74%) assumptions in Ashworth and Feachem 1985c); and
   (iv) average annual diarrhoea mortality is 14 per 1000.

Table 9.6 *Cost-effectiveness of diarrhoea prevention and other health interventions*

Intervention	Cost ($US 1982) per diarrhoea episode averted in children under 5 years of age ( ) = (median)	Cost ($US 1982) per death averted in children under 5 years of age * ( ) = (median)
Measles vaccination	3–60 (10)	70–1160 (140)
Rotavirus vaccination	3–30 (10)	140–1400 (220)
Cholera vaccination (in Bangladesh)	90–1450 (170)	1070–16710 (2000)
Breast-feeding promotion	3–140 (20)	90–10750 (1190)
Improved weaning practices (nutrition aspects)	—	70–1700 (800)
Hygiene promotion	5–500 (10)	N/A
ORT	—	100–8000 † (220)
Other health programmes in developing countries	N/A	100–12000 ‡ (2000)

* For all the interventions except 'other health programmes' this refers to death from diarrhoea.

† Based on data from 13 projects summarised in Shepard and Brenzel (1985) and converted in $US 1982 assuming an inflation rate of 10%.

‡ Cost per infant death averted. Based on data summarised in Walsh and Warren (1979) and Cochrane and Zachariah (1983) and converted to $US 1982 assuming an inflation rate of 10%.

N/A = Not available.

programmes and the estimated cost per infant death averted by a variety of other health interventions. The results indicate that none of the diarrhoea interventions can, on present evidence, be dismissed as clearly inefficient approaches to reducing childhood mortality. None, except for cholera vaccination, have upper estimates of cost per death averted that are higher than for some ORT or other health interventions, and the median results for both measles and rotavirus vaccination lie below that for ORT. Furthermore, several of the six interventions (for instance measles vaccination and breast-feeding promotion) reduce mortality from causes other than diarrhoea. If this were taken into account it would reduce the estimates of cost per child death averted, an important point which is discussed further below.

With the exception of weaning education designed to reduce weaning-age malnutrition, the six interventions also play a role in reducing diarrhoea morbidity. Measles and rotavirus vaccination and breast-feeding and hygiene promotion can all be implemented for probably less than $50 per diarrhoea episode averted.

While measles and rotavirus vaccination both appear to be particularly promising, the results do not suggest that any one intervention is unambiguously superior to the others in terms of its efficiency in reducing either diarrhoea episodes or deaths. The ranges of results overlap, and the number of observations from which the averages are derived is generally too small for confident generalizations.

Factors influencing cost-effectiveness ratios

The results of this study to assess the cost-effectiveness of alternative strategies for diarrhoeal disease control reveals the importance of local circumstances in determining relative efficiency, and the difficulty – in the light of present knowledge – of making universal recommendations. A framework for exploring those factors likely to influence cost-effectiveness is presented here. This is followed in the next section by a discussion of some of the parameters of decision-making not explicitly addressed by comparisons of cost per diarrhoea episode or death averted: population coverage, health impacts other than diarrhoea, and equity in the distribution of costs and benefits.

Some of the variation in cost-effectiveness estimates for any given intervention may be due to inaccuracies in the data. Methodological problems in measuring both impact (for example, a failure to take account of confounding factors), and costs (for example, a failure to specify resource requirements accurately) may give rise to spurious differences in cost-effectiveness between individual projects. Some of the variation – at least for those interventions whose costs are based on actual resource use – may reflect differences between countries in the price of inputs relative to the official exchange-rate.

However, much of the observed variation in cost-effectiveness can probably be attributed to real differences in efficiency, and not simply to data inconsistencies or to price differentials. It is important to understand these sources of variation in order to predict which interventions or strategies are likely to be appropriate in a given country, and to design cost-effective strategies accordingly. Unfortunately, the data are woefully inadequate for such modelling of the relationships between cost-effectiveness results and most key variables, although the relationships can be discussed in general terms. Broadly, the factors underlying difference in cost-effectiveness for a particular intervention can be categorized as:

- the characteristics of the educational and health targets;

- the characteristics of the existing infrastructure;

- technical features of the intervention itself;

- the scale of the intervention; and

- the mix of interventions (i.e. the combined production function).

Target characteristics

The prevalence of risk factors such as the failure of mothers to breast-feed or to wash hands, poor nutritional status, and the incidence of measles, rotavirus, or cholera in children, may be important in deciding what type of intervention would be the most efficient in preventing diarrhoea in any particular country or location. Some risk factors do not appear to show much variation (for example, measles and rotavirus prevalence), while others (for example, cholera prevalence, breast-feeding rates) do show significant variation, although this is not always captured in the estimates.

For example, cholera vaccination is likely to be considerably less cost-effective in most countries than the estimates here, based on the particular case of Bangladesh, suggest. In the analysis of weaning education, the examples explored had pre-intervention malnutrition levels of around 35 per cent. One report suggested that the proportion of malnourished children can be as high as 50 per cent (INCS 1981). Where this is the case, the estimated impact on diarrhoea mortality would be some 30 per cent higher than our estimates (all other things being equal).

Prevalence of a risk factor is not the only characteristic of the target population likely to influence cost-effectiveness: accessibility and responsiveness of the target to the intervention, and the strength of the association between the risk factor and diarrhoeal disease, are also important, and indeed have led to a focus on mothers as the primary target of most educational strategies. Care should be taken, however, in using these criteria to be even more selective in targeting these interventions. Firstly, the criteria are not always unrelated, and may be negatively correlated. For example, populations which are least accessible may well be populations with a higher incidence of the risk factor and of diarrhoea mortality. Secondly, identifying high-risk groups and targeting messages at them can be costly. For example, to deal with families of *Shigella* cases selectively and effectively required a rapid marshalling of educational resources and intensive small-group education, both of which have significant cost implications (Khan 1982). Thirdly, there is considerable scope with some interventions for adapting educational messages and approaches to the specific circumstances of the particular population. This may be a more efficient approach than selecting populations on the basis of their likely responsiveness to recommendations on some 'ideal' behaviour.

Infrastructure characteristics

The characteristics of the existing infrastructure may have an important influence on cost-effectiveness for two reasons. Firstly, the existence of other activities may reinforce or moderate the impact of a programme. For example, weaning education may be particularly successful when attached to supplementary feeding programmes. Secondly, the more resources that are already in place and can be deployed, the cheaper it will be to mount any new programme. For example, it might be possible to build on existing systems of outreach (for example, agricultural extension workers) to convey educational messages concerning weaning.

Intervention characteristics

Technical aspects of the design of a strategy clearly have important implications for cost-effectiveness. The impact of education, for example, is influenced by the choice of media, message design and content, location and timing of sessions, and incentives for teachers to teach and teach well, and for educational targets to attend, learn, and act. Some consensus is now emerging as to the characteristics of educational activities that appear to be particularly important determinants of effectiveness (see Hornik 1985; Manoff 1985; and Gatherer *et al.* 1979). However, there have been few attempts to consider such issues in relation to budgetary constraints. In many instances, effectiveness and costs move in the same direction: for example, the longer the exposure to messages or the better designed the messages (and the more background research done), the more effective and the more costly is the strategy. Without data which describe the nature of this relationship it is impossible to determine the optimum levels of investment.

Scale

Scale can be an important determinant of cost-effectiveness for some interventions. Strategies involving mass media, for example, require a high initial investment but carry comparatively little extra cost for each additional person exposed to the message: cost-effectiveness is consequently likely to increase with the size of the population exposed. Vaccination programmes also exhibit such increasing returns to scale (Creese *et al.* 1982), though there are good reasons for expecting that beyond a certain point the costs of reaching the more remote communities or less willing individuals would reverse this pattern (Over 1986).

Because the cost-effectiveness of any one strategy and the priority ordering of strategies with respect to cost-effectiveness can change with size, the choice between different interventions or strategies may well depend on coverage objectives or budgetary constraints. For example, if limited funds are available, the most cost-effective option for reducing diarrhoea may well be to promote changes in hospital routine for women giving birth. This requires relatively little investment in order to achieve good results. The same small investment devoted to, say, a mass-media campaign may, in contrast, be largely wasted, absorbed by central administration or preliminary research, with few funds remaining for implementation. A larger budget could make mass media a more competitive option. Where the total budget for diarrhoea prevention is fixed, assessment of efficiency must take into account the cost-effectiveness of the investment of all the funds. For example if the preferred option is changing hospital routine, but this only uses up half the allocated budget, it will be necessary to assess the cost-effectiveness of alternative uses of the remaining funds.

Combinations of interventions

This chapter has focused on separate interventions, exploring their likely cost-effectiveness as independent activities. In practice, the range of potential options also includes various combinations of interventions. There has been little research devoted to investigating their impact; but there are some clues which help to predict the likely consequences of joint implementation. There are three levels at which interactions between interventions may occur.

Firstly, there may be cost savings associated with joint provision. For example, delivering more than one educational message at any one contact with the target may have important cost-saving implications, particularly for face-to-face education. Secondly, the impact of an intervention on the risk factor through which it changes diarrhoea incidence may be influenced by the presence of other interventions. For example, educational campaigns which incorporate related messages in a package (for example, breast-feeding and weaning) may be more successful than the evidence from separate campaigns would suggest.

A third possibility, and one for which there is somewhat more evidence, is that the strength of the association between the risk factor and diarrhoea incidence may be altered by combining interventions. For example, interventions targeted at the same age-group or diarrhoea aetiology may not be additive in their effects. There is some evidence that breast-feeding protects against rotavirus (see, for example, Chrystie *et al.* 1978), cholera (Gunn *et al.* 1979), and *Shigella* (Stoll *et al.* 1982), suggesting that the impact of the combination of breast-feeding promotion with either rotavirus, cholera, or measles vaccination may be less than additive. However, the major impact on diarrhoea of any given increase in breast-feeding rates is on infants under 6 months, with no evidence of any effect beyond 12 months (Feachem and Koblinsky 1984). The scope for overlap is therefore limited if rotavirus vaccine is given at 6 months, measles vaccine at 9 months, and cholera vaccine in the second year. For most other combinations of interventions (except those involving hygiene education) the aetiologies of the diarrhoea prevented and the age-group affected suggest that there is unlikely to be major overlap, and that the impact of these interventions would be additive.

ORT is already a well-established approach to diarrhoea control, and the task of decision-makers is likely to be one of determining which interventions best complement ORT. With the exception of weaning education restricted to improving nutrition, all the interventions are potentially effective in preventing diarrhoea morbidity – an advantage ORT does not share to any significant degree. ORT is largely ineffective in averting deaths from dysenteric or chronic diarrhoeas. Interventions such as measles vaccination, breast-feeding promotion, and hygiene education, which appear to be effective against dysenteric or chronic diarrhoeas, are therefore particularly attractive.

The limits to cost-effectiveness analysis

Cost-effectiveness analysis is a useful tool for exploring the efficiency of resource-allocation patterns. It has, however, a number of limitations in its scope, three of which are of particular relevance here. They relate to (i) the potential population coverage of different strategies; (ii) the significance of costs and benefits other than those relating to diarrhoea; and (iii) the distribution of costs and benefits between individuals and groups.

Population coverage

High coverage is likely to be an important objective for most diarrhoeal disease-control activities. It is therefore useful to recognize the natural boundaries to the coverage that can be achieved with a particular strategy; boundaries delineated by the proportion of children that could potentially be affected if the strategy were fully exploited.

Community-based activities can in theory be targeted at the whole population. Most other strategies are more circumscribed: strategies relying on health facilities, for example, will in general reach only those mothers who utilize these facilities – a high proportion of women in some countries such as China, The Gambia, and Vietnam, but very low, for instance, in Honduras and Nigeria. Hospital-based activities for breast-feeding promotion are unlikely to have much impact beyond those mothers hospitalized for childbirth – a relatively high proportion in a number of Latin American and Caribbean countries, but low in many Asian and African countries (WHO 1979*b*). Only women in the formal sector will be affected by legislation concerning conditions for working women. A primary school education programme has the potential to affect indirectly a considerable proportion of young children: demographic patterns suggest that over 50 per cent of under-five-year-olds will have primary-school-age siblings in most developing countries, and primary school enrolment averages between 60 per cent and 80 per cent (UNESCO 1984). Access to mass media is variable – highest in Latin America (on average 324 licensed radio receivers per 1000 population) and lowest in Asia (UNESCO 1984).

Other costs and benefits

If optimal resource-allocation is to be achieved, it is important that all the ramifications of an intervention should be taken into account. It is possible to measure different outcomes in different units, and leave the decision-makers to make the necessary trade-offs using the disaggregated data. The danger with this approach is that the complexity of the process may obscure the nature of implicit value judgements adopted. Cost-effectiveness analysis is a technique which is most readily applied when a single indicator is used to measure outcome.

Finding a single indicator which captures the main dimensions of the effects of health interventions is, however, not easy. Measures such as infant mortality rate, life expectancy, or nutritional status, which are sometimes used as proxies for general health status, are generally both insufficiently sensitive to specific interventions and insufficiently broad. Other approaches, such as composite indices or weighted scores of health characteristics, for instance 'quality-adjusted life years' and 'healthy days of life lost' (Ghana Health Assessment Project Team 1981), provide broader measures of health status or impact, but make substantial data demands, and embody important (and debatable) assumptions about the equivalence of a year of illness or death at any age (Barnum 1986). The translation of outcomes into money terms would be a useful way of facilitating comparisons between programmes. However, the one aspect that can most feasibly be measured in financial terms, savings in treatment costs, provides only a partial measure of outcome, and one which is highly dependent on the nature of the existing distribution of services.

The unit chosen here, 'provider cost per diarrhoea episode or diarrhoea death averted', fails to capture some important dimensions of the interventions discussed. This is not necessarily a problem unless the alternative strategies differ in the scale and scope of these 'uncaptured' costs and benefits. Unfortunately they do. Some of the differences are noted below.

'Quality' of diarrhoea events. Diarrhoea episodes are not all alike. Cholera and rotavirus diarrhoeas, for example, appear to be of above-average severity (de Zoysa and Feachem 1985*a*), and measles-associated diarrhoeas have been found to be of significantly longer duration than other diarrhoeas (Koster *et al.* 1981). The age-distribution of diarrhoea prevention varies among interventions: the diarrhoeas prevented through a breast-feeding campaign are likely, on average, to be in a younger age-group than for most other interventions. This may have health consequences, since there is evidence that the younger the infant, the more serious the long-term consequences of an episode of diarrhoea of any given immediate severity.

Even mortality measures may not be truly comparable. Firstly, the age-distribution of diarrhoea deaths prevented is different for the interventions. This could be significant for two reasons; the value placed on the life saved may depend either on the age at death itself (are four-year-olds valued more than four-month-olds?), or on the length of life saved by the average under-five death prevented. For example, it has been suggested that measles-associated diarrhoea selectively kills the weakest, whose chances of survival, even if they avoid measles, are low (O'Donovan

1971). Secondly, quality of life expectancy may differ between the interventions for reasons other than those related to age.

The interventions are also different in their impact on diarrhoea mortality and morbidity in the over-five group, both the target group themselves as they grow older, and children who are already over five when the intervention takes place. Weaning and breast-feeding promotion and rotavirus and measles vaccination will have little or no impact on diarrhoea in those over five years of age. Cholera vaccinations and hygiene education, on the other hand, may have a significant impact on diarrhoea in older age-groups – an added bonus not captured by the measures of effectiveness used here.

Non-diarrhoea effects. The interventions differ, too, in their impact on health variables apart from diarrhoea. Some of the interventions are quite specifically targeted at diarrhoea (for example, rotavirus and cholera vaccinations). Others have broader health effects: hygiene education on skin disease, hepatitis A, and intestinal worms; measles vaccination on measles and on complications of measles other than diarrhoea; and breast-feeding on morbidity and mortality from a range of causes (Winikoff and Baer 1980) and on child-spacing (Population Reports 1981). In some cases there are negative health consequences: vaccinations can cause fever or local reactions, and sometimes more serious complications (for example, encephalitis and encephalopathy in the case of measles vaccine: Willems and Sanders 1981).

Privately-incurred costs. Individuals as well as implementing agencies bear costs that are not taken into account in the cost measure used here. Mothers may incur costs in time and travel to attend educational or vaccination sessions, or in the form of batteries to operate radios. The behaviours that the interventions promote frequently imply further costs: forfeited wages or time and fees for vaccination, purchase of soap and perhaps water for handwashing, and purchase of more, or more expensive, weaning foods and time to prepare them. It is difficult to generalize about the relative significance of private costs among the different interventions: the magnitude of private costs for any given intervention will be highly dependent on the form in which the interventions are provided and current practices. For example, the private costs associated with vaccination may well depend on whether mobile or fixed facilities are provided. And the private costs of improved weaning will depend on how much change is required in weaning practices. Private costs are seldom measured, though it is clear from some studies (such as that by Zeitlin (1981) on weaning foods) that they can be substantial.

In some cases there can be financial savings for individuals, such as those associated with breast-feeding: the total cost for proper feeding with breast-milk substitutes has been estimated to be of the order of $US 200–300 for the first year of life (Population Reports 1981). Furthermore, bottle-feeding can be more time-consuming (Greiner *et al.* 1979). On the other hand this has to be set against the lost work opportunities that breast-feeding women may face, and their extra nutritional requirements.

Other costs. In some cases it is extremely difficult to predict the ramifications of interventions and the incidence of costs and benefits, particularly for those interventions involving legislation. For example, legislation against breast-milk substitutes imposes costs on manufacturers, with the loss of lucrative markets or the imposition of penalties for breaking the law. If these costs are substantial, and the manufacturers influential, governments may be taking political risks in implementing legislation. Industries asked to shoulder the costs of facilitating breast-feeding by working women may well shift some of these costs to women. In Malaysia, it has been reported that women in the electronics industry were required to resign on marriage, so that the firm could avoid payment of the maternity benefits required by law (Lim 1978).

Equity

Even if it were possible to identify a suitable effectiveness measure to encapsulate all the consequences of the various strategies, cost-effectiveness results are not in themselves sufficient to guide decision-making. For one thing, the results say nothing about the distribution of the costs and benefits within society. The most cost-effective option may be a programme in a more accessible geographical area which disproportionately benefits the better-off. In a country with a policy of favouring the poor (and most countries pay at least lip-service to the notion of equity) there may be good reasons for choosing a less cost-effective but more equitable programme.

To some extent, equity objectives can be served at the same time as efficiency goals are met: the incidence of diarrhoea and of risk factors associated with diarrhoea (two important determinants of cost-effectiveness) are both likely to be negatively correlated with income. For example, less wealthy people are likely to have a higher incidence of poor hygiene and malnutrition. There are instances, however, where the prevalence of risky behaviour and income levels are positively correlated. For example, in some countries bottle-feeding, a risk factor for diarrhoea in any setting, is more common in upper income groups. There are other factors also which may work against the tendency for efficiency and equity goals to be realized by the same programme: poorer people may be less likely to own radios, to have hospital births, and to attend health education sessions; and, consequently, may be more costly to reach.

Conclusions

The analysis in this chapter leads to conclusions at three different levels: it has identified some strategies for diarrhoeal disease control which appear to be worth promoting, it has highlighted areas for further research, and it has elaborated on the difficulties of using cost-effectiveness analysis as a tool for guiding decision-making in this field.

The inadequacy of many of the data and the considerable variation that exists between the regions and countries of the world makes for difficulty in proposing global priorities for action in diarrhoea control. There are a few specific strategies, however, which appear to be strong candidates for implementation in most countries: changing hospital routine to encourage breast-feeding by mothers hospitalized for delivery; incorporating measles vaccine (and possibly, in the future, rotavirus vaccine) into ongoing vaccination programmes and devoting resources to improving vaccination take-up, particularly in geographical areas already served by the programme; and linking hygiene-promotion activities to commercial efforts to sell soap. Education concerning breast-feeding, improved weaning practices, and hygiene has considerable potential for reducing diarrhoea; but the exact form the education should take is unclear, and will probably vary greatly, depending on particular country circumstances.

Recommendations for research are rather easier to make. The analysis in this chapter reveals substantial gaps in knowledge concerning the cost-effectiveness of alternative ways of controlling diarrhoeal diseases. These exist for both cost and effectiveness, and for all interventions discussed. More cost data based on actual experience, particularly in developing countries, are required for all interventions. Researchers investigating the impact of interventions on diarrhoea or associated risk factors should supplement their epidemiological research with cost studies. Educational strategies, particularly for hygiene, and combinations of different interventions are two areas which require special attention.

Before deciding on priorities for diarrhoeal disease control it is clearly desirable to be aware of the potential effectiveness and costs of the alternatives. How broadly one defines effectiveness can be crucial. Choices based solely on criteria such as cost per diarrhoea death or episode averted are not necessarily efficient choices for society when the alternatives differ dramatically in the scale and nature of other effects. Nevertheless, for those concerned primarily with diarrhoeal disease control this information can provide a useful basis for collaboration and negotiation: for example, identifying how much diarrhoeal disease-control programme-managers should be prepared to contribute to interventions partially justified on other grounds.

The limitations of global analyses are even more acute. There are dangers in making crude comparisons of different interventions which are implemented in different countries. It is important, though difficult, to sort out how much of the difference in cost-effectiveness is due to the nature of the interventions and how much is particular to the circumstances of the countries (prices, population distribution, existing infrastructure). Analysing the average of results for a particular intervention and comparing it with the average for other interventions can be misleading when so many factors vary. Ranges of results, while more comprehensive, can mask the significance of differences between interventions where these ranges are large and overlapping. A series of country-based comparisons is needed to determine whether there is a pattern which indicates which interventions are consistently most cost-effective. These studies should clearly spell out the conditions that pertain, so that their relevance elsewhere can be judged.

References

Ashworth, A. and Feachem, R. G. (1985*a*). Interventions for the control of diarrhoea among young children: weaning education. *Bulletin of the World Health Organization*, **63**(6), 1115–27.

Ashworth, A. and Feachem, R. G. (1985*b*). Interventions for the control of diarrhoea among young children: prevention of low birth weight. *Bulletin of the World Health Organization*, **63**(1), 165–84.

Ashworth, A. and Feachem, R. G. (1985*c*). *Interventions for the control of diarrhoea among young children: improving lactation*, Document CDD/85.2. WHO, Geneva.

Ashworth, A. and Feachem, R. G. (1986). *Interventions for the control of diarrhoea among young children: growth monitoring programmes*, Document CDD/86.1. WHO, Geneva.

Austin, J. E., Mahin, M., Pyle, D., and Zeitlin, M. (1978). *Annotated directory of nutrition programmes in developing countries*. Harvard Institute for International Development, Cambridge, Mass.

Baer, E. C. (1981). Promoting breast-feeding: a national responsibility. *Studies in Family Planning*, **12** (4), 198–206.

Barnum, H. (1986). *Evaluating healthy days of life gained from health projects*. Paper prepared for the Scientific Working Group on Epidemiology and Social and Economic Research: Informal Consultation on Cost-Effectiveness Analysis of Health Interventions in Developing Countries. World Health Organization, Geneva, July 21–24. [Mimeo].

Beaton, G. H. and Ghassemi, H. (1982). Supplementary feeding programme for young children in developing countries. *American Journal of Clinical Nutrition*, **35** (4, supplement), 863–914.

Black, R. E., Dykes, A. C., Anderson, K. E., Wells, J. G., Sinclair, S. P., Gary, G. W., *et al.* (1981). Handwashing to prevent diarrhoea in day-care centres. *American Journal of Epidemiology*, **113**, 445–51.

Black, R., Brown, K. H., Becker, S., Alim, A. R. M. A., and Merson, M. (1982). Contamination of weaning foods and transmission of enterotoxigenic *Escherichia coli* diarrhoea in children in rural Bangladesh. *Transactions of the Royal Society of Tropical Medicine and Hygiene*, **76**, 259–64.

Black, R. E., Brown, K. H., and Becker, S. (1984). Malnutrition is a determining factor in diarrhoeal duration, but not incidence, among young children in a longitudinal study in rural Bangladesh. *American Journal of Clinical Nutrition*, **39**, 87–94.

Chen, L. C., Chowdhury, A., and Huffman, S. L. (1980). Anthropometric assessment of energy-protein malnutrition and subsequent risk of malnutrition among pre-school aged children. *American Journal of Clinical Nutrition*, **33**(8), 1836–45.

Chrystie, I. L., Totterdell, B. M., and Banatvala, J.E. (1978). Asymptomatic endemic rotavirus infections in the newborn. *Lancet*, **i**, 1176–8.

Cochrane, S. H. and Zachariah, K. C. (1983). *Infant mortality as a determinant of fertility: the policy implications*, World Bank Staff Working Paper No. 556. The Bank, Washington, DC.

Creese, A. L., Sriyabbaya, N., Casabal, G., and Wiseso, G. (1982). Cost-effectiveness appraisal of immunization programmes. *Bulletin of the World Health Organization*, **60**(4), 621–32.

de Wit, J. C. and Kampelmacher, E. H. (1982). Microbiological aspects of washing hands in slaughterhouses. *Zentralblatt für Bakteriologie und Hygiene*, I Abt. Orig. B., **176**(5/6), 553–61.

de Zoysa, I. F. and Feachem, R. G. (1985a). Interventions for the control of diarrhoeal diseases among young children: rotavirus and cholera immunisation. *Bulletin of the World Health Organization*, **63**(3), 569–83.

de Zoysa, I. F. and Feachem, R. G. (1985b). Interventions for the control of diarrhoeal disease among young children: chemoprophylaxis. *Bulletin of the World Health Organization*, **63**(2), 295–315.

Dingle, J. H., Badger, G. F., and Jordan, W. S. (1964). *Illness in the home*. Press of Case Western Reserve, Cleveland, Ohio.

Durongdej, S. and Israel, R. C. (1986). Using educational strategies to promote breast-feeding: a case study of Thailand. In *Using communications to solve nutrition problems: a compendium* (ed. C. Hollis). International Nutrition Communication Service, Newton, Mass.

Elmendorf, M. and Buckles, P. (1980). *Sociocultural aspects of water supply and excreta disposal*. The World Bank, Washington, DC.

Esrey, S. A. (1991). Interventions for the control of diarrhoeal diseases among young children: fly control. Unpublished document WHO/CDD/91.37. WHO, Geneva.

Esrey, S. A. and Feachem R. G. (1989). Interventions for the control of diarrhoeal diseases among young children: food hygiene. Unpublished document WHO/CDD/89.30. WHO, Geneva.

Esrey, S. A., Feachem, R. G., and Hughes, J. M. (1985). Interventions for the control of diarrhoeal diseases among young children: improving water supplies and excreta disposal facilities. *Bulletin of the World Health Organization*, **63** (4), 757–72.

Feachem, R. G. (1983). Interventions for the control of diarrhoeal disease among young children: supplementary feeding programme. *Bulletin of the World Health Organization*, **61**(6), 967–79.

Feachem, R. G. (1984). Interventions for the control of diarrhoeal disease among young children: promotion of personal and domestic hygiene. *Bulletin of the World Health Organization*, **62**(3), 467–76.

Feachem, R. G. (1986). Preventing diarrhoea: what are the policy options? *Health Policy and Planning*, **1**(2), 109–17.

Feachem, R. G. (1987). Vitamin A deficiency and diarrhoea: a review of inter-relationships and their implications for the control of xerophthalmia and diarrhoea. *Tropical Diseases Bulletin*, **84**(3), R1–R16.

Feachem, R. G. and Koblinsky, M. A. (1983). Interventions for the control of diarrhoeal diseases among young children: measles immunization. *Bulletin of the World Health Organization*, **61**(4), 641–52.

Feachem, R. G. and Koblinsky, M. A. (1984). Interventions for the control of diarrhoeal diseases among young children: promotion of breast-feeding. *Bulletin of the World Health Organization*, **62**(2), 271–91.

Feachem, R. G., Hogan, R. C., and Merson, M. H. (1983). Diarrhoeal disease control: reviews of potential interventions. *Bulletin of the World Health Organization*, **61**(4), 637–40.

Gatherer, A., Parfit, J., Porter, E., and Vessey, M. (1979). *Is health education effective? Abstracts, bibliography and overview of evaluated studies*. The Health Education Council, London.

Ghana Health Assessment Project Team (1981). A quantitative method of assessing the health impact of different diseases in less developed countries. *International Journal of Epidemiology*, **10**(1), 73–80.

Gilmore, J., Adelman, C., Meyer, A., and Thorne, M. (1980). *Morocco: food aid and nutrition education*, Project Impact Evaluation No. 8. US Agency for International Development, Washington, DC.

Greenough, W. B. (1985). Specific public health measures. In *Good health at low cost. Proceedings of a conference held at Bellagio Conference Centre, Bellagio, Italy, April 29–May 3*. Rockefeller Foundation, New York.

Greiner, T., Almroth, S., and Latham, M. C. (1979). *The economic value of breast-feeding (with results from research conducted in Ghana and the Ivory Coast)*. Programme on International Nutrition, Cornell University, Ithaca, New York.

Gunn, R. A., Kimball, A. M., Pollard, R. A., Feeley, J. C., Feldman, R. A., Dutta, S. R., et al. (1979). Bottle-feeding as a risk factor for cholera in infants. *Lancet*, **ii**, 730–2.

Hales, D. J. (1981). Promoting breast-feeding: strategies for changing hospital policy. *Studies in Family Planning*, **12**, 157–72.

Hornik, R. C. (1985). *Nutrition education: a state of the art review*, ACC/SCN Nutrition Policy Discussion Paper No. 1. United Nations, New York.

INCS (International Nutrition Communication Service) (1981). *Maternal and infant nutrition reviews: a guide to the literature* (ed. R. Israel et al.) INCS, Newton, Mass.

Jones, E. M. and Munger, S. T. (1978). *Applications of a field guide for evaluation of nutrition education programmes in the Philippines*. Agency for International Development, Washington, DC.

Khan, M. U. (1982). Interruption of shigellosis by hand-washing. *Transactions of the Royal Society of Tropical Medicine and Hygiene*, **76**, 164–8.

Koopman, J. S. (1978). Diarrhoea and school toilet hygiene in Cali, Colombia. *American Journal of Epidemiology*, **107**(5), 412–20.

Koster, F. T., Curlin, G. C., Aziz, K. M. A., and Hague, A. (1981). Synergistic impact of measles on nutrition and mortality in Bangladesh. *Bulletin of the World Health Organization*, **59**(6), 901–8.

Lim, L. (1978). *Women workers in multinational corporations: the case of the electronics industry in Malaysia and Singapore*, Occasional Papers in Women's Studies, 9. University of Michigan, Michigan, USA.

Manoff, R. K. (1985). *Social marketing: new imperative for public health*. Praeger, New York

O'Donovan, C. (1971). Measles in Kenyan children. *East African Medical Journal*, **48**, 526–33.

Over, M. (1986). The effect of scale on cost projections for a primary health care programme in a developing country. *Social Science and Medicine*, **22**, 351–61.

Phillips, M. A., Feachem, R. G. and Mills, A. (1987). *Options for diarrhoeal disease control: the cost and cost-effectiveness of selected interventions for the prevention of diarrhoea*, EPC Publication No. 13. Evaluation and Planning Centre, London School of Hygiene and Tropical Medicine.

Population Reports (1981). *Breast-feeding, fertility and family planning*, Population Report No 24, November-December. Washington University Medical Centre, Washington D. C.

Rohde, J. E. and Sadjimin, T. (1980). Elementary school pupils as health educators: role of school health programmes in primary health care. *Lancet*, **i**, 1350–2.

Shepard, D. S. and Brenzel, L. E. (1985). *Cost-effectiveness of the mass media and health practices project*. A Report from Stanford University to USAID prepared by Applied Communication Technology. Stanford University, Palo Alto.

Smart, J. L. and Bamford, F. N. (1976). Breast-feeding: 'spontaneous' trends and differences. *Lancet*, **ii**, 42.

Snyder, J. D. and Merson, M. H. (1982). The magnitude of the global problem of acute diarrhoeal disease: a review of active surveillance data. *Bulletin of the World Health Organization*, **60**(4), 605–13.

Stoll, B. J., Glass, R. I., Huq, M. I., Khan, M. V., Banu, H., and Holt, J. (1982). Epidemiologic and clinical features of patients infected with *Shigella* who attended a diarrhoeal diseases hospital in Bangladesh. *Journal of Infectious Diseases*, **146**, 177–83.

Torun, C. (1982). Environmental and educational interventions against diarrhoea in Guatemala. In *Diarrhoea and malnutrition: interactions, mechanisms and interventions* (ed. L. C. Chen and N. S. Scrimshaw), pp. 235–66. Plenum Press, New York.

UNESCO (United Nations Educational, Scientific and Cultural Organization) (1984). *1984 statistical year book*. UNESCO, Paris.

Walsh, J. A. and Warren, K. S. (1979). An interim strategy for disease control in developing countries. *The New England Journal of Medicine*, **301**(18), 967–74.

WHO (World Health Organization) (1979*a*). *Expanded programme on immunisation: costing guidelines*, EPI/GEN/79/5. WHO, Geneva.

WHO (World Health Organization) (1979*b*). *Coverage of maternity care: a tabulation of available information*. WHO, Geneva.

Willems, J. S. and Sanders, C. R. (1981). Cost-effectiveness and cost-benefit analyses of vaccines. *Journal of Infectious Diseases*, **144**(5), 486–93.

Winikoff, B. and Baer, E. C. (1980). The obstetricians' opportunity: translating 'breast is best' from theory to practice. *American Journal of Obstetrics and Gynecology*, **138**, 105–17.

Zeitlin, M. F. (1981). Upper Volta case study of home-based community level weaning food development. In *Nutrition intervention in developing countries. Studies IV. Formulated foods* (ed. J. Heimendinger), pp. 79–165. Oelgeshlager, Gunn and Hain, Cambridge, Mass.

Zeitlin, M. F. (1984). *Indonesia Nutrition Development Programme. Volume IV, Household evaluation. Nutrition communication and behaviour change component.* Report by Manoff International Inc. to Department of Health, Republic of Indonesia, June.

Zeitlin, M. F. and Formacion, C. S. (1981). *Study II: Nutrition education.* Prepared for the Office of Nutrition Development Support Bureau, US Agency for International Development, Washington, DC.

Author's note

This paper is drawn from research, funded by the Diarrhoeal Diseases Control Programme, WHO, which benefited from the contributions of a number of individuals, including J. S. Akin, A. Creese, R. Feachem, D. Helitzer-Allen, R. Hogan, M. Merson, A. Mills, F. Orivel, D. Shepard, and B. Winikoff.

10

The determinants of hospital costs: an analysis of Ethiopia

Ricardo Bitran-Dicowsky and David W. Dunlop

Introduction

The problem of financing health care in poor countries has become increasingly acute since Alma Ata. In the context of health financing, hospitals are viewed with scepticism as facilities which are not cost-effective in the provision of primary health-care services. Given this view, some analysts suggest that such institutions should become financially independent from government subsidies, and find other ways to finance both their recurrent and capital costs.

In order to ensure that scarce resources are used to best effect and to develop a financing strategy package which will help to cover all or some of the costs involved in operating such institutions, it is necessary to know how hospital costs are influenced by output levels and other variables. This chapter analyses the determinants of hospital costs in a poor country, namely Ethiopia. To the best of our knowledge, this case study and analysis was the first to explicitly address the issue of economies of scale and scope in the delivery of hospital-based health-care services in a poor country. This chapter also attempts to ascertain whether an improved policy insight can be obtained in the process, particularly with respect to the development of a financing strategy.

A translog-like cost function specification similar to the one employed by Grannemann *et al.* (1986) was used in the analysis. This specification enables an explicit determination of the marginal expenditure of care, given the structure of output and other factors, such as input prices, that might affect the structure of expenditures. Thus the specification provides a more theoretically appropriate framework of analysis than that of the overworked 'unit cost' approach (see below).

The analytical approach followed in this paper recognizes that hospitals in all countries are multi-product firms. As such, they produce a number of different types of both in- and outpatient curative services, such as surgery, laboratory examinations, and X-rays, and of preventive care, such as family planning, maternal and child health, and immunizations. The empirical specification of this production process allows for output heterogeneity, and thereby permits an analysis of whether there are efficiency advantages to be derived from producing these services individually or jointly, i.e. whether economies of scale and scope exist.

The following sections describe the cost-function model used in this analysis; define all the dependent and independent variables; describe the data; discuss the methodological approaches taken to address the econometric problems encountered in the empirical estimation; and present the empirical results of the analysis of the determinants of total hospital cost in Ethiopia. The results from several analyses are shown: the determinants of total costs; the marginal and average incremental costs of providing health services; and an analysis of economies of scale and scope. The implications of the empirical results for financing and other policy issues in Ethiopian hospitals are explored in the concluding section.

Models of hospital costs

This chapter draws its theoretical framework from a recent set of papers by Cowing and Holtmann (1983), Conrad and Strauss (1983) and Grannemann *et al.* (1986), in which a translog-like cost specification is employed. The approach represents a departure from the previous analyses of hospital costs built upon the work of Martin Feldstein (1967), the Lave's (1970 and 1972), Rafferty (1972), and Bays (1979), which specified the dependent variable in terms of the average cost or 'unit cost' of a hospital inpatient day and/or stay, and employed a set of independent variables thought to determine or be correlated with average cost. There are several disadvantages of the Feldstein and Lave approach to hospital cost analysis. These include: the use of a single output measure for a multi-product firm; the problem of including output as the dependent variable (in the denominator) and as an independent variable; and the lack of underlying economic rationale for the inclusion of certain independent variables in the cost function.

The econometric analysis employed in this chapter assumes that total hospital costs are an exponential function of: input prices (the

'P variables'); output types and volume (the 'Y and Z variables'); and other factors assumed to be determinants of fixed costs (the 'X variables'). The marginal cost of each of the output vector (Y) variables can be computed, given the level of the other set of X, P, and Z variables included in the analysis. This functional form of the cost function is homothetic, in the sense that the cost-minimizing input mix remains constant as the output level changes. This characteristic also means that as input prices change, cost estimates are affected only by a scale factor, and that the relationships between marginal and average incremental cost or measures of economies of scale are not affected.

This approach explicitly allows for the use of separate measures of as many important hospital outputs as may exist in any given situation, including a disaggregation of output according to case type defined by disease and/or other characteristics. For example, in the context of Ethiopia, the hospital is an important producer of ambulatory as well as inpatient care. Thus, in this instance, both in- and outpatient measures of service were included, as well as measures of laboratory and X-ray tests and surgical procedures.

Issues in modelling hospital costs

Assumptions of hospital behaviour

Econometric studies of hospital costs – such as those cited above – have assumed that hospitals are cost minimizers. Such behaviour implies that the cost function is homogeneous of degree one in input prices, and can be tested econometrically (Friedlander 1977) if adequate information on both output levels and input prices is available. Unfortunately, the Ethiopian data, like the data set employed by Grannemann *et al.* (1986), do not contain adequate input-price information. Consequently, it was not possible to estimate a general, more flexible translog cost function, let alone to test for cost-minimizing behaviour or other theoretical features of cost functions.

Cost-minimization analysis is also thwarted in this study by the way in which hospital resource-allocation decisions were made in Ethiopia. The Ministry of Finance allocated all financial resources to each health facility, with the agreement of the central Ministry of

Health, so that in practice most hospitals had very little discretion over the quantity of inputs available to them for the provision of health services. Thus, responsibility for decision-making about the use of hospital resources was withheld from facility administrators, and was retained by the Ministries of Finance and Health in their control over specific line-item budget allocations for each facility.

Costs and expenditure analysis

Although the language of 'cost function' is used throughout this paper, our dependent variable is hospital expenditure rather than cost. While the distinction between these two terms is, generally, semantic, in this case there is a more fundamental distinction. First, total expenditure data underestimate actual resources used, since there were a large number of unrecorded gifts in kind provided by international organizations such as UNICEF or by private groups. The amounts of these gifts varied from year to year and from facility to facility, and there was no information system in place which monitored these flows. On the basis of the limited available data Donaldson and Dunlop (1987) estimated that, in some Ethiopian hospitals, donated resources amounted to at least 15 per cent of total government-allocated expenditures. More importantly, such donations accounted for a large share (in some cases, over 50 per cent) of certain drugs and other supplies. Thus, the actual total recurrent expenditure requirements of providing health services to the population in Ethiopia were higher than the recorded level of official Ministry of Health-monitored expenditures, particularly with respect to drugs and repair and maintenance supplies. In addition, the analysis here does not include an estimate of the depreciation of the capital stock, which constitutes an important cost element. Finally, budgetary expenditure flows are seldom valued on the basis of the opportunity cost of the resources made available via government allocations. Thus, although the terms cost function and cost analysis are used throughout the paper, the empirical study presented here is an analysis of government hospital expenditures, and not of total hospital cost, the former being an underestimate of the latter. However, if in-kind gifts and depreciation costs represented a similar share of total costs in all hospitals, then the use of government expenditure, as opposed to total cost, does not affect the interpretation of our study results.

Capital stock adjustments

Initial capital costs represent a major component of total hospital expenditure. Since it is difficult to adjust capital inputs quickly as desired levels of output change, the amount of capital used is unlikely to be set at the cost-minimizing level for the output produced in any given year. This is true even though there are examples of hospitals in East Africa operating at occupancy levels that exceed 100 per cent. This is particularly the case in maternity wards of large urban hospitals (see Dunlop 1984).

In the longer term adjustments may be made to a hospital's capital stock; but in the Ethiopian case, that adjustment period may be long, given resource scarcities and the general lack of alternative domestic private philanthropic resources which a facility in other contexts may tap. It is unlikely that the period of time is under the control of the facility, or even under that of the Ministry of Health. Even Ethiopia's National Committee for Central Planning was not able to predict easily if it might be able to adjust hospital capital stocks during any given time-period, owing to the macroeconomic problems facing the country. This problem was highlighted in Ethiopia in the mid 1980s, when it had to adjust downward its planned health-sector capital budget by over 50 per cent in three years on account of adverse economic performance (see Donaldson and Dunlop 1987).

The implication is that, in contradistinction to the situation in many more affluent countries, where capital stocks cannot be considered exogenous, it is possible – in the case of Ethiopia at this time – to consider decisions regarding the size of the capital stock in the hospital sector as outside the purview of the decision-makers. Thus, in this instance, it is possible to estimate a total cost function that includes measures of the capital stock in the equation without risking simultaneous equation bias. Measures of the 'quality' of the capital stock – in the sense of its level of maintenance and repair – have been included in several specifications in order to assess the extent to which the condition of buildings and equipment affected the level of total recurrent expenditure. These, and other findings, are reported below.

Specification of the empirical total cost model

As was stated earlier, there are four types of independent variables in the cost function: 'X' variables, which are a vector of factors that affect the level, but not the shape, of the expenditure function with respect to the outputs; 'Y' variables, which are a vector of primary outputs, such as the number of outpatient visits, inpatient admissions, and inpatient days; 'P', or input-price variables; and 'Z' variables, which include a vector of other outputs produced in the hospital, such as surgical procedures, X-ray tests, laboratory tests, and normal deliveries.

The total cost function employed in the analysis is an exponential and multiplicative function of its arguments. Such a functional form is characteristic of a translog (transcendental logarithmic) specification. Thus the cost function is as follows:

$$C = e^{(m_0 + m_1 \cdot BEDS)} \prod_i P_i^{a_i} e^{f(Y)} \qquad (1)$$

where C is total hospital cost; e is the base of the natural exponential function; $\prod_i$ denotes the product of i terms of the form $P_i^{a_i}$; m_0, m_i, and a_i are coefficients to be estimated; BEDS is the total number of beds in the hospital, and has been included as a proxy measure for capital stock (i.e. an X variable); P_i is the price of the ith input; and $f(Y)$ is a function linear in output levels. Using the properties of multiplicative and exponential functions, the expenditure function can be linearized by taking the natural logarithm on both sides of expression (1):

$$\ln C = m_0 + m_1 \cdot BEDS + \sum_i (a_i \ln P_i) + f(Y), \qquad (2)$$

where

$$\sum_i (a_i \cdot \ln P_i) = a_1 \cdot \ln PHY/PER + a_2 \cdot \ln MILES, \qquad (3)$$

and

$$f(Y) = b_{11} \cdot IP + b_{12} \cdot OP + b_{13} \cdot DELIV + b_{14} \cdot XRAY + b_{15} \cdot SURG \\ + b_{16} \cdot LAB + C_{11} \cdot IP_2 + c_{12} \cdot OP^2 + d_{11} \cdot IP^*OP. \qquad (4)$$

In expression (3) the variable *PHY/PER* is used as a proxy for input prices. It represents the proportion of physicians in relation to the total personnel employed in a hospital, and is intended to capture relative average labour costs in different hospitals. A second input price proxy, the variable *MILES*, reflects the distance from the hospital to the capital city of Addis Ababa. It is included to capture the tendency for important inputs such as drugs and gasoline to become more expensive when the hospital is farther away from the capital, as a result of additional transport and storage costs.

In expression (4) the variables *IP* and *OP* represent the volumes of in- and outpatient activity respectively (i.e. *Y* vector variables). As is explained later, several alternative indicators were used to measure these. The '*Z*' variables *DELIV, XRAY, SURG*, and *LAB* represent respectively the number of deliveries, X-rays, surgical procedures, and laboratory examinations performed at the hospital. The terms *IP²* and *OP²* represent the squares of the variables *IP* and *OP*. The variable *IP*OP* is an interaction term which corresponds to the product of the variables *IP* and *OP*.

The above specification corresponds neither to a general multiple-output translog function nor to a structural function; rather, it combines features of both. The lack of adequate measures of input prices thwarted the inclusion of interaction terms between input prices and output levels. In addition, given the limited number of observations, it was thought that a gain in flexibility from including those terms would not offset the loss in terms of degrees of freedom. Finally, the above specification is linear in both the variables and the coefficients, and therefore can be estimated using the technique of ordinary least-squares regression (OLS).

Expressions for the marginal cost of in-and out patient services (*MCIP* and *MCOP*) can be derived from the above cost function by taking the partial derivatives with respect to the variables *IP* and *OP*:

$$MCIP = \frac{\partial C}{\partial IP} = \left(\frac{\partial C}{\partial \ln C}\right) \cdot \left(\frac{\partial \ln C}{\partial IP}\right) = C \cdot \left(\frac{\partial f(Y)}{\partial IP}\right), \qquad (5)$$

and

$$MCOP = \frac{\partial C}{\partial OP} = \left(\frac{\partial C}{\partial \ln C}\right) \cdot \left(\frac{\partial \ln C}{\partial OP}\right) = C \cdot \left(\frac{\partial f(Y)}{\partial OP}\right). \qquad (6)$$

Given the specification of the $f(Y)$ function, the marginal expenditure functions become:

$$MCIP = C.(b_{11} + 2 \cdot c_{11} \cdot IP + d_{11} \cdot OP), \qquad (7)$$

and

$$MCOP = C.(b_{12} + 2 \cdot c_{12} \cdot OP + d_{11} \cdot IP). \qquad (8)$$

The cost specification also enables one to compute the average incremental cost (AIC). AIC indicates how much average total cost will increase if output Y_i is produced rather than not produced at all. To illustrate, consider a hospital with two types of output: days of inpatient service and of outpatient visits. The AIC of the inpatient care produced at the hospital measures the increase in hospital average cost per unit of inpatient care that would result if the hospital added that service relative to the situation where no inpatient care was produced at the facility. AIC is specified for a given level of output for all variables. More formally, AIC is defined in the following way:

$$AIC \ Y_i = \{C(Y_1, Y_2, \dots ,Y_i \dots Y_n) - C(Y_1,Y_2 \dots ,0, \dots ,Y_n)\}/Y_i \qquad (9)$$

A final useful measure to compute is an indicator of product-specific economies of scale (EOS). Product-specific economies of scale measure the effect of a proportional increase in all inputs on the output of a particular product when the level of output of all other products remains constant. The product-specific EOS indicator can be computed as the ratio between the AIC and the MC for any given output. Where economies of scale exist, the ratio between the AIC and the MC is greater than one. Where diseconomies of scale exist the ratio is less than one. This concept is equivalent to the ratio of average and marginal cost in the single-output case.

Variable definition

The dependent and independent variables included in the analysis are presented in Table 10.1 by variable type.

Table 10.1 *List of variables, definition, and data sources for an analysis of total hospital costs*

Acronym	Definition	Data source	Expected sign
I. Dependent Variable			
1. *EXPEND*	Total Expenditure in Thousands of *birr*	(1)	N/A
II. Independent Variables			
'*X*' *vector variables* — those which affect level but not shape of cost function			
2. *BEDS*	Number of hospital beds	(2)	POS
3. *BDGA*	Maintenance condition of buildings is 'A', i.e. in good condition relative to 'D' condition, which needs replacement.	(2)	NEG
4. *BDGB*	Maintenance condition of building is 'B', i.e. requires some minor repair relative to 'D' condition, which needs replacement.	(2)	NEG
5. *BDGC*	Maintenance condition of building is 'C', i.e. requires major repair relative to 'D' condition, which needs replacement.	(2)	NEG
'*Y*' *vector variables* — those which are measures of 'primary outputs'			
6. *IPDAYS*	Number of inpatient days	(2)	POS
7. *NIP*	Number of inpatients	(1), (2)	POS
8. *NFOP*	Number of first outpatient visits	(1), (2)	POS
9. *NOP*	Total number of out patient visits (first and repeat)	(2)	POS
10. *NROP*	Number of repeat out patient visits	(2)	POS

Table 10.1 (*cont.*)

Acronym	Definition	Data source	Expected sign

'Z' vector variables — those which are measures of 'other' hospital outputs

Acronym	Definition	Data source	Expected sign
11. *DELIV*	Number of normal deliveries	(2)	POS
12. *LAB*	Number of lab tests performed	(2)	POS
13. *XRAY*	Number of X-ray tests performed	(2)	POS
14. *SURG*	Number of surgical procedures performed	(2)	POS

'P' or input-price vector variables – those which measure input-price variations between hospitals

Acronym	Definition	Data source	Expected sign
15. *MILES*	Miles from Addis Ababa to facility (a proxy measure for input-cost differentials between Addis Ababa and other locations)	(2)	POS
16. *PHY/PER*	Physician share of total employment	(2)	POS

Sources: (1) Donaldson and Dunlop (1987).
(2) Ministry of Health (1982, 1986).

Dependent variables

In this analysis the dependent variable is total annual government recurrent hospital expenditure. This variable specification excludes provision for capital replenishment, although repair and maintenance of the capital stock are included. As has been indicated, the variable specification does not include in-kind gifts.

Independent variables

'X' variables. This set of variables comprises indicators of the hospital capital stock. These include the number of hospital beds and the physical condition of the hospital buildings, as measured by a periodic Ministry of Health survey of all health facilities. The expected hypothetical relationships between total hospital cost and '*X*' vector variables are presented in Table 10.1. It is postulated that total hospital cost will rises with a larger capital stock, as measured by the number of beds, and that newer, or more carefully maintained facilities, will require lower maintenance costs.

'*Y*' *variables*. The '*Y*' vector variables comprise indicators of primary hospital output. They include measures of in-and out-patient activity, such as: the number of hospital admissions; the number of inpatient days; the total number of outpatient visits; the number of first outpatient visits; and the number of repeat outpatient visits. The sum of first plus repeat visits is equal to the total number of outpatient visits. The hypothesized relationship between these independent variables and total hospital cost is summarized in Table 10.1. It is expected that as the total volume of patient activity increases, so too does total cost.

'*Z*' *variables*. '*Z*' vector variables comprise other hospital outputs such as the number of normal deliveries, laboratory tests, X-ray tests, and surgical procedures. These output indicators further define the complexity of the ambulatory and inpatient care provided, and the skill level of the staff employed at each facility. It is hypothesized that all these outputs are positively related to total cost.

'*P*' *Variables*. '*P*' vector variables comprise a set of input-price indicators which are included to control for possible differences in costs among facilities because of input-price differences. Input-price differences across facilities are frequently the result of wage differences between various labour markets. Although wage information for each hospital was not available from our data set, there was little wage variation in Ethiopia within personnel categories, because wage-scales were nationally defined by the civil service system. However, average labour costs may have differed across facilities because of differences in personnel mix, as well as differences in the experience and length of service of the personnel employed in each facility. Further, it was expected that there would be a tendency for a larger share of skilled health workers – particularly physicians – to work in those facilities which produced the more complex set of services, particularly those embodied in the '*Z*' set of output indicators. Thus it is hypothesized that the ratio of physicians to total personnel employed in any facility is positively related to total cost.

Price data on inputs other than labour were not available.

The only other input-price proxy included was an indicator of transportation cost differentials measured as the distance (in miles) from Addis Ababa to the hospital. The assumed relationship is positive, reflecting the additional transport costs associated with increased distance from Addis Ababa.

Description of Ethiopian data

As Table 10.1 indicates, two principal data sources were used in our analysis: the three Ministry of Health Service Directories compiled in 1976, 1982, and 1984 (Ministry of Health, 1982, 1986), and the World Bank-supported health financing study conducted by Dayl Donaldson and David Dunlop in 1986. The three MOH Directories provided a complete listing for the year specified of all health facilities operating in the country, excluding those operated by and on behalf of the military. They also provided information about location; date of initiating service; service utilization; number of personnel by staff cadre; vehicle numbers and states of repair; hospital building states of repair; and approved hospital budgets. The health financing study drew upon the information provided in the Directories, but added certain specific information about the actual hospital operating expenditures and other health facilities for the 1983–5 period. The actual expenditure data were obtained from the accounting division of the Ministry of Health, which monitored all hospital data, which were verified by information obtained from each hospital's accounting records. In addition, the study used utilization data for the same period of time. With these two sources of information it was possible to develop a pooled cross-section, time-series data set of 38 observations for fifteen of the country's eighty-three hospitals for the variables specified in Table 10.1. Table 10.2 contains the data set descriptive statistics.

Observations were pooled across hospitals and over time. Annual expenditure data were adjusted for inflation, and all expenditures are in 1985 *birr*. Time-series pooling tests are important in determining whether hospital cost behaviour changes over time. However, the limited number of observations per hospital (between one and three) precluded us from statistically checking for the validity of the time-series pooling.

The hospitals in our sample were either large or small, with no medium-sized hospitals. It was therefore thought that the

Table 10.2 *Descriptive statistics: total cost function values*

Variable	N	Mean	Standard deviation	Minimum value	Maximum value	Std error of mean
EXPEND	38	1150.07	1177.87	218.00	4908.00	191.07
REXPEND	38	1373.38	1394.42	281.43	5011.66	226.20
BUDGET	38	1434.10	1299.84	264.00	4931.00	237.31
BEDS	38	152.52	138.47	26.00	495.00	22.46
BDGA	38	0.23	0.43	0.00	1.00	0.06
BDGB	38	0.34	0.48	0.00	1.00	0.07
BDGC	38	0.31	0.47	0.00	1.00	0.07
NIP	38	3136.89	2199.43	200.00	7423.00	356.79
ALOS	38	9.62	5.28	2.20	24.60	0.85
NFOP	38	25520.39	10413.45	7993.00	45202.00	1689.28
NROP	38	28667.78	16098.10	10601.76	73049.00	2611.45
NOP	38	54188.18	23936.10	25748.00	116019.00	3882.94
DELIV	38	1016.13	1339.99	0.00	4190.00	217.37
LAB	38	46691.28	43158.25	2912.00	155673.00	7001.19
XRAY	38	4781.63	6776.86	0.00	28438.00	1099.35
SURG	38	1758.02	1595.33	0.00	5540.00	258.79
LMILES	38	3.04	2.51	0.00	5.69	0.40
LPHYPER	38	-3.35	0.48	-4.57	-2.65	0.07

behaviour of small and large hospitals might differ, so observations were sorted in ascending order of total annual expenditure. The sample was then divided into two sub-samples, each containing one-half (19 observations) of the sorted sample. The first sample contained small hospitals, with an annual expenditure ranging from 281000 to 727000 *birr*; while the second exhibited a range of 789000 to 4908000 *birr* per year.

OLS regressions were run on each of the two samples and on the aggregate sample. An F-test, known as the 'Chow test' (Chow 1960), was constructed to test the hypothesis that hospitals in both half-samples exhibited the same type of cost behaviour. A value of 2.92 for the F-test suggested that the hypothesis should be rejected at the 95 per cent confidence level. In other words, the test implied that the cost function coefficients were significantly different for each sample. Nevertheless, the data were pooled in order to increase the robustness of the estimates. Thus the coefficient estimates cannot be interpreted as representing the expenditure behaviour of hospitals in either sample, but rather that of a representative hospital of average size, i.e., with 152 beds and a total annual expenditure of 1373000 *birr*.

Empirical results

Total cost function

The results of the regression model of the determinants of total hospital cost are presented in Table 10.3. The original regression included the variable *XRAY* and the logarithm of the two input-price proxy variables *PHY/PER* and *MILES*. All three variables were excluded from the basic regression, for reasons discussed later in this section. The exclusion of the variables resulted in a better statistical fit, as measured by $\bar{R}$ (i.e. R^2 adjusted for the number of degrees of freedom). Results from three other regression equations are presented in Bitran-Dicowsky and Dunlop (1989). As shown in Table 10.3, both the intercept and the number of *BEDS* variable – which can be interpreted as measures of fixed cost – were positive and statistically significant. An estimate of the fixed costs of an average-size hospital can be obtained by evaluating the estimated cost function at a zero output level and by using an average value for the number of beds. When outputs are set to zero, the total expenditure function defined in (1) becomes:

$$C = e^{(m_0 + m_1 \cdot BEDS)}$$

When this equation is evaluated at the average value of *BEDS* = 152, and using the estimates for m_0 and m_1 from Table 10.3, we obtain a fixed-cost estimate of 476240 *birr*. This fixed cost represents approximately 34.7 per cent of the total annual expenditure for the average hospital of nearly 1373000 *birr*. The main expenditure item going to make up the fixed component is wages and salaries. Other fixed costs are staff housing, some transport costs for supplies and drugs, utility costs, and certain equipment-maintenance costs.

As was indicated earlier, ambulatory care output can be measured by several alternative indicators, including the total number of outpatient visits (*NOP*), the number of first outpatient visits (*NFOP*), and the number of repeat visits (*NROP*). In most instances, the first visit per illness episode is more resource-intensive than repeat visits, since the diagnosis and initial treatment are performed then. Thus, from a resource-use perspective, both *NFOP* and *NROP* are more homogeneous measures of ambulatory

Table 10.3 *Empirical results of the determinants of Ethiopian total hospital costs, 1983–1985*

Variable name	Abbreviation	Regression statistics coefficient	t–statistic
Intercept	m_0	5.45	22.51**
BEDS	m_1	4.71×10^{-3}	8.89**
IPDAYS	b_{11}	2.18×10^{-5}	3.44**
NFOP	b_{12}	1.91×10^{-6}	0.08
DELIV	b_{13}	1.68×10^{-4}	5.39**
SURG	b_{15}	3.21×10^{-6}	0.11
LAB	b_{16}	7.63×10^{-6}	7.97**
IPDAYS²	c_{11}	-1.65×10^{-12}	–0.02
NFOP²	c_{12}	1.42×10^{-10}	0.26
IPDAYS–NFOP	d_{11}	-7.50×10^{-10}	–2.42*

Total number of observations: 38, Degrees of freedom: 28, Adjusted R^2: 0.963, F=107.5

Notes: * statistically significant at the 0.05 level.
** statistically significant at the 0.01 level.

care than *NOP*, and should be entered as individual variables in the cost equation.

Each of these indicators of ambulatory output was empirically investigated both singly and in various combinations. The results presented in Table 10.3 include *NFOP* as the indicator of ambulatory care, with the estimated coefficient being positive but not statistically significant. Alternative model specifications which included both *NFOP* and *NROP*, as well as ones which included only *NOP*, did not provide better statistical results than the model specification that used only *NFOP*. Since *NOP* includes both resource-intensive and relatively non-intensive visits, it is understandable that it did not perform as well as a more disaggregated indicator such as *NFOP*. Also, since repeat visits (*NROP*) are less resource-intensive, it was expected that their impact on cost would not be as great. Hence, from an empirical perspective, *NFOP* was the preferred outpatient indicator.

In investigating differences in the determinants of total expenditures between small and large hospitals, it was observed that in small hospitals *NFOP* was both consistently positive and statistically significant. This finding suggests that when more observations are available the sample should be segmented into larger and smaller hospitals and analysed separately. This could yield additional insights into the determinants of hospital expenditures as the output mix changes with increasing service and patient complexity in larger hospitals as against the smaller (and more rural) facilities.

From an inpatient-care perspective, two measures of output were investigated. These were the number of inpatients (*NIP*) and the number of inpatient days (*IPDAYS*). These indicators were highly and negatively correlated with one another, with a partial correlation coefficient of -0.83. This finding can only be explained by assuming that the disease mix differed between the hospitals. This possibility is supported by evidence that the average length of stay across the sample of hospitals for the various years included in the sample varied from a low of 2.2 days in a hospital known for its high volume of deliveries and other obstetrical care to a high of 24.6 days in a hospital with many accidents and injuries and other long-term-care patients.

Since *NIP* and *IPDAYS* are highly correlated, multicolinearity was suspected. When *NIP* was also included in an estimated equation, its sign was negative, though not statistically significant.

The variable *IPDAYS* appeared to be the most consistently significant and positive, as expected. Thus, it was used in most of the empirical analyses conducted. In Table 10.3, *IPDAYS* is positive, and statistically significant at the 0.01 level.

In the preliminary analysis of the differences in the determinants of hospital cost between large and small hospitals, inpatient indicators of hospital output were not as often statistically significant as was the outpatient indicator, *NFOP*. This suggests that the output-structure differences between large and small facilities will bear further investigation when a larger sample is available.

Four other output variables were included in the empirical analysis: *DELIV*, *LAB*, *XRAY*, and *SURG*. It was found that three of the four – *DELIV*, *LAB*, and *SURG* – consistently had the expected positive sign and that two – *LAB* and *DELIV* – were consistently statistically significant. It was unclear from the analysis why the variable *XRAY*, contrary to expectations, had a negative sign, and was often statistically significant. This result may be attributed to the fact that the *XRAY* variable was correlated with both *DELIV* (0.69) and the interaction term, *DAY-NFOP* (0.72). In addition, the sample data show that certain small hospitals (in terms of beds) reported performing a large number of X-rays, while some large hospitals reported few X-rays. This reflects output-mix specialization, and could explain the seemingly puzzling result.

The empirical performance of the two '*P*' variables *MILES* and *PHY/PER* was disappointing. They were generally statistically insignificant. The variable *MILES*, which was intended to capture the positive effect that distance from the capital city to a given facility had on input costs, turned out to have a negative sign, suggesting that total hospital cost was reduced as the distance between hospitals and Addis Ababa increased. This result may reflect a characteristic of the sample rather than any cost behaviour, and may reflect the smaller size of hospitals outside Addis Ababa rather than lower travel costs. It is also likely that rurally-based hospitals were not fully billed for the transport cost of all items shipped to them from Addis Ababa.

The variable *PHY/PER* was statistically insignificant, and is therefore dropped from the results presented in Table 10.3. Furthermore, the exclusion of both proxy variables resulted in a better statistical fit as measured by $\bar{R}$. If we assume that input prices were relatively similar across hospitals within the sample, then the omitted variable bias is unimportant. The fact that salaries, which were a major cost component, are set at the central level in Ethiopia supports this assumption.

The impact on total hospital costs of the physical condition of the hospital buildings was also assessed. The tested hypothesis was that the poorer the physical condition of the buildings, the larger would be the costs of repairs and maintenance. Thus the three grades of building condition A,B, and C should be associated with lower cost levels than building condition D. The results of this test (presented in Bitran-Dikowsky and Dunlop 1989) showed that two of the three conditions relative to the poorest condition appeared to have an effect on total cost, but not in the expected negative direction. Building conditions B and C appeared to have a significantly positive impact on total costs, and building condition A had the hypothesized impact, but was not statistically significant.

The data may help to explain this unexpected finding. Most of the large (in terms of beds) hospital buildings were classified as condition B or C. Since their expenditure levels tended to be greater than those of other facilities, the statistical finding may be only reflecting an artefact of the data rather than any behavioural relationship of interest to the policy-maker. The finding may also reflect the fact that Ethiopian decision-makers only allocated their scarce resources to maintenance once a minimum period of time had elapsed since construction.

Marginal and average incremental cost

The marginal and average incremental cost for the principal outputs with statistically significant estimated parameters (i.e. *IPDAYS*, *DELIV*, and *LAB*) were calculated using equations similar to (7), (8), and (9), as specified earlier. The calculations were done using the mean values for all variables (see Table 10.2), and are presented in Table 10.4 along with the calculated product-specific economies of scale index (EOS). For purposes of comparison with MC and AIC, the table also provides information on fees charged for these services in 1985, and the ratio of 1985 fees in comparison to their respective marginal cost.

The results in Table 10.4 reveal several important findings. First, for those services enumerated in the table, the data show that the services' marginal cost was always greater than average incremental cost (i.e. the EOS index was less than one for all three services). This indicates that the representative hospital was operating slightly within the diseconomies of scale range of output for these three services. Given the statistical variation in the sample, it can be concluded that the sample of hospitals is best characterized by nearly constant (slightly decreasing) economies of scale.

Table 10.4 *Estimates of marginal and average incremental cost, product–specific economies of scale index, and prices changed at Ethiopian hospitals in 1985 (Expenditures in 1985* birr)

	Output		
	Inpatient days (IPDAYS)	Delivery (DELIV)	Laboratory exams (LAB)
1. Marginal cost (MC)	2.58	169.1	7.7
2. Average incremental cost (AIC)[a]	2.53	155.4	6.5
3. Product–specific economies of scale index (EOS)	0.98	0.92	0.84
4. Range of fees charged at Ethiopian hospitals, 1985[b],[c],[d],[e]			
High	30.0	100.0	10.0
Low	1.0	5.0	0.25
Median	2.0	15.0	1.5
5. Ratio of median price to (MC)	0.78	0.09	0.19

Notes: a. See Bitran–Dicowsky and Dunlop (1989) for method of calculation.
b. Bed–day fee only.
c. Normal delivery fee only.
d. All types of laboratory tests.
e. Each hospital has the jurisdiction to establish its own fee structure. Typically the inter-hospital differences in fees are based on rural–urban distinctions and on the historical management of the hospital, i.e. mission *vs* government. For further information about fees see Donaldson and Dunlop (1987).

Source: Donaldson and Dunlop (1987).

Public goods pricing theory recommends that prices should be set according to the marginal cost of production in order to achieve economic efficiency. In certain instances, discussed in greater detail by de Ferranti (1985), departures from marginal cost pricing may be justified either for equity reasons or where positive externalities may accrue to society. A comparison of fees actually charged at Ethiopian hospitals with the computed marginal costs show that these fees were generally lower than marginal cost. The median fee charged per bed-day was about two *birr* in 1985, or 25 per cent below the estimated marginal cost figure. The median laboratory fee of around one and one half *birr* was only one-fifth of the estimated marginal cost for a laboratory test.

The median delivery fee was well below the estimated marginal cost for a normal delivery. Society may obtain positive externalities from health-facility-based normal deliveries. To the extent that the infant mortality rate is reduced below the level it would otherwise be, over time the demand for additional children may be reduced, which may possibly lead to slower rates of population growth. This argument is discussed in greater detail in the 1984 *World development report* (World Bank 1984). However, it is unclear whether the positive social externality per normal delivery would justify the differential between the median fee charged in Ethiopia in 1985 and the estimated marginal cost. Some upward adjustment in this and other fees appeared warranted.

Conclusions

Several points emerge from this analysis. First, it provides greater insight into the various factors which influence the cost of providing hospital-based health services in Ethiopia. Second, the theoretical approach employed in conducting this empirical investigation has provided results which appear plausible and robust over several alternative empirical specifications of the theoretical model. Most if not all principal hospital outputs had a positive effect on total cost. Third, the results themselves are of interest. The volume of outpatient activity, as measured by the number of first outpatient visits to the hospital's clinic, had a positive impact on total costs. The marginal costs slightly exceeded average incremental costs, suggesting that hospitals in our sample had reached the point of constant economies of scale for the inpatient days, laboratory examinations, and delivery outputs. A negative and statistically significant coefficient associated with the output-interaction term indicated the existence of economies of scope between the number of inpatient days and first outpatient visits. The total number of beds in a hospital appeared to have a positive and significant independent effect on total hospital cost. Neither of the input-price proxy variables indicated a statistically significant impact on total cost. Finally, the estimated marginal expenditure on an inpatient day was around 3 *birr*, and on a laboratory test, 8 *birr*.

This analysis is viewed by the authors as preliminary. Additional empirical investigation is warranted; however, it must await further information from additional facilities. When this is available, it will be important to disaggregate the sample by hospital size and to estimate separately the equations of cost determinants: both the output and input structure may be sufficiently different between small and large facilities to warrant a separate analysis. Improved measures of input prices are also required. With such additional data, other statistical tests can be conducted to ascertain whether the typical assumption of cost or expenditure minimization behaviour applies.

In spite of data deficiencies, the approach taken here and its results appear promising, and have important policy implications for pricing hospital services in poor countries.

References

Bays, C. (1979). Specification error in the estimation of hospital cost functions. *The Review of Economics and Statistics*, **61**(3), 302–5.

Bitran-Dicowsky, R. and Dunlop, D. W. (1989). *The determinants of hospital costs. An analysis of Ethiopia*, Working Paper Series 249. Population and Human Resources Department, The World Bank, Washington, DC.

Chow, G. (1960). A test of equality between sets of observations in two linear regressions. *Econometrica*, **28**, 591–605.

Conrad, R. and Strauss, R. P. (1983). A multiple-output multiple-input model of the hospital industry in North Carolina. *Applied Economics*, **15**, 341–52.

Cowing, T. G. and Holtmann, A. G. (1983). Multiple short run hospital cost functions: empirical evidence and policy implications from cross-section data. *Southern Economic Journal*, **49**(4), 637–53.

de Ferranti, D. (1985). *Paying for health services in developing countries: an overview*, World Bank Staff Working Paper No. 721. World Bank, Washington, DC.

Donaldson, D. S. and Dunlop, D. W. (1987). *Sector review Ethiopia: a study of health financing: issues and options*, Report No. 6624-ET, 2 vols. World Bank, Washington, DC.

Dunlop, D.W. (1984). *Cost implications of selected health care components and programs*, Paper prepared for the PHN Department, World Bank. The Bank, Washington, DC.

Feldstein, M. (1967). *Economic analysis for health service efficiency*. North Holland, Amsterdam.

Friedlander, A. (1977). Estimation of the translog cost function. In *Alternative scenarios for federal transportation policy*, Vol. III pp 85–142, prepared for the US Department of Transportation, Washington, DC.

Grannemann, T., Brown, R., and Pauly, M. (1986). Estimating hospital costs: a multiple-output analysis. *Journal of Health Economics*, **5**, 107–27.

Lave, J., and Lave, L. (1970). Hospital cost functions. *American Economic Review*, **60**, 379–95.

Lave, J., Lave, L., and Silverman, L. (1972). Hospital cost estimation controlling for case mix. *Applied Economics*, **4**, 165–80.

Ministry of Health (1982). *Comprehensive health service directory, 1974 EC (1981/82 GC)*. Government of Ethiopia, Addis Ababa.

Ministry of Health (1986). *Comprehensive health service directory, 1976 EC (1983/84 GC)*. Government of Ethiopia, Addis Ababa.

Rafferty, J. (1972). Measurement of hospital case mix: a note on alternative patient classifications. *Applied Economics*, **4**, 301–5.

World Bank (1984). *World development report*. World Bank, Washington, DC.

Author's note

This paper was prepared for the Population, Health, and Nutrition Department, World Bank, Washington, DC. The authors acknowledge the important contributions made to the paper by Dayl S. Donaldson, Harvard University, throughout its development. We are responsible for any errors which might remain.

11

Cost-effectiveness analysis of chemotherapy regimes of schistosomiasis control

Nicholas Prescott

Introduction

Schistosomiasis is one of the most widespread human parasitic infections, and is generally regarded as second only to malaria in terms of public health importance in developing countries. More than 200 million rural people are infected in Asia, Africa, South America, the Caribbean, and the Middle East, and prevalence is increasing with agricultural development and the expansion of the irrigated land area. These considerations have justified implementation of several national control programmes (WHO 1985).

Ideally, the policy decision to allocate scarce resources to schistosomiasis control would be based on an analysis of both external and internal efficiency (Prescott and Warford 1983). External efficiency is concerned with the broad question posed in cost-benefit analysis: is schistosomiasis control worth while by comparison with expenditure on alternative projects within the health sector or in other sectors? Internal efficiency is concerned narrowly with the question posed in cost-effectiveness analysis: what is the most efficient choice among alternative methods of achieving schistosomiasis control? In practice, however, external efficiency criteria are hard to apply because of the complexities associated with valuation of the health benefits of schistosomiasis control (Prescott 1979; Weimer 1987). Thus, for operational purposes, it appears more useful to emphasize cost-effectiveness criteria, which can facilitate project design once schistosomiasis control has already been judged socially worth while on the basis of intangible considerations instead of on that of a formal cost-benefit analysis.

The design of any schistosomiasis control programme entails the selection of one of a number of alternative interventions or of a combination of several of them: control of snails through molluscicides, biological control, or engineering methods; or control of host–parasite contact through chemotherapy or improved water supplies and sanitation. Despite this diversity, there has been little previous research into the cost-effectiveness of these alternatives. The earliest contribution was made by Rosenfield *et al.* (1977), who developed a model of schistosomiasis transmission in Iran in order to simulate the effectiveness of applying different control techniques – molluscicides, engineering methods, chemotherapy, and a combination of these controls – subject to a given budget constraint over a seven-year planning horizon. Their analysis indicated that a combination of chemotherapy and mollusciciding was most cost-effective where the programme objective was specified in terms of maximizing the reduction in prevalence achieved after seven years. This mix of interventions reduced the prevalence rate from 64 per cent to 20 per cent, whereas the next best alternative – chemotherapy – achieved a terminal prevalence rate of 60 per cent. However, this measure of effectiveness did not take into account the prevalence reductions achieved during the planning period. Specifying effectiveness differently, in terms of maximizing the total number of cases prevented during the seven-year period, changed the ranking of alternatives. With this objective, chemotherapy was the most cost-effective intervention, at a cost per case prevented of US $1.26, followed by the combination of interventions, at a unit cost of US $1.29.

More recently, Korte *et al.* (1986) have analysed the most cost-effective choice between two alternative antischistosomal drugs: metrifonate and praziquantel. The unit cost of metrifonate is substantially lower than that of praziquantel. But the standard drug regimen for metrifonate requires three doses at two-week intervals, whereas praziquantel can be administered in a single dose. Their illustrative analysis for Africa showed that praziquantel was more cost-effective than metrifonate in achieving the objective of reducing prevalence from 50 per cent to less than 5 per cent, for the following reasons. First, attrition due to the low rates of compliance with, and cure by, each round of the multiple-dosage regimen necessitated four separate rounds of the three-dose treatment with metrifonate to achieve the prevalence objective, compared with only two rounds of administration of the single dose of praziquantel. For metrifonate, compliance was assumed to be 100, 75, and 50 per cent with the first, second, and third doses respectively. Corresponding cure rates with each successive dose were 5, 15, and 60 per cent (Table 1 in Korte *et al.* 1986). Thus only 46 per cent of infected persons could be cured with each round of the three-dose regime of metrifonate. By contrast, it was assumed that compliance with the single dose of praziquantel was 100 per cent, and the cure rate was 85 per cent. Second, much higher transport and personnel costs were associated with metrifonate. Each round of the three-dose regime for metrifonate required three field trips to the target population, as against only one for praziquantel. Taking into account the number of complete rounds of treatment required to achieve the prevalence objective, twelve separate field trips were needed for administration of metrifonate, as against only two for praziquantel. As a result, the lower drug costs of metrifonate were substantially outweighed by its higher delivery-system costs.

Recent advances in antischistosomal therapy mean that treatment is now generally considered to be the most cost-effective way of controlling schistosomiasis (WHO 1985). However, opinions differ as to which of the different operational approaches to delivering chemotherapy is best. At one extreme, the development of safe and effective single-dose oral drugs such as oxamniqine and praziquantel has made mass chemotherapy a practical option. At the other extreme, there has been a revival of advocacy for some form of selective treatment (Anderson and May 1982; Warren 1981). Each of these different delivery systems has different costs and levels of effectiveness. The question of which is the most cost-effective has emerged as the most important issue in the design of efficient schistosomiasis control programmes, yet has not been addressed in previous cost-effectiveness analyses. This chapter therefore presents a resource-allocation framework designed to analyse the optimal choice of delivery system for schistosomal treatment.

Specification of the analytical framework

This analysis models four alternative delivery regimes for single-dose chemotherapy described (with different nomenclature) by the World Health Organization (WHO 1985) as follows. First, mass population chemotherapy: treatment is given to an entire population without prior individual diagnosis. Second, screened population chemotherapy: urine or stool specimens from the entire population are examined, and only persons excreting schistosoma eggs are treated. Third, mass group chemotherapy: since peak prevalence, intensity, and morbidity are generally found in the younger age-groups, treatment is offered to all persons in these selected groups. Fourth, screened group chemotherapy: treatment is offered only to those found to be infected among the selected groups. Another variant, targeted chemotherapy, is discussed later.

It is assumed throughout that the objective of schistosomiasis control is to maximize the number of cases cured. With no budget constraint, the optimal choice will depend upon a combination of both behavioural and epidemiological parameters. With a budget constraint, the optimal choice will also depend upon economic parameters. The next section models the cost and effectiveness of each of the alternative regimes described above. The definition and illustrative values of the model parameters are given in Table 11.1.

Then it is shown how the optimal choice of regime is derived with and without a budget constraint. The entire analysis models the cost-effectiveness of interventions applied for one year. Since a control programme implemented continuously for several years consists of a sequence of discrete one-year interventions, the same framework can be used to identify the optimal choice for each year within the multi-year period. The required extension would be a transmission model linking prevalence rates from one year to the next. This approach might identify a mixture of chemotherapy regimes that would be more cost-effective than continued repetition of the same regime for several years.

The cost and effectiveness of four chemotherapy regimes

Mass population chemotherapy

Chemotherapy is offered to a proportion, Z_m, of the population eligible for treatment, N_e. This proportion represents the intensity at which the intervention is applied, and may vary between 0 and 1. Those eligible exclude the significant number who are contraindicated (young children and pregnant and lactating women). Only a proportion, π_m, of the target group $z_m N_e$ will comply with the offer of mass chemotherapy. Assuming a fixed unit cost c_t per treatment (delivery system plus chemotherapy costs), the cost per capita of mass population chemotherapy will be:

$$(C_m/N) = c_t \pi_m Z_m (N_e/N) \qquad (1)$$

If the treated group $\pi_m z_m N_e$ is an unbiased sample of the eligible fraction, then the proportion who actually have schistosomiasis will equal the prevalence rate in the eligible population, p_e. With an efficacy rate e for chemotherapy, the number of cases cured by mass population chemotherapy K_m, expressed as a proportion of total cases pN, will be:

$$(K_m/pN) - e\pi_m z_m (p_e/p) (N_e/N) \qquad (2)$$

Table 11.1 *Definitions and values of model parameters*

	Symbol	Value
Economic		
Unit cost per treatment	c_t	2.50
Unit cost per screening test	c_s	0.50
Budget per capita (US$)	C/N	—
Behavioural		
Compliance rate for mass chemotherapy	π_m	0.90
Compliance rate for screening	π_s	0.75
Compliance rate for screened chemotherapy	π_c	0.95
Epidomiological		
Total population	N	—
Eligible fraction	N_e/N	0.80
High-prevalence fraction	N_h/N	0.40
Proportion of eligible population offered chemotherapy	z_m	—
Proportion of screen-positives offered treatment	z_s	—
Prevalence rate in N	p	0.45
Prevalence rate in N_e	p_e	0.50
Prevalence rate in N_h	P_h	0.70
Efficacy of chemotherapy	e	0.90
Sensitivity of screening test	s	0.90

Screened population chemotherapy

Screening is offered to the entire fraction of the population that is eligible for treatment. Assuming that only a proportion π_s of the eligible fraction will comply with the screening procedure, then the number of persons screened will be $\pi_s N_e$. With a unit cost c_s per screening test, the total cost of screening will be $c_s \pi_s N_e$. According to the World Health Organization description, this represents a lumpy fixed cost which must be incurred before any treatments are given. Assuming that the screened group is an unbiased sample of the eligible fraction, then the number of screen-positives identified by a screening test with sensitivity s will be $s\pi_s p_e N_e$. Note that this implies the use of a test with perfect specificity, otherwise the number of screen-positives will be augmented by a certain number of false-positives. A proportion z_s of screen-positives are offered treatment, of which π_c will comply at the unit cost c_t per treatment. The total cost per capita of screening plus treatment will therefore be:

$$(C_s/N) = c_s\pi_s \, (N_e/N) + c_t\pi_c z_s s\pi_s p_e \, (N_e/N) \qquad (3)$$

If the treated group is also an unbiased sample of the eligible fraction, then the number of cases cured will be the number of true-positives offered and complying with treatment of efficacy e. Expressed as a proportion of total cases:

$$(K_s/pN) - e\pi_c z_s s\pi_s \, (p_e/p) \, (N_e/N) \qquad (4)$$

Mass group chemotherapy

The difference between this regime and mass population chemotherapy lies simply in the selection of a sub-group, N_h, with a higher than average prevalence rate, P_h. This approach seeks the epidemiological advantage of a direct screening procedure while avoiding its cost disadvantage by substituting a costless indirect screening test and selecting high-risk groups, typically the young. The cost and effectiveness functions are identical to those for mass population chemotherapy, except for the substitution of P_h and N_h for P_e and N_e:

$$(C_{mg}/N) = c_t \pi_m z_m (N_h/N) \qquad (5)$$

$$(K_{mg}/pN) = e\pi_m z_m (p_h/p)(N_h/N) \qquad (6)$$

Screened group chemotherapy

The justification for this regime as an alternative to screened population chemotherapy is analogous to that given for mass group chemotherapy. Consequently, the cost and effectiveness functions are similar to those developed for screened population chemotherapy:

$$(C_{sg}/N) = c_s \pi_s (N_h/N) + c_t \pi_c z_s s \pi_s p_h (N_h/N) \qquad (7)$$

$$(K_{sg}/pN) = e \, \pi_c z_s s \pi_s (p_h/p)(N_h/N) \qquad (8)$$

Targeted chemotherapy

The term targeted chemotherapy has been used to describe field experiments in which treatment is limited to those individuals demonstrating a high egg output. Polderman and Manshande (1981) and Warren (1981) describe two such regimes that limit treatment to cases excreting more than 100 eggs/g faeces and 400 eggs/g respectively. Superficially, this approach appears to be a variant of screened chemotherapy, with the difference that screening is used to differentiate levels of infection intensity as distinct from the mere presence of infection. Essentially, the essence of the targeted approach is to redefine the planning objective as the maximization of the number of high-intensity cases cured. This objective is intrinsically neutral as to the optimal method of achieving it, which, as will be shown below, will tend to depend upon particular circumstances. From a modelling point of view, therefore, targeted chemotherapy can be represented simply by respecifying p as the prevalence rate of high-intensity cases, and should not be regarded as a different delivery regime.

Optimal choice with no budget constraint

We consider first the simplest case, when no budget constraint binds the optimal solution. Here, the planning problem is to choose the delivery regime which maximizes the proportion of total cases cured regardless of cost. The effectiveness of each regime is estimated for the maximum intensity of each intervention, that is when z_m (the proportion of the eligible population offered chemotherapy) and z_s (the proportion of screen-positives offered treatment) equal 1 in equations (2), (4), (6), and (8). This specification represents the maximum capacity of each regime to cure cases. The results obtained with the illustrative parameter values given in Table 11.1 are shown in Table 11.2.

In this example, mass population chemotherapy easily dominates the other regimes in terms of the proportion of total cases cured. This accords with expectation, because its coverage of the entire eligible population is modified by only one parameter, the compliance rate for chemotherapy. In contrast, the maximum impact of screened population chemotherapy is modified by three coverage-related parameters: the willingness of the eligible population to comply with the initial screening test; the sensitivity of the screening test itself; and the willingness of the screen-positives to present themselves for subsequent treatment. A low value for any one or more of these parameters necessarily produces a commensurately low overall impact for screened population chemotherapy. The same observations apply to the group variants of these basic approaches. The overall effectiveness of these interventions tends to be low because the pre-selection of a population subgroup automatically limits their coverage, and hence their potential impact, to only a proportion of the total cases.

In general, however, the optimal choice is sensitive to extreme variations in parameter values. Table 11.3 provides a sensitivity analysis for the comparison of mass population chemotherapy with the three alternative regimes. For each comparison, the table shows the decision inequality which must be satisfied for mass population chemotherapy to dominate. These inequalities enable

Table 11.2 *Maximum effectiveness: no budget constraint*

Delivery regime	Proportion of total cases cured	Cost per capita (US$)
Mass population	0.72	1.80
Screened population	0.51	0.94
Mass group	0.50	0.90
Screened group	0.36	0.60

us to calculate the switching value for key parameters needed for mass population chemotherapy to be the preferred regime.

For example, the first equation shows that mass population chemotherapy will produce a greater proportion of cases cured than screened population chemotherapy if the compliance rate for mass chemotherapy, π_m, exceeds the compliance rate for screening, π_s, weighted both by the sensitivity of the screening test, s, and by the compliance rate with chemotherapy among screen-positives, π_c. Using the illustrative parameter values in Table 11.1, this condition will hold true for any compliance rate with mass chemotherapy which is greater than the switching value of 0.64. By contrast, the second equation indicates that mass population chemotherapy will not be preferred to screened population chemotherapy if the prevalence rate in the selected group (p_h) is more than twice the prevalence rate in the eligible population (P_e). The third equation indicates that screened group chemotherapy would be preferred only if the prevalence ratio (p_h/p_e) is greater than 2.80.

Optimal choice with a budget constraint

Now we consider the general planning problem of choosing the most effective chemotherapy regime subject to a budget constraint. In this case, the effect of the budget constraint is to determine the intensity at which an intervention can operate, that is the proportion z_m or z_s of the target group which can be offered treatment. This in turn determines the number of cases cured under each regime. By setting the per capita cost of each regime equal to the budget constraint $(\bar{C}/N)$, and then substituting this constraint into the cost equations, we obtain the proportions offered treatment as a function of the budget constraint. Substituting these functions into the effectiveness equations then enables us to express the

Table 11.3 *Decision inequalities with no budget constraint*

$(K_m/pN) > (K_s/pN)$	requires π_m	$> \pi_c s \pi_s$
$(K_m/pN) > (K_{mg}/pN)$	requires 1	$> (P_h/p_e)(N_h/N_e)$
$(K_m/pN) > (K_{sg}/pN)$	requires π_m	$> \pi_c s \pi_s (p_h/p_e)(N_h/N_e)$

effectiveness of each intervention as a function of the budget constraint.

Mass population chemotherapy:

$$z_m = (\bar{C}/c_t \pi_m N_e) \tag{9}$$

$$(K_m/pN) = (e/c_t) \, (p_e/p) \, (\bar{C}/N) \tag{10}$$

Screened population chemotherapy:

$$z_s = (\bar{C} - c_s \pi_s N_e) \, / \, (c_t \pi_c s \pi_s p_e N_e) \tag{11}$$

$$(K_s/pN) = (e/c_t p) \, [(\bar{C}N) - c_s \pi_s (N_e/N)] \tag{12}$$

Mass group chemotherapy:

$$z_m = (\bar{C}/c_t \pi_m N_h) \tag{13}$$

$$(K_{mg}/pN) = (e/c_t) \, (p_h/p) \, (\bar{C}/N) \tag{14}$$

Screened group chemotherapy:

$$z_s = (\bar{C} - c_s \pi_s N_h) \, / \, (c_t \pi_c s \pi_s p_h N_h) \tag{15}$$

$$(K_{sg}/pN) = (e/c_t p) \, [(\bar{C}/N) - c_s \pi_s \, (N_h/N)] \tag{16}$$

The effectiveness functions simulated using the illustrative parameter values are shown in Table 11.4 and graphed in Figs 11.1 and 11.2. The outer envelope of these functions as shown in Fig. 11.3 indicates the maximum proportion of cases cured attainable for any given budget.

As the budget constraint increases from zero, mass group chemotherapy is initially the most effective intervention, until the proportion of cases cured reaches 0.28 at US$0.50 per capita. Then screened group chemotherapy takes over briefly, until the proportion of cases cured reaches 0.36 at US$0.64 per capita. The optimal choice then reswitches to mass group chemotherapy when the proportion of cases cured reaches 0.50, at a budget of US$0.93 per capita. Thereafter, screened population chemotherapy is the most effective intervention up to a per capita budget level of

Table 11.4 *Simulated effectiveness of alternative delivery regimes*

Budget per capita	Proportion of cases cured			
	Mass population	Screened population	Mass group	Screened population
0.00	0.00	0.00	0.00	0.00
0.10	0.04	0.00	0.06	0.00
0.15	—	—	—	0.00
0.20	0.08	0.00	0.11	0.04
0.30	0.12	0.00	0.17	0.12
0.40	0.16	0.08	0.22	0.20
0.50	0.20	0.16	0.28	0.28
0.60	0.24	0.24	0.34	0.36
0.70	0.28	0.32	0.39	—
0.80	0.32	0.40	0.45	—
0.90	0.36	0.48	0.50	—
0.94	—	0.51	—	—
1.00	0.40	—	—	—
1.10	0.44	—	—	—
1.20	0.48	—	—	—
1.30	0.52	—	—	—
1.40	0.56	—	—	—
1.50	0.60	—	—	—
1.60	0.64	—	—	—
1.70	0.68	—	—	—
1.80	0.72	—	—	—

US$1.28, when the proportion of cases cured is only slightly higher at 0.51. Finally, mass population chemotherapy takes over at higher budget levels up to a maximum of US$1.80 per capita, at which the maximum attainable proportion of cases cured, 0.72, is reached.

Five important features emerge from this illustration. The first, and the most important, is that the optimal choice of chemotherapy regime tends to be very sensitive to the level of the budget constraint. Second, the group regimes tend to be more effective at the lower budget levels than the population regimes. Third, the screening regimes tend to be less effective than their mass counterparts because, at any given budget level, the initial lumpy cost of screening has to be covered before residual resources can be devoted to treating screen-positives. Fourth, at higher budget

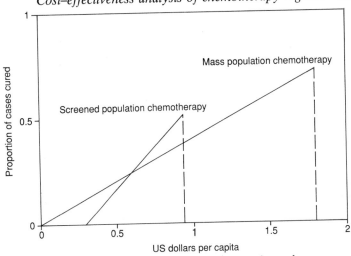

Fig. 11.1 Mass versus screened population chemotherapy.

levels, the population-based regimes tend to be more effective because the group approaches quickly exhaust their inherently limited capacity to cure cases. And fifth, the capacity limits of each regime produce some discontinuities in the envelope of the effectiveness functions. For example, the horizontal portion of the envelope between budget levels US$0.94 and US$1.28

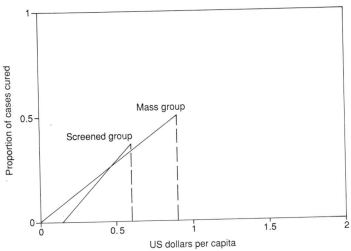

Fig. 11.2 Mass group versus screened group chemotherapy.

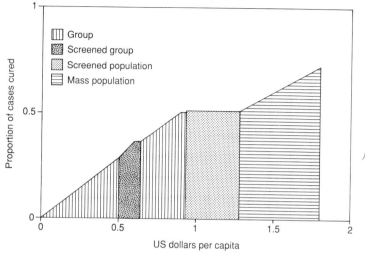

Fig. 11.3   Optimal choice of delivery regime.

indicates that screened population chemotherapy remains the preferred intervention in this range, even though its maximum output is produced at US$0.94 per capita. Thus, there is no need for additional expenditure until a higher level of output is produced with mass population chemotherapy at a cost of US$1.28 per capita.

The sensitivity of the optimal choice of regime to variations in the budget constraint can be derived analytically from the effectiveness functions (10), (12), (14), and (16). Table 11.5 provides as an example the decision inequalities which must be satisfied for mass population chemotherapy to dominate its alternatives. In this case, there are two inequalities. The first applies to lower levels of the budget constraint where each intervention is producing below its

Table 11.5 *Decision inequalities with a budget constraint*

$(K_m/pN) > (K_s/pN)$	requires	$(\bar{C}/N) < [(c_s\pi_s)/(1-p_e)](N_e/N);$
	and	$(\bar{C}/N) > c_t\pi_c s\pi_s (N_e/N).$
$(K_m/pN) > (K_{mg}/pN)$	requires	$P_h < P_e;$
	and	$(\bar{C}/N) > c_t\pi_m(P_h/P_e) (N_h/N).$
$(K_m/pN) > (K_{sg}/pN)$	requires	$(\bar{C}/N) < [(c_s\pi_s)/1-p_e)](N_h/N);$
	and	$(\bar{C}/N) > c_t\pi_c s\pi_s(p_h/p_e)(N_h/N).$

maximum output shown in Table 11.2. The second applies to higher budget levels where the dominated regime has already attained its maximum output.

The interpretation of these inequalities is easily illustrated using the parameter values in Table 11.1. Mass population chemotherapy is preferred to its screened population counterpart when the budget constraint is lower than US$0.60 and higher than US$1.28. Mass population chemotherapy is never preferable to mass group chemotherapy at low budget levels, because that would require the prevalence rate in the high-prevalence group to be lower than in the entire eligible fraction, which is impossible by definition. However, at budget levels higher than US$1.26, it does dominate. Finally, mass population chemotherapy dominates screened group chemotherapy at budget levels lower than US$0.30 and greater than US$0.90.

The same inequalities can be used to examine the sensitivity of the choice of optimal strategy to variations in the other parameters. Of special interest here are two key parameters: the prevalence rate, and the unit cost of the screening test. Both of these affect the comparisons between mass population chemotherapy and its screened alternatives. Figure 11.4 provides a sensitivity analysis of the optimal choice between mass population chemotherapy and screened population chemotherapy. The straight line shows for each unit cost per treatment the combination of prevalence rates and screening costs for which planners would be indifferent between the two alternatives: that is, both decision inequalities given in Table 11.5 are simultaneously satisfied. The equation for the indifference line is:

$$p_e = 1 - [c_s/(c_t \pi_c s)] \qquad (17)$$

For combinations lying above the indifference line, mass population chemotherapy always dominates, and conversely.

First, suppose that the unit treatment cost, c_t is US$2.00. At that cost, mass population chemotherapy will be preferred at any budget level or prevalence rate if the unit screening cost, c_s, is greater than US$1.71. If the unit screening cost is only US$1.50, mass population chemotherapy will be preferred only if the prevalence rate, p_e, in the eligible fraction exceeds 0.12. But if the unit screening cost drops to only US$0.50, screened population chemotherapy would be preferred at any prevalence

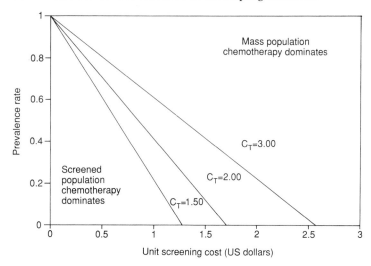

Fig. 11.4 Trade-offs between prevalence and screening costs (mass versus screened population chemotherapy).

rate below 0.70. In general, the lower the screening cost, the higher the prevalence rate required to justify mass population chemotherapy. Conversely, the higher the cost of drug treatment, the lower screening costs will have to be for screened population chemotherapy to be preferable at any given prevalence rate.

Conclusions

The main conclusion of this analysis is that the optimal choice of chemotherapy regime is very sensitive to behavioural and economic parameters which are usually neglected in the consideration of schistosomiasis control strategies. An important implication of the analysis is, therefore, that no single chemotherapy regime is necessarily the best choice in all circumstances. In the absence of a budget constraint, rates of compliance with treatment and screening play an important role in determining the effectiveness of different regimes. When budget constraints are present, as is usually the case, the optimal choice will depend not only on the level of the budget constraint but also on the unit costs of screening and treatment. The lack of attention given to these factors is evident in the virtual absence of published data on, or discussion of, compliance rates and costs in schistosomiasis control programmes. Systematic attention to these factors is a high priority for the future design of cost-effective chemotherapy programmes for schistosomiasis control.

References

Anderson, R. M. and May, R. M. (1982). Population dynamics of human helminth infections: control by chemotherapy. *Nature*, **297**, 557–63.

Korte, R., Schmidt-Ehry, B., Kielmann, A. A., and Brinkmann U. K. (1986). Cost and effectiveness of different approaches to schistosomiasis control in Africa. *Tropical Medicine and Parasitology*, **37**, 149–52.

Polderman, A. M. and Manshande, J. P. (1981). Failure of targeted mass treatment to control schistosomiasis. *Lancet*, i, 27–8.

Prescott N. M. (1979). Schistosomiasis and development. *World Development*, **7**, 1–14.

Prescott N. M. and Warford J. (1983). Economic appraisal in the health sector. In *The economics of health in developing countries*. (ed. K. Lee and A. Mills), pp. 127–45. Oxford University Press.

Rosenfield, P.L., Smith, R. A., and Wolman, M. G. (1977). Development and verification of a schistosomiasis transmission model. *American Journal of Tropical Medicine and Hygiene*, **26**, 505–16.

Warren, K. S. (1981). The control of helminths: nonreplicating infectious agents of man. *Annual Reviews of Public Health*, **2**, 101–15.

Weimer, C. (1987). Optimal disease control through combined use of preventive and curative measures. *Journal of Development Economics*, **25**, 301–19.

WHO (World Health Organization) (1985). *The control of schistosomiasis: report of a WHO Expert Committee*, Technical Report Series No. 728. WHO, Geneva.

Author's note

This chapter is based on an earlier article on 'The economics of schistosomiasis chemotherapy', published in *Parasitology Today*. The views and interpretations expressed are those of the author, and should not be attributed to the World Bank, to its affiliated organizations, or to any individual acting on their behalf.

12

Economic aspects of the production and use of pharmaceuticals: evidence and gaps in research

Susan D. Foster

Introduction

Most developing countries do not have enough of the right drugs in the right places to meet the health needs of their populations. A WHO report estimated that some 2 billion people, nearly half the world's population, have no access to even essential basic drugs (WHO 1988a). The problem is as much one of poor economic and political choices as one of scarcity. Most countries are already spending significant amounts on drugs; but for a number of reasons the shortages persist. That the issue of pharmaceuticals has become highly politicized is not surprising, given that the international market for pharmaceuticals was estimated to be worth $100 billion in 1987, and the pharmaceutical industry is one of the world's most profitable (Wyke 1987). Political considerations often spill over into the economics of pharmaceuticals, and economic analysis is often pressed into the service of political or commercial interests, or used to defend a point of view. The characteristics of the research are sometimes closely linked to the source of its financing. Interest groups which have a stake in any move towards more rational use of drugs in developing countries include the government and ministry of health; the medical profession; the political élite; the pharmaceutical industry; and the industrialized countries (Yudkin 1980).

Much of the field-work done by economists working in teams alongside pharmacists, physicians, and other specialists has found practical application in drug policy. Indeed the Essential Drugs Policy promoted by WHO since 1977 resulted from debate and discussion between economists and medical specialists. An eminent group of experts concluded, to their surprise, that medical needs and the proper use of drugs were consistent with economic rationality.

An interesting case study in the application of economics to drugs policy is provided by Bangladesh. A review of the situation prior to 1982, when a major revision of the drugs policy was undertaken, found that a third of the drugs on the market were useless or even harmful; that the pharmaceutical market was dominated by a few multinational companies; and that some of the multinationals' practices, including incomplete transfer of technology and the charging of inflated prices for raw materials, were detrimental to the economy (Islam 1984). The government set about reviewing every drug on the market, and over a third were withdrawn. Multinationals were no longer permitted to produce 'simple' drugs that could be produced by local firms. Other reforms were introduced that were designed to reduce prices and to introduce rationality into the production and use of drugs. The whole policy was hotly contested, especially by the pharmaceutical industry, and significant pressure was brought to bear on Bangladesh to abandon the policy.

Several years after this controversial policy was implemented, two studies were carried out by groups representing opposite sides. The Pharmaceutical Manufacturers' Association (PMA) of the United States commissioned a study to show that the policy had failed dismally (Jayasuriya 1985). A few months later, the International Organization of Consumers' Unions (IOCU) presented their own study to show that the policy had succeeded admirably (Tiranti 1986). The studies were in agreement that the policy alone did not improve the availability of drugs to the rural population, although this was never a stated goal of the policy. That was the only point of agreement, however. The PMA study focused on the problems with quality control, the smuggling of banned drugs, and continued lack of access to drugs in rural areas. It pointed out the impact on the multinationals, and cited as evidence the 'considerable' losses of $101000 (Glaxo) and of $218000 (Hoechst). But on estimated sales of $12.4 million and $4 million respectively, these losses do not appear to deserve the term 'considerable'. In contrast, the IOCU study pointed out that local producers' share of the market had increased significantly, and the market share of the 45 most essential drugs had increased from 30 per cent to 65 per cent by 1984. Prices for raw materials had dropped by 20–88 per cent. But, most importantly, prices of essential drugs had dropped, in some cases by significant margins (Tiranti 1986). There was, in fact, little evidence that the multinationals had suffered: none had left, and sales had increased, because the market had expanded. One more multinational has since entered the market (WHO 1988a). The Bangladesh experience illustrates the limitations of an essential drugs policy implemented without supporting measures to improve drug access and other measures to strengthen the health system and the drug control authority in particular. It was, however, a courageous and necessary first step, and Bangladesh has provided an example to many countries of what can be done to rationalize drug production and use.

The existing literature on some aspects of drug economics is ample, on others less so. Several useful bibliographies and review articles are available (Mamdani and Walker 1985 and 1986; WHO 1988b). The European Community has looked into the export of pharmaceuticals to developing countries (Banotti 1986), and consumer groups (in both industrialized and developing countries) have examined the practices of the pharmaceutical industry, particularly with regard to exporting, pricing, advertising, and promotion (Chetley 1985). Concerned with the sustainability of their investments, international organizations and donors have focused on policy and financing aspects (World Bank 1987). And in developing countries themselves research has also focused on means of financing drug supplies, pricing policies, and ways of increasing domestic drug production.

The complex chain of events leading a drug from the production site to its prescription and consumption by a patient involves economic choices, either explicit or implicit, at almost every step of the way. After reviewing expenditure on pharmaceuticals, this chapter will consider evidence on six main aspects of drug supply and use: selection and cost-effectiveness considerations; local production; drug prices and procurement; distribution and logistics; prescription and compliance; and financing. The focus of much drugs-related economic research is on the practical application of economics to urgent problems. A special concern is that of equity, which has proved an elusive goal, leading some economists working on drug-supply issues in developing countries to take a normative approach to their work. The economics of the pharmaceutical industry in industrialized countries, and in the more advanced industrializing countries, present a separate set of issues which is beyond the scope of this chapter.

Expenditure on pharmaceuticals

Drug shortages are often ascribed to low spending levels for drugs. Analysts frequently estimate expenditure on drugs as a percentage of health expenditure or as a percentage of GNP, and then assess the expenditure level as 'satisfactory' or 'unsatisfactory.' But essential basic drugs cost the same for a given disease whether the patient is poor or rich. Likewise, annual drug-needs estimates (the figure of $1 per head has been frequently cited) are highly dependent on the number of treatment episodes a person seeks annually, which is in turn influenced by access to health care – a highly variable factor. Furthermore, international drug prices fluctuate. In 1981 UNICEF began tendering for large quantities of bulk generic drugs and publishing the prices it obtained, thereby bringing competition into the field of bulk generic drugs. The resulting prices were as little as a tenth of brand-name equivalents. In the following few years, the strong downward pressure exerted on drug prices resulted in a dramatic change in the pharmaceutical market. UNICEF's tender prices fell by 50 per cent from 1981 to 1985, but then rose again by about 25 per cent in 1986 owing to the fall in the dollar, and by another 25 per cent again in 1987.

How much should be spent on drugs? Evidence on drug costs from Kenya shows that in 1984, at dispensary and health-centre levels, provision of about 40 drugs cost an average of $0.30 per treatment (Ministry of Health, Kenya, DANIDA, SIDA, and WHO 1984). At outpatient facilities in the district and provincial hospitals, drugs cost about $0.50 per average treatment episode in 1985; this included treatment for such chronic diseases as hypertension and diabetes (WHO 1985a). Similar figures have been obtained in Gambia, Morocco, and Benin. It seems that in 1985 an annual expenditure of $1, therefore, would have sufficed for three health-centre or dispensary visits, or two hospital outpatient visits.

Virtually all countries were already spending at least $1 per head on drugs in the mid 1980s, and most spent considerably more (Catsambas and Foster 1986). So, in theory at least, there should be enough money for basic drugs in all but the most desperately poor countries. Why, then, are there never enough drugs available to treat the major diseases? In many countries, under pressure from the economic crisis, health budgets have stagnated. Few governments found themselves able to reduce the intake of new medical and nursing graduates. It is even more difficult to reduce expenditure on existing personnel; growth or preservation of the share of personnel in the budget has often been at the expense of allocations for drugs and supplies, which have at best remained stagnant in real terms. With inflation and population growth, public-sector drug availability per person has declined steadily in many countries.

Other factors have aggravated an already difficult situation, and prevented countries from making the best use of available funds. First of all, many countries are buying the wrong drugs, or not enough of the drugs needed for their health problems. Secondly, procurement is done very poorly, and many countries pay too much for the drugs they buy, either from overseas suppliers or from inefficient and heavily protected local industry. Thirdly, in many countries the distribution of available drugs is inefficient and inequitable, with virtually none reaching the rural health facilities which serve the majority of the population. Fourthly, inefficient prescription and poor compliance by patients further reduce the benefit from available drugs. And finally, in some countries foreign exchange problems and reliance on donated drugs have made rational procurement impossible. These problems will be reviewed in sequence.

Selection of drugs and cost-effectiveness considerations

In 1975 the World Health Assembly called upon the WHO to advise member states on the selection and procurement of essential drugs, and a committee met in 1977 to draw up the first Model List of Essential Drugs (WHO 1977). The report of that committee noted that 'cost represents a major selection criterion'. Some 90 per cent of the drugs selected for the Model List were older drugs whose safety and efficacy had been proved, and whose patents had expired. Even cimetidine, now recognized as a truly valuable new drug, was excluded from that first list on the grounds that data on the safety of long-term use were lacking. At about the same time, an important article on the cost-effectiveness of drug therapy appeared: on the basis of experience in a developing country, the author argued that Western prescribing habits were extravagant and wasteful, especially in low-income countries, and that cost should be one of the factors to be considered in making a therapeutic decision (Speight 1975).

While the cost of drugs has received more attention recently, considerations of low cost are often confused with cost-effectiveness. Evidence on compliance, ease of use, and mode of administration, in addition to the price of the drug, needs to be more fully included in comparisons of drug therapies. In a West African country, for the treatment of urinary tract infections preference was given to sulphadimidine, a 'cheap' antibiotic, over cotrimoxazole, a relatively more expensive drug. However, although the course of treatment with sulphadimidine cost slightly less, it required 86 tablets to be taken. Good compliance under such a regimen cannot be expected of a semi-literate (or even a literate) patient. Study of the cost-effectiveness of pharmaceuticals, through comparisons either between different drugs or between drug and non-drug therapies, remains a neglected area, even in major disease-control programmes, where a change of drug can have a major impact on costs and benefits. A review of over a hundred cost-effectiveness studies of parasitic disease-control programmes found only a few studies which compared the cost-effectiveness of a given drug therapy with that of other control measures; and only seven which compared different drug treatments (or routes of administration) for a given disease (Barlow and Grobar 1986).

Cost-effectiveness studies done for tuberculosis control demonstrate the potential value of this type of analysis. It is, of course, most useful where the different drug therapy regimens produce comparable results. One study of alternatives for tuberculosis control in a southern African country showed that the more expensive drugs (rifampicin or ethambutol) used in shorter outpatient regimens would result in a lower cost per case effectively treated than would a regimen using cheaper drugs (thiacetazone and isoniazid), because of improved compliance, elimination of the need for hospitalization, and improved case-holding (Barnum 1986).

Once drugs and standard treatments have been determined, it is possible to quantify drug needs and to estimate the overall cost: this figure can then serve as a basis for budgeting. WHO has developed a methodology to estimate drug needs on the basis of carefully selected drugs, standardized treatment schedules, past consumption patterns, and epidemiological data (WHO 1988c). The validity of such estimates depends on prescribers adhering to the treatment schedules, which in turn requires that the drugs should be made available. Countries are making efforts to inform prescribers about the cost of the drugs they prescribe, and to implement standardized treatment schedules.

Domestic drug production

The developing countries' share of world drug production is still relatively small – under 12 per cent in 1982. They imported 32 per cent of the world's total imports, or about $4.5 billion worth, while they exported only about $600 million, or 4.4 per cent of the world total. They represent an important export market for industrialized countries' pharmaceuticals (*Scrip* 1985). Faced with seemingly endless dependence on the industrialized countries for drug supply, most developing countries have attempted some form of local production or formulation of finished dosage forms from imported intermediates. However, only a few (India, China, Mexico, Brazil, Argentina, and Egypt) have achieved a high level of independent local production, defined by UNIDO as the local manufacture of intermediates and production of the plant and equipment required.

Local production is an area where political considerations have frequently overshadowed economic ones. Since economic analysis relies on forecasting future trends, uncertainty is a major problem, and this provides all the more reason to be particularly prudent in estimating economic parameters and avoiding bias that is encouraged by political considerations. UNIDO and bilateral donors in the past financed a number of plants which have turned out to be only marginally economic. Many factories are operating at 10–20 per cent of capacity, unable to sell their products on even their domestic market. A major constraint has been management: running a modern pharmaceutical plant requires technical and managerial skills which are scarce in developing countries. Furthermore, the decision to begin local production was frequently made on the basis of faulty economic assumptions.

Domestically produced products were expected to replace brand-name imports, and it was assumed that they would simply displace the imported brand-name drugs. Therefore, if feasibility studies were carried out, the reference price used to analyse whether local production would be economic was that of the brand-name drug. Before 1980, there was little trade in generic drugs, and consequently there were no international benchmark prices. With the growth of the institutional market led by UNICEF's competitive tenders, generic drug prices declined by about 50 per cent in US dollar terms between 1980 and 1985. While this was a godsend to poor countries, who could benefit from very low prices for basic drugs, it put great pressure on marginal local production units, which sometimes could not buy the raw materials for the prices of the finished products offered on the international market. Domestic products not only were no cheaper than imported drugs; they often failed to displace the brand-name imports because they were perceived to be of lower quality.

A second common assumption was that local production would save foreign exchange. In many countries, the main local input is unskilled labour – virtually everything else is imported. But pharmaceutical production is not labour-intensive. Raw materials, moreover, are only one part of the foreign exchange component of a drug. Packing materials are often imported, as is the machinery used for production, spare parts, repair services, quality-control equipment, and maintenance. Training of staff abroad and expatriate manpower may be required. Technology must often be purchased in the form of patent and licence fees; transfer prices may be a further source of leakage of foreign exchange. An effective export strategy requires advertising, and a network of distribution points and agents must be developed; these too must be paid for in foreign exchange. Even electricity production and water purification may require imported fuel. The case for foreign exchange savings, therefore, is not as clear as it might first appear.

A third assumption was that pharmaceutical chemicals – raw materials and intermediates – would be cheaper than finished products, and would be readily available to developing-country manufacturers. But production of most pharmaceutical chemicals is highly concentrated; intermediates for some of even the most common drugs are produced by only four or five suppliers. A UNIDO study found that 10 of 26 essential drugs studied were manufactured by six or fewer firms at one or more stages in their production process (PAHO 1984). Quantities required by small developing-country firms are often so small that suppliers simply ignore the order; these small firms lack the power to negotiate a good price. They may pay more for the intermediates than they would for the finished product procured through a competitive tender. Unlike prices for finished products, international price information on pharmaceutical chemicals is difficult to obtain, and, as a result, countries may pay significantly more than they need to.

Larger countries have a different problem, in that they often have subsidiaries of multinational companies operating on their territory. The subsidiaries are often required to buy raw materials and intermediates from the parent company or from another subsidiary. The 'transfer price' which then applies may be excessive. Where the product is internationally traded, there is evidence that transfer prices are substantially higher than the world market price. The Colombian government estimated that the weighted average of overpricing for a range of imports between 1967 and 1970 was 155 per cent of the international price; for individual products the overpricing was up to 6500 per cent. In Mexico, a hormone (progesterone) was imported by one firm at $2490 per kg and exported by another firm at $110 per kg (UNCTC 1983). Transfer prices were a major factor in the decision of the Bangladesh government to implement its new drug policy in 1982 (Islam 1984). Wider dissemination of price information for pharmaceutical chemicals would assist developing countries to produce more economically by allowing even small plants to negotiate better prices for raw materials and intermediates.

A fourth assumption that many countries made was the possibility of drug exports. In Africa, for example, several countries established local production facilities with the idea of exporting to their neighbours, while many of those neighbours were thinking along the same lines and creating similar facilities. In other countries, preferences for established brand-name drugs from Europe were so strong that lower prices were not enough to secure a share of the market. Some countries have reached an unhappy compromise by producing drugs of questionable therapeutic value for their domestic market.

Uncertainty is inherent in feasibility studies. But sound economic analysis of the realistic possibilities of local production still has much to contribute in assisting countries to make the best use of their resources. Research is needed to help countries find the best entry points into pharmaceutical production, and to decide what to do with uneconomic production units. Countries need better advice than they are currently getting from international organizations and the international financial community; short-term economic feasibility considerations, based on a somewhat static 'snapshot' view of an economy, need to be balanced with long-term, but realistic, industrial development goals.

Drug prices and procurement

The price-differential between branded and generic drugs is considerable. One study found that, on average, the prices of branded products were 10 times those of the generic equivalent (Szuba 1986a). The purchase of branded drugs in some developing countries is responsible for the observed drug shortages. Costs of production typically account for about 40 per cent of the ex-factory cost of drugs; distribution and promotion for 17 per cent; and research, for 10 per cent (Cooper and Culyer, cited in Patel 1983). One author estimates, however, that for branded drugs the costs of production account for 10 per cent, and for generic products, closer to 70 per cent of the ex-factory price including profit (Szuba 1986a). In fact, raw-material price information shows that generic finished products are often priced relatively close to the costs of production, while brand-name drug prices are determined by market conditions (WHO 1984). There is no international price for brand-name drugs, and prices vary considerably from country to country. Prices of the same branded drug produced by the same manufacturer and sold on different European markets and in the United States vary by an average factor of 1 to 5 (Szuba 1986b). Furthermore, prices of a single product may vary on a given market by a wide margin. In Thailand, 60 different forms of ampicillin were on the market; the highest price was more than 17 times the lowest available price (Sepulveda-Alvarez 1985).

Until 1981, when UNICEF published the results of its tenders, price information for generic drugs was not widely available. The main source of information on branded drugs was the drug manufacturers themselves. It was difficult for a procurement agency to know whether it was paying a fair price; and this created opportunities for corruption. Yet the availability of information alone has not been sufficient to change procurement habits, and countries continue to spend more than they need on drugs. Partly this is the result of many years of habit and of pressure from the medical profession, the pharmaceutical industry, and the industrialized countries. Reliance on established supply sources, often from the former colonial power, may be reinforced by currency arrangements such as prevail in French-speaking West Africa. The CFA franc is fully convertible with regard to transactions in France and other CFA franc countries, and is pegged to the French franc at a fixed rate; but countries outside the franc zone and France are considered 'foreign'. Conversion to other currencies involves a lengthy procedure plus payment of a commission. The dissuasive effect of such controls can be significant. In Mali, for example, a study showed that a large percentage of the drugs budget was spent on ampicillin; at one health centre, it accounted for 30 per cent of the total health-centre drugs budget. Yet the government continued to procure a French brand of ampicillin at a retail price of about $1 per vial; a generic equivalent could have been procured elsewhere for less than $0.20 (ex-factory). Allowing 100 per cent for shipping and handling, the price would still have been only $0.40. This centre could have saved up to 15 per cent of its drug budget if it had purchased a generic equivalent form of ampicillin (WHO 1985*b*).

Procurement of drugs provides many opportunities for private gain at public expense, and corruption may explain many observed drug shortages. Yudkin was one of the first to describe the mechanism of corruption and its effect on the health services (Yudkin 1980). Van der Geest approached the problem of corruption from an anthropologist's viewpoint, and drew attention to the interests preventing a change in the system (van der Geest 1982). Corruption may explain the continued reluctance to purchase generic drugs in some countries; generic manufacturers operate on a thin profit margin that leaves no scope for payment of bribes. In one country, a company had bribed procurement officials to purchase quantities of the company's brand-name drugs which would have sufficed for 10–13 years of normal consumption. In another country, 46 years' supply of a drug had been purchased (Yudkin 1980). Clearly, such practices make it impossible to buy enough drugs with a limited budget.

Distribution and logistics

Once the drugs have been procured and delivered, problems of storage and distribution to health facilities arise. Drugs have specific characteristics which call for special storage and handling.

They are high-value, low-bulk items, and their 'portability' makes special security measures essential. They are fragile and have a limited life, so good stock-management techniques and storage conditions are needed. Drugs continue to have market value (as distinct from therapeutic value) even after they have expired, since they can be removed from the packaging which indicates the date of expiry. Proper disposal of expired stocks is therefore essential. And finally, special knowledge is required to use them properly; improper use can be dangerous and, in some cases, fatal.

Storage and management have been neglected in the past, resulting in such anomalies as $1 million worth of expired drugs on the shelves of a drug agency in a low-income West African country, and storage of valuable stocks under leaky roofs or even outdoors. The wastage which results constitutes a severe drain of resources. Other countries have their funds tied up in excessive inventories of slow-moving drugs, while fast-moving drugs are out of stock because of shortage of funds.

Distribution poses a different set of problems. Where drugs are scarce, a common difficulty is that available drugs 'stick' at higher levels, where politically influential people are more likely to be treated. This is especially true in health facilities that are used as drug depots and on-shipping points; health staff keep what they need, and send what may be left over down to the next level. One African country had a national per capita drug expenditure of $1.20. At the national teaching hospital, however, the average expenditure was $9 per patient – in the general medical wards, expenditure was $5.90 per patient, but for private patients and senior officials, it was $13. It could not be shown that more serious conditions requiring more costly drugs accounted for this discrepancy. More disturbing was the fact that in the rural dispensaries only $0.02 was spent per patient (Yudkin 1980).

Another widespread problem is pilferage; some estimates are that as many as 70 per cent of drugs are diverted (WHO 1987a). Pilferage of drugs is not only a waste of public resources and an indication of the scarcity value of drugs, but a significant source of income for health staff in many countries. When the parallel market is a thriving and profitable one, incentives for improving logistics are removed, and the possibility that staff may deliberately resist improvements must be dealt with (van der Geest 1982).

The debate over the public versus private provision of health services has been carried over into the question of drugs distribution, with a major industry which depends heavily on the private consumption of drugs in developed countries weighing in on the side of 'privatization'. As health-care costs have risen in the public sector, pressure has grown for cost-containment measures, such as limited lists of drugs, which are seen as a threat by the 'research-based' pharmaceutical industry. In the private sector, where costs are borne by consumers or by insurance companies which simply pass on their costs, cost-containment is more difficult to organize and implement. Especially in developing countries, problems with public-sector distribution channels have led some observers to conclude that the private sector is more efficient, and there has been a gradual privatization of the drug-supply function in a number of countries. Some have made it part of an explicit policy, promoted by the World Bank and International Monetary Fund, to divest the government of government-owned and parastatal enterprises, including those responsible for drug importation and distribution. In other countries, it has become the tacit policy of a government that is unable to provide drugs within its budgetary constraints, yet for political reasons cannot reverse a policy of free drugs.

Privatization is a superficially attractive solution. In fact, however, the two sectors have different objectives; the public sector is charged with providing low-cost drugs to all persons who need them, regardless of income, status, or place of residence, and is at least nominally concerned with equity. The private sector, in contrast, is not burdened with such expectations, and simply sells drugs to those who can pay. Prices charged in private pharmacies are often extremely high, and a comparison of costs per tablet delivered might call into question the efficiency of the private sector.

Furthermore, the private sector in developing countries rarely provides low-cost drugs in remote areas. In most of West Africa, for example, almost all the private pharmacies are in the capital cities and larger towns. Incentives would be needed to induce them to extend their services to remote areas and to people with low purchasing power, and to carry a line of low-cost essential drugs. In Norway, for instance, special remuneration is provided by the government to pharmacists established in rural areas with low turnover (WHO 1987*b*). No adequate assessment has been made of the cost of the shift to private-sector distribution in terms of equity and access of the poorest income-groups to low-cost drugs; nor of the efficiency of such a shift.

Some observers have recommended that drugs should be distributed through commercial channels such as market traders. But not all drugs could be safely distributed in this way, without prescription or medical guidance. Turning over part of the distribution to private-sector traders would thus solve only part of the problem. In some cases self-medication, especially when it involves antibiotics, can be dangerous; so, while this solution may save money for patients and reduce the burden on health services, it also carries a number of risks (Fassin 1986).

Much of the developing world's population turns first to traditional medicine, especially for the cure of illnesses that are not perceived as serious (Ladinsky *et al*. 1987). Some very interesting sociological and anthropological work has been done in this area; but its economic importance remains to be fully explored, as does its potential role in drug distribution.

The public-sector system can be made to work. Storage and distribution of drugs require good planning to prevent shortages and oversupply of limited-life drugs. Up-to-date management techniques are now being applied to drug-supply issues (MSH 1981). One example is the concept of a 'pipeline', useful to visualize the flow of drugs through a supply system: the diameter is the volume of consumption per month, and the length is the time between commitment of funds and availability of proceeds to purchase more drugs. It is possible to quantify and cost the drugs needed to fill the pipeline and prevent shortages (Cross *et al*. 1986).

Another technique is the 'kit system' developed in Kenya and now in use in Tanzania and several other countries, which has proved especially useful in limiting wastage and pilferage. It involves careful selection of drugs and estimation of needs on the basis of past consumption and patient-load. On a regular basis, each health centre receives a sealed carton containing the drugs it will need for a specific number of patients or length of time (Moore 1982). The kit is shipped, unopened, to the final destination, and is designed to make it easy to determine whether it has been opened en route. Responsibility for on-shipping is clearly determined, and it is possible to detect where breaks in the kit occurred. The system has reduced pilferage and waste from an estimated 25 per cent to around 5 per cent (Ministry of Health, Kenya, DANIDA, SIDA, and WHO 1984).

Prescription practices

Drug prescription in developing countries is often characterized by excessive and inappropriate prescribing. Drugs may be prescribed which are not necessary for the condition, or too many drugs are prescribed (WHO 1987*b*). Typical prescriptions in developing countries include 5 or more drugs; in Mali a prescription survey found as many as 10 or 12 drugs were routinely prescribed per prescription, which would cost some 10–15 per cent of the annual per capita income. Sometimes the same generic drug was included under several different brand names; it was not clear that the prescriber was aware that they were the same drug. Often the drug prescribed does not correspond with the diagnosis, or is simply ineffective for the diagnosis. A study carried out in Ghana found that prescriptions contained an average of 3.9 items, and that 96 per cent of visits received at least one injection, in most cases either an antimalarial injection or penicillin. When compared with 'best practice' prescriptions, the cost of the actual prescriptions was over 3 times that of the appropriate prescription (Barnett *et al.* 1980).

The reasons for this situation include the limited diagnostic equipment available to many prescribers, and the fact that objective information is often not available. Patients often demand, or are perceived by the prescriber to demand, a large number of drugs. Prescribers yield to pressure from patients to prescribe drugs other than the ones medically indicated; a common example is the use of injectible preparations where oral preparations (or no drug at all) would have been appropriate. Furthermore, prescribers often do not have the time (or fail to take the time) to assess the patients adequately. Data from an East African country indicated that only 45 per cent of patients were actually examined, and the diagnosis was correct in 64 per cent of cases. The prescription was correct in 85 per cent of those cases. Only 30 per cent of the patients were judged to have been correctly managed. Although the study did not measure compliance, it is likely to have been low as well, since only 23 per cent of patients were told anything about the drug they were prescribed (Ministry of Health, Tanzania, UNICEF, and AMREF 1985).

Prescription drugs are different from other goods in that it is often neither the seller (the pharmacist or dispenser) nor the buyer (the patient) who makes the decision about which product to buy and what price to pay, but rather a third person (the prescriber) who makes this decision. The industry directs major efforts at the prescriber in order to create demand for prescription drugs, using medical journals, meetings, promotional travel, and gifts. The information that industry provides to prescribers is often incomplete. Contraindications and side-effects may be downplayed, while sometimes exaggerated claims of efficacy are made.

In industrialized countries there is a specific, separate group of products which are authorized to be sold without prescription 'over the counter' (OTC). Demand-creation for these products is focused on consumers themselves, and the primary means used is advertising in the form of radio spots, posters, etc. In developing countries, however, the distinction between prescription and OTC drugs is blurred, and in some of them virtually all drugs are available without prescription, including drugs which have been withdrawn from the international market for safety reasons. The prescriber's role is limited in such a situation.

Prescribers may also (perhaps unintentionally) reduce their own importance in the prescription process. A prescriber who fails to take account of the patient's economic situation, or of the prices of drugs, may write a prescription which is too expensive for the patient. Similarly, a patient may feel that the time or other costs of waiting for health care are excessive, and bypass health facilities altogether by going directly to a private pharmacy (Igun 1987). In both cases, either the patient himself or the storekeeper, who often has no training or qualifications, decides which drug to administer. To some extent self-medication of this type is 'poor man's health care'. In Thailand, it was found that, as people's incomes rose, not only did demand for health services rise, but there was a consumption shift as well: households substituted professional health care for self-treatment with drugs (Myers *et al.* 1985). Another study, however, found a negative correlation between GNP per capita and the rate of use of a medical doctor for childhood diarrhoea (John Snow Inc. 1986). Poor mothers tended to visit a physician first, perhaps because the children were already quite ill when mothers decided to seek treatment.

Compliance with drug therapy

Patient compliance with therapy – the extent to which the patient follows instructions about taking the medicines prescribed – has not been thoroughly investigated in developing countries, except in the context of disease-control programmes for leprosy and tuberculosis. Major efforts are put into getting drugs to where they are needed, with the assumption being that the patient will do the rest. However, studies from industrialized countries show that an average compliance rate of about 50 per cent is not unusual. It is unlikely, given overprescription, low literacy rates, conflicting beliefs about Western medicine, poor packaging, and lack of communication between prescriber and patient, that compliance in developing countries is better than 50 per cent. It may be significantly worse. In the Dominican Republic, the average length of the physician–patient encounter was 3 minutes; the study concluded that compliance was perhaps less than 25 per cent (Ugalde *et al.* 1986). A study of mothers' responses to childhood diarrhoea in five countries found that 75 per cent of mothers who had been prescribed medicine other than the easily recognizable oral rehydration salts were unable to say what drug had been prescribed for their child, or how to use it (John Snow Inc. 1986). In a leprosy control project in India, only 30 per cent of doses were taken as prescribed (G. Ellard, personal communication 1986). When attractive drugs are provided free to destitute patients, the patient may prefer to sell some or all of the medication rather than consume it as the prescriber intended; non-compliance becomes an income-generating behaviour. The economic rationality of this behaviour is clear, especially considering the benefit a destitute leprosy patient might obtain from the proceeds.

If little is known about patients' compliance in developing countries, even less is known about the economic consequences. If diagnosis and prescription are correct in 80 per cent of cases, dispensing is correct in a further 80 per cent of those cases, and patients' compliance is 50 per cent on average, the likelihood that the treatment objective (control, cure, prophylaxis, or relief) will be attained is just over 30 per cent ($0.8 \times 0.8 \times 0.5 = 0.32$). The economic costs of the 70 per cent of cases for whom the treatment objective was not attained are significant, and include resources wasted on health facilities, staff time, and drugs. Non-compliance can also lead to re-treatment with more expensive drugs, spread of infection and treatment of new cases, and the need to develop new antibiotics and anti-infectives to keep up with patterns of resistance. These costs are seldom taken into account – which is virtually tantamount to assuming compliance to be 100 per cent. One study which did link compliance with other economic parameters found that compliance significantly influenced the outcome of treatment (Barnum 1986).

More research is needed into causes of poor compliance in developing countries, means of improvement, and the costs of non-compliance. Promising areas would include measures to improve information exchange between the patient, the prescriber, and the pharmacist or dispenser. Research into simplification and shortening of treatment regimens, provision of information to patients, and reduction of the economic obstacles to compliance through rational prescribing and an improved availability of low-cost drugs could also make a significant contribution to improved compliance.

Financing and foreign exchange considerations

If the most important of the economic aspects of rational drug use has been left to last, it was to show that significant improvements in the efficiency, and equity, of drug supply are still possible. Much recent research has focused on 'paying for health'; but too often existing possibilities for reducing costs are neglected. This has left the impression that cost-recovery is the only option open to governments wishing to improve resource availability. Yet changes in resource allocation and use can significantly increase the availability of resources. Only when such improvements are being implemented should cost-recovery be envisaged: emphasis should be placed on improving the system before asking people to pay for inefficiency and waste.

Equity

Discussions of financing and cost-recovery always raise – but seldom answer – the question of equity. Little is known about how user charges affect the poorest income-groups. The World Bank has recently suggested that a 'modest' fee would be 1 per cent of annual income, which should suffice for two annual visits (World Bank 1987). Another point of reference may be what people have paid in the past, and thereby demonstrated themselves 'willing' to pay. But people often make expenditures on drugs in what are perceived (rightly or wrongly) to be life-or-death situations. Since economic barriers to seeking care are greater for poor people, they may tend to delay seeking care until the situation really is life-threatening. They may go into debt or sell important possessions (cattle, etc.) in order to purchase drugs and medical care in an emergency. 'Willingness to pay' data, therefore, must be used carefully, with the understanding that the poorer the person, the more likely it is that the expenditure recorded reflects an extraordinary situation, and cannot be taken to represent an amount he or she would be willing (or able) to pay on a regular basis. Special caution must be exercised when using such data to predict revenues from fees or utilization of routine health services when fees are introduced.

The considerable inequality of income-distribution patterns in many developing countries, with income highly concentrated in the upper 10 per cent or 20 per cent of the population, is another cause for concern when setting a fee. Data for nine low-income countries showed that on average, the top quintile (i.e. the richest 20 per cent of the population) had about 52 per cent of total income; the second quintile, 20 per cent; the third quintile, 12 per cent; the fourth quintile, 10 per cent; and the lowest quintile, 6 per cent (World Bank 1985). Taking for illustrative purposes a West African country where average per capita income was estimated at $170, if income distribution followed this pattern, the lowest income quintile would have an average per capita income of $50. Roughly half the population would have less than $100 per year, and the highest quintile would have about $425. If the World Bank proposal were adopted in setting the fee, the level would be set at $1.70 for two visits. Imposition of such a fee would represent over 3 per cent of per capita income for the lowest quintile, but only about 0.4 per cent for the highest quintile. Furthermore, per capita income usually includes goods which are not traded (such as home-consumed produce), and thus are not converted into cash; but user fees must usually be paid in cash. Again, this is likely to hit hardest at the lowest-income groups, who engage in subsistence agriculture.

Time costs, travel expenses, and lost income are other costs which are often not taken into account. Each visit for which a theoretical 0.5 per cent of income would be charged could easily represent a much higher percentage of income when travel costs, loss of a day's wages, and other factors are taken into account. A final equity consideration is that in many countries even the poor pay taxes, often calculated as a proportion of income – the proportion remaining the same regardless of income level; taxes therefore, although neutral in impact, impose a heavy burden on poorer groups, who spend a high proportion of their income on essentials such as food, shelter, and medical care (WHO 1984). User fees imposed at lower-level health facilities which are not intended to cover the cost of drugs are in part supplementing the salaries of government employees, for which people have already paid taxes, and are therefore highly inequitable. Further operational research into how equity considerations can be accommodated within cost-recovery schemes is urgently needed.

Some experience with drug-financing schemes

Financing schemes for drugs can be classified into three basic types. The first exists at local level, where it often takes the form of community drug funds or banks. The second type, implemented usually on a national scale, involves direct user charges in health facilities, to be paid at the time of receiving care. These charges include prescription fees, fees-for-service, and laboratory fees. A third type involves shifting the burden of payment in time, either to before or to after the illness episode; it may also involve spreading the risk over a larger number of people. A range of alternative mechanisms has been designed for this approach to financing drug supplies, including insurance schemes, excise taxes, and lotteries.

There are many examples of community financing schemes, often started with external donor support and technical assistance (Carrin 1987). Some have been quite successful; one example is the Bhojpur drug scheme in Nepal. The mechanism often used is a revolving fund, which is to recover all costs associated with the running of the scheme and permit replacement of the drugs; these schemes have been amply documented, and excellent guidelines are available (Cross *et al.* 1986; MSH 1981). Common pitfalls include lack of support (or active opposition) from interest groups such as private pharmacists. Authoritarian governments may oppose community-based drug-supply initiatives, which can catalyse community action around other issues (Foster and Drager 1988). Lack of management experience and poor control over funds plague even successful programmes: in Thailand, community drug banks were started in 18000 villages, yet a detailed survey could account for less than half, and not all were operating at a satisfactory level (Myers *et al*. 1985).

Experience with user fees in government facilities is less well-documented, partly because political resistance to charging for health care is only now diminishing, and such policies are relatively new in many countries. Since it is politically difficult to introduce fees in urban areas, they are often introduced first in rural areas. This is not only inequitable, since urban hospitals primarily serve higher-income populations, but also inefficient, since charges in low-income areas often reduce utilization, with resulting high collection costs relative to fee income. In Indonesia, a study concluded that the cost-recovery scheme was inequitable (Meesook 1983). Poorer households received less than their share of health-care subsidies, since they used lower-level facilities more, where cost-recovery through user charges was higher (12 per cent of overall costs at hospital level, 39 per cent at public health-centre level). Despite having paid a fee of 150 Rp (US$0.25), which was supposed to include drugs, they frequently had to pay more for the drugs or buy them elsewhere. The average direct cost of a health-centre visit was found to be Rp 209; the average daily per capita income was Rp 202. Transportation costs and loss of income for patients were not included. Use of facilities may fall off sharply when fees are introduced. In Nigeria's Imo State, steep fees were introduced before the quality of services was improved, and drugs were still unavailable despite the fees; the result was severe underutilization of the health services (Attah 1986).

Other approaches have been tried, especially in Latin America, to finance the basic drugs needed for the poorest segments of the population. Examples are lotteries, earmarked taxes on alcohol and tobacco, taxes on casino revenues, etc. These too may be somewhat regressive in impact, but it seems unlikely that the very poor are able to spend significant amounts of their income on alcohol, tobacco, or casino gambling; although the case for high expenditure by the poor on lotteries could probably be made. The concern about regressivity might be mitigated by the fact that participation in these activities is voluntary (unlike user fees, for example), and, if properly administered, such a scheme would be one of the few mechanisms which ensure that the funds recovered from the poor are really spent on benefits for the poor.

Foreign exchange considerations

Drug shortages are often attributed to foreign exchange scarcity; but drug imports must be kept in perspective in relation to other imports. Typically, drugs do not account for a significant share of imports when compared with other items such as fuel and food-grains: drugs accounted for less than 2 per cent of imports in 60 per cent of 97 countries studied, and less than 3 per cent of imports in 90 per cent of the countries studied (WHO 1984).

There is no 'magic bullet' when it comes to solving the problem of foreign exchange for drug imports. Domestic drug production is not always the answer. It is a question of establishing and respecting priorities, planning for and justifying foreign exchange needs, and striking a balance between expenditure for basic essential drugs and for less essential products and cosmetics. The ministry of health must co-ordinate its efforts with the ministry of finance, and health authorities must rationalize their foreign exchange expenditure on drugs and plan carefully. When Zimbabwe presented a carefully quantified and costed list of needed drugs to the financial authorities, it received authorization for the entire foreign exchange requirement. Procurement officials must seek out the best price through efficient procurement. The ministry of finance, in turn, is responsible for supporting these efforts by making required foreign exchange available when needed, and ensuring that the basic drug needs of the public sector are met. International competitive bidding – the most advantageous method of procurement – is out of the question unless the ministry of finance undertakes to make the necessary foreign exchange available. It is especially important for the public sector to avoid the need for emergency purchases from local traders who have had access to foreign exchange, since their prices are typically as much as three times the international market price (Catsambas and Foster 1986).

Drug donations and tied supplier credits pose particular problems. Donations are often made of useless drugs, or drugs close to their expiry date. In almost all cases they are overvalued. In some countries the drug agency must pay customs fees (in some countries as much as 35 per cent of the declared value of the donation) and port handling charges (typically 5–10 per cent of their value). Tied credits impose constraints on which products may be purchased and what prices are paid; and prices are often excessive. In one West African country which relies heavily on donations and tied credits, donated drugs and those purchased with tied credits cost up to 9 times the prevailing international prices. In addition, in this country, some 40 per cent of the drugs budget was transferred to other parts of the government in the form of port fees, bank fees, and customs duties.

Foreign exchange auctions instituted under adjustment programmes may have a negative impact on public-sector drug supplies in countries where the public sector competes with private-sector importers on the same terms. Private-sector bidders can simply pass on their extra costs to their consumers, who are often wealthier than the patients who must rely on public health services. The public sector does not usually have the option of passing its costs straight on, and the result is a decline in the availability of drugs. Research is needed to assess the impact of adjustment programmes and to find ways in which economic reforms can be made compatible with improving the health status of the majority of the population.

Conclusion

Much remains to be done to rationalize the production, purchase, and use of drugs. Good economic research is needed to help decision-makers select from the available options for rationalization, and improve efficiency without sacrificing equity. The advent of AIDS, a new disease which will consume large amounts of scarce health resources in many countries, adds urgency to research into ways of improving the use of existing resources. Promising areas would be the conditions under which domestic production of drugs can contribute to economic development; pricing issues and ways to lower costs and improve procurement of both finished products and raw materials; improved distribution and incentives for improving logistics in both public and private sectors; and cost-effective ways to rationalize prescription and improve compliance. Another set of issues relates to cost-recovery and the financing of drugs; how can additional funds be generated without discouraging use by the most disadvantaged groups in society? The impact of different financing approaches on the availability of drugs for poor people needs to be assessed, as well as the impact of privatization on health. Important variables such as the distance to the nearest private drug outlet, its price levels and range of products, and the availability of low-cost generic drugs need to be included in any assessment.

Powerful interests are involved in virtually all aspects of the production and use of drugs. Economically rational decisions are not always taken as soon as convincing evidence is available; but the clear trend is in the direction of more rational use of drugs. Additional evidence provided by economic research could do much to speed the pace of change.

References

Attah, E. B. (1986). *Underutilization of public sector health facilities in Imo State, Nigeria*, PHN Technical Note 86–1. World Bank, Washington, DC.

Banotti, M. (rapporteur) (1986). *Report on the export of pharmaceutical products from the European Community to the countries of the Third World*. European Parliament doc. A 2–36/86, Brussels.

Barlow, R. and Grobar, L. M. (1986). *Costs and benefits of controlling parasitic diseases*, PHN Technical Note 85–17. World Bank, Washington, DC.

Barnett, A., Creese, A. L., and Ayivor, E. C. K. (1980). The economics of pharmaceutical policy in Ghana. *International Journal of Health Services*, 10(3), 479–99.

Barnum, H. (1986). Cost savings from alternative treatments for tuberculosis. *Social Science and Medicine*, 23(9), 847–50.

Carrin, G. (1987). Community financing of drugs in sub-Saharan Africa. *International Journal of Health Planning and Management*, 2, 125–45.

Catsambas, T. and Foster, S. D. (1986). Spending money sensibly: the case of essential drugs. *Finance and Developement*, 23, 29–32.

Chetley, A. (1985). *Cleared for export: an examination of the European Community's chemical and pharmaceutical trade*. Coalition against Dangerous Exports, London.

Cross, P. N., Huff, M. A., Quick, J. D., and Bates, J. A. (1986). Revolving drug funds: conducting business in the public sector. *Social Science and Medicine*, 22, 335–43.

Fassin, D. (1986). La vente illicite des médicaments au Senegal: conséquences pour la santé des populations. *Bulletin de la Societé de Pathologie Exotique*, 79, 557–70.

Foster, S. D. and Drager, N. (1988). How community drug sales schemes may succeed. *World Health Forum*, 9(2), 200–6.

Igun, U. A. (1987). Why we seek treatment here: retail pharmacy and clinical practice in Maiduguri, Nigeria. *Social Science and Medicine*, **24**, 689–95.

Islam, N. (1984). On a national drug policy for Bangladesh. *Tropical Doctor*, **14**, 3–7.

Jayasuriya, D. C. (1985). *The public health and economic dimension of the new drug policy of Bangladesh*. Pharmaceutical Manufacturers Association, Washington, DC.

John Snow Inc. (1986). *Report on a knowledge, attitude, and practice survey of mothers, physicians, and pharmacists in 5 developing countries: use of anti-diarrhoeal drugs and infant formula*. John Snow Inc., Boston.

Ladinsky, J. L., Volk, N. D., and Robinson, M. (1987). The influence of traditional medicine in shaping medical care practices in Vietnam today. *Social Science and Medicine*, **25**(10), 1105–10.

Mamdani, M. and Walker, G. (1985). *Essential drugs and developing countries: a review and selected annotated bibliography*. Evaluation and Planning Centre, London School of Hygiene and Tropical Medicine.

Mamdani, M. and Walker, G. (1986). Essential drugs in the developing world. *Health Policy and Planning*, **1**, 187–201.

Meesook, O. A. (1983). *Financing and equity in the social sectors in Indonesia*, CPD Discussion Paper no. 1983–5. World Bank, Washington, DC.

Ministry of Health, Kenya, DANIDA, SIDA, and WHO (1984). *Evaluation of management of drug supplies to rural health facilities in Kenya*. The Ministry, Nairobi.

Ministry of Health, Tanzania, UNICEF, and AMREF (African Medical and Research Foundation) (1985). *Tanzania essential drugs programme: report of a study on patient management, essential drugs, and equipment supplies in rural health facilities: summary of findings* (unpublished).

Moore, G. D. (1982). Essential drugs for Kenya's rural population. *World Health Forum*, **3**, 196–9.

MSH (Management Sciences for Health) (1981). *Managing drug supply*, MSH, Boston.

Myers, C. N., Mongkolsmai, D., and Causino, N. (1985). *Financing health services and medical care in Thailand*. United States Agency for International Development (USAID), Bangkok.

PAHO (Pan American Health Organization) (1984). *Policies for the production and marketing of essential drugs*, Scientific Publication 462. PAHO, Washington, DC.

Patel, M. S. (1983). Drug costs in developing countries and policies to reduce them *World Development*, **11**, 195–204.

Scrip (Scrip World Pharmaceutical News) (1985). Various issues. London.

Sepulveda-Alvarez, C. (1985). In search of pharmaceutical health: the case of Thailand. *Development Dialogue.*, **2**, 56–68.

Speight, A. N. P. (1975). Cost effectiveness and drug therapy. *Tropical Doctor*, **5**, 89–92.

Szuba, T. J. (1986*a*). *Drugs for all: propaedeutics of pharmaceutical economics* [mimeo]. Warsaw.

Szuba, T. J. (1986*b*). International comparison of drug consumption: impact of prices. *Social Science and Medicine* **22**, 1019–25.

Tiranti, D. J. (1986). *The Bangladesh example – four years on*. New Internationalist Publications, Oxford, UK.

Ugalde, A., Homedes, N., and Collado Urena, J. (1986). Do patients understand their physicians? prescription compliance in a rural area of the Dominican Republic. *Health Policy and Planning*, **1**, 250–9.

UNCTC (United Nations Centre on Transnational Corporations) (1983). *Transnational corporations in the pharmaceutical industry of developing countries*. UNCTC, New York.

van der Geest, S. (1982). The efficiency of inefficiency: medicine distribution in south Cameroon. *Social Science and Medicine*, **16**, 2145–53.

World Bank (1985). *World development report, 1985*. World Bank, Washington, DC.

World Bank (1987). *Financing health services in developing countries: an agenda for reform*. World Bank, Washington, DC.

WHO (World Health Organization) (1977). *The selection of essential drugs*, Technical Report Series 615. WHO, Geneva.

WHO (World Health Organization) (1984). *Report of a WHO meeting on drug policies and management: procurement and financing of essential drugs*, DAP/84.5. WHO, Geneva.

WHO (World Health Organization) (1985*a*). *Study of hospital drug supply system in Kenya*. WHO, Geneva.

WHO (World Health Organization) (1985*b*) *Mali: soutien de l'OMS à la réforme pharmaceutique: rapport d'une mission OMS, 12–17 août 1985* (unpublished). WHO, Geneva.

WHO (World Health Organization) (1987*a*). *Economic support for national Health for All strategies*, Doc.no.A40/tech.disc./2. WHO, Geneva.

WHO (World Health Organization) (1987*b*). *The rational use of drugs: report of the conference of experts, Nairobi, 25–29 November 1985*. WHO, Geneva.

WHO (World Health Organization) (1988*a*). *The world drug situation*. Action Programme on Essential Drugs, WHO, Geneva.

WHO (World Health Organization) (1988*b*). *Selected annotated bibliography on essential drugs*. Action Programme on Essential Drugs, WHO, Geneva.

WHO (World Health Organization) (1988*c*). *Estimating drug requirements: a practical manual*. Action Programme on Essential Drugs, WHO, Geneva.

Wyke, A. (1987). Pharmaceuticals. *The Economist*, 7 February 1987.

Yudkin, J. S. (1980). The economics of pharmaceutical supply in Tanzania. *International Journal of Health Services*, **10**, 455–77.

13

The productivity of manpower and supplies in public health services in Java

Peter Berman and Suomi Sakai

Introduction

Public-sector health services in developing countries are widely perceived to be inefficient. Observers often note the evidence of inefficiency, such as low productivity with low patient loads, and staff idle during working hours; and poor practices in use of pharmaceuticals. A World Bank policy study on health-care financing in developing countries reinforced this perception when it identified 'internal inefficiency – wasteful public programs of poor quality' as one of the 'three main problems in the health sector' (World Bank 1987).

While such inefficiences are often criticized, there has been little substantive effort in most countries to analyse their causes, measure their size, or develop approaches for their reduction. Inefficiency implies an opportunity cost in wasted resources; resources which could be used to increase health, or to secure other benefits. Despite concerns about how best to finance the health sector, there has been little effort to estimate the size and consequences of such costs, and their importance in financing.

This chapter develops some measures of operating efficiency in the use of manpower and expendable supplies in rural health services in Java, Indonesia. The first section reviews briefly some issues in studying efficiency in the production of public-sector outputs. This is followed by background information on Indonesia and a description of the data. The main sections of the paper describe the current levels and variability of productivity of health manpower and supplies relative to health outputs for curative care (CC), maternal and child health and family planning (MCH/FP), and immunization (IMM) services. Factors associated with different levels of productivity are assessed, and estimates are given of potential resource gains through improving productivity. The final section discusses these results and possible strategies for improving operating efficiency in the rural health system.

Conceptual framework and objectives

Operating efficiency

In assessing the efficiency of health services, it is crucial to ask: 'efficiency relative to what?' This study is concerned with the internal operating efficiency of public-sector primary health-care services. It aims to describe and assess the quantities of health-care manpower and supplies that are typically used to produce certain service outputs, in this case contacts of various kinds with patients.

From a public policy perspective, this approach accepts as given certain decisions already made by society and reflected in the current structure of health programmes. Public health services are assumed to be desirable on the grounds of social welfare. This study does not provide information on the social benefits of improving the efficiency of health-service delivery, nor of reallocating resources to other uses. Nor will analysis of operating efficiency indicate whether a particular mix of services is the most desirable one in terms of health benefits to the population. Such questions are the subjects of cost-benefit and cost-effectiveness analysis (Mills 1985). For this study, we take the current level of health-care investment and the current mix of programmes as given. The underlying assumption is that more health outputs of the kinds now provided are desirable, and that one should try to maximize the quantity of services provided with the available resources, within acceptable levels of quality of care.

The focus on manpower and supplies reflects the fact that these inputs account for most of the cost of health services. An earlier paper showed that these two items can account for more than 95 per cent of the annualized total cost of outpatient services at rural facilities (Berman 1986). Fortunately, such inputs are also amenable to changes from improved management, making them the most likely targets of efforts to increase efficiency.

Measures of operating efficiency

The assessment of operating efficiency in a health-care programme can be approached by measuring actual units of input (such as personnel days or ampoules of vaccine) or their monetary value (i.e. the costs of those inputs). Measuring actual units of inputs is cumbersome, and may be impossibly complex if – as is usually the case – more than one type of input is required in producing output. However, in some instances it is useful to be able to measure the productivity of a specific input, for example the number of immunizations per day given by field-workers. It is important in making such measurements to control for the effects of other inputs which may be complements or substitutes, such as use of transportation or availability of vaccine in the example just given.

In general, measurement in monetary (cost) terms is more flexible. It allows for the combination of many different types of inputs into a single measure. Since monetary resources can be used to purchase many different types of inputs, the least-cost combinations of inputs can be considered the most efficient. However, in interpreting results care must be taken to control for differences in the quality of outputs and for price differences in inputs.

The most useful indicator of operating efficiency is average or unit cost. This is the total cost per unit of output or, for specific inputs, the total cost of that input per unit of output. Average costs can be compared across similar facilities to determine typical levels of productivity, and the degree to which facilities in different locations deviate from these levels.

Determinants of operating efficiency and the problem of standards

There are two main dimensions to operating efficiency in public-sector health services: those related to the organization of health-care delivery, and those related to the management of resources. One example of the former is 'economies of scale': that is, the ability to achieve lower costs for similar outputs in larger facilities than in smaller ones. Our concern in this chapter is mainly with efficiencies related to the management of resources. This requires that operating efficiency should be compared across similar health-care delivery units, in this case rural health centres.

A major problem in analysing the operating efficiency of public-sector services lies in identifying a standard for comparison. While the optimum may be the least-cost combination of resources, it is unlikely that this ideal state will be observed empirically. How can one determine the most desirable level of productivity for rural health resources?

The neoclassical economic theory of production and costs neatly solves this problem when dealing with the private sector. The theory posits that the competitive market exerts a substantial pressure on firms to operate at economically efficient levels and in economically efficient ways. With these and other assumptions, empirical estimation of production and cost functions from large numbers of producers can be expected to approximate to the least-cost optima. Unfortunately, such assumptions are clearly not justified in analysing public-sector services. Individual providers of public services may not easily be able to add or subtract inputs, such as staff, as needed. They do not depend on generating an economic surplus for their survival. And they are often required to operate in the least economically advantageous conditions, serving poor and remote populations.

One approach to identifying efficiency standards for public-sector health services has been to apply the operations-research techniques used in industry. Some examples of this can be found in studies from India and Kenya (Department of International Health 1976; Vogel *et al.* 1976). Such methods can provide insights into the relationship between the process of service-delivery and efficiency. But the standards often reflect the environment of a service-delivery 'laboratory', which may be of limited relevance to the routine operations of the vast majority of facilities.

An alternative approach is to define efficiency standards using expert opinion. Adequate-quality care, for example, may require that a health worker should see no more than 12 curative-care outpatients per hour, thereby setting an upper limit to productivity. This approach focuses more on assuring a minimal quality of care in high-output units than on increasing the output of low-productivity resources.

Numerous studies have been made of the cost of rural health services in developing countries (Robertson 1984). However, most have been used to estimate cost levels for planning purposes. In general, cost data have not been used as a management tool to assess operating efficiency (Berman 1986).

The present approach and its applications

In this study, the problem of setting absolute efficiency standards was avoided by focusing on the comparative efficiency of the facilities. The first step in this process was to estimate the current average level of efficiency for key inputs in functioning health units. It was widely recognized that the average efficiency was low and needed to be improved, although there was also substantial variation across facilities. The second step was to demonstrate the range of efficiency within the existing (low) level. Even where institutional constraints impeded improved levels of efficiency in the short run, there would still be substantial room for improvement through raising the efficiency of the poorest performers within that low average level.

In the analysis below, the efficiency of manpower and supply use in providing CC, MCH/FP, and IMM contacts is measured both in terms of real resources (for example, patient-contacts per full-time staff equivalent) and costs (for example, personnel cost per contact). Our objectives were:

- To estimate the current average level of efficiency in the use of key resources and the range of variation around that level.

- To identify and discuss important organizational and management determinants of the current level of efficiency and its variability across facilities.

- To estimate the opportunity cost to the public sector of the low efficiency of the worst-performing facilities, and to assess its importance in the overall financing of rural health services.

- To identify and discuss strategies for improving the efficiency of service-delivery in rural health facilities.

More broadly, we hoped to stimulate and justify further interest in improving the efficiency of rural services, and to encourage the measurement of operating efficiency in other environments.

Study environment, data sources, and methods

The organization of rural health services in Java

Health centres are the main health facility in each rural sub-district in Java. Headed by a physician, they provide a variety of service functions, including curative care, maternal and child health, family planning, nutrition, hygiene and sanitation, dental care, and school health services. Two types of smaller satellite facilities are also common in Java. Sub-centres are fixed facilities with a permanent resident staff – usually of 1 to 3 paramedicals. Health posts are also fixed facilities, but are only opened on certain days when staff from the health centre or sub-centre visit. Vehicles used as mobile health centres also make periodic visits to villages. Sub-district health personnel may number from 10 to 50 staff. Individuals are often assigned responsibility for one of several service functions. Generally, curative care and MCH/FP outpatient services are routinely provided at the health facilities, and some immunizations are also provided there. Most other services are provided in outreach visits to households or communities. In some areas of Java, single-function malaria workers are posted to rural villages. In endemic areas, these malaria workers make up the largest health-centre programme, often accounting for over half the salaried staff. In addition, volunteer community-based health and nutrition workers have also been established in most areas. These workers provide simple treatments for common illness, growth monitoring, and nutrition education, and assist health-service personnel in other community-based activities.

While these types of health-service organization are fairly uniform throughout Java, they are combined in different ways at the sub-district level. For example, in this study of 26 sub-districts, ten different combinations of health centre, sub-centre, health post, and community health worker were found. Personnel assignments also vary by sub-district, although there are some basic patterns. Health-centre physicians spend the bulk of their time in administrative work. Curative care is usually provided by several nurses and assistant nurses, with the physician available for consultation. A clerk and an assistant pharmacist may also help. MCH/FP services are provided by one or several midwives and assistant midwives. One paramedical is usually assigned full-time to immunization, with activities divided between immunizing clinic visitors and village outreach. Additional paramedicals may be assigned to hygiene and sanitation, school health, health and education, and other programmes. Responsibility for community nutrition programmes often falls on the MCH staff, and they may also provide immunizations.

Data sources and methods

The data presented here were collected from 26 rural sub-districts – *kecamatan*, each with a population of between 30000 and

50000 – in Central Java and Yogyakarta provinces in late 1982. The sub-districts were selected randomly in three rural regencies or *kabupaten*, with populations between 300000 and 800000: Wonosobo, Kulon Progo, and Bantul, representing mountainous, hilly, and coastal plain areas respectively.

Data were collected from sub-district statistics, health-service records and reports, and informal interviews with health-service personnel. The information included the following:

- physical, demographic, and socio-economic information on each sub-district;

- health-service resources, including the number and size of facilities, the number and type of personnel, drugs, supplies, equipment, vehicles, etc.;

- health-service outputs over four quarters, including outpatient contacts for curative care, and maternal and child health and family planning services, the number and type of immunizations, and community-based health and nutrition activities;

- costs of health-care inputs, including salaries and non-salary payments to all personnel (data on drug prices and capital costs were collected separately at provincial and central levels); and

- allocation of personnel time and capital inputs to specific service functions.

To estimate the time-allocation of health-service personnel, staff present at the time of our visits to the sub-districts were asked to identify the first, second, and third most important health-service functions to which their activities belonged. They were then asked to estimate, on average, what proportion of their time they devoted to each function over the last year. For personnel who were not present, group discussions of health-service staff were used to allocate their time. In some cases, there was no consensus about staff time, and these data were left missing. This type of information is, at best, an approximation to true time-allocation. No account is given of non-productive time, although previous studies have shown that this may account for more than 50 per cent of official working hours in Indonesian health centres. However, in health-service cost analysis, it is common practice to allocate personnel costs according to the proportion of *active* service-time staff devote to specific functions. Thus, what is deemed most important is not the absolute time spent on each function, but whether the relative proportions of time reported for functions accurately reflect the proportions of active service-time devoted to those functions. We feel that this is a reasonable assumption.

Personnel inputs were presented as full-time staff equivalents (FTSE). FTSE's were calculated by adding up the proportion of individual staff time allocated to specific functions. For example, if a nurse reported 50 per cent of his time spent on curative care and a midwife 25 per cent of her time, that would be counted as 0.75 FTSE. Almost all staff time allocated to specific clinical functions was for trained health workers, not for ancillary staff such as cleaners.

Data on expendable supplies were collected from each facility's monthly report. These reports listed all supplies used for outpatient care, but did not include items such as the vaccines used in the immunization programme or fuel for vehicles. Drugs accounted for the vast majority of supplies, but items such as bandages, cotton, and alcohol were also included. Almost all of these items were used primarily for curative care services.

For each sub-district, supply reports were copied for four months during 1982: February, May, August, and November, representing four quarters. These reports listed the initial supply available for that month, the amount received, the amount used, and the remaining stock. Prices (i.e. the cost to the government) for most of these inputs were recorded from the official bids of successful vendors. When those prices were not available, 60 per cent of the retail price reported in *Data Obat Indonesia 1982*, a locally published physicians' reference, was used. There were still some items for which prices could not be found, and these were omitted from the analysis. They were usually locally purchased drugs used in small quantities. Thus the supply cost figures were underestimates, with an unknown – and hopefully small – amount of error.

Total supply costs for the four months sampled for each sub-district were calculated. Annual costs were then estimated by multiplying these totals (of four months) by three, for comparison with annual utilization figures for CC. This multiplication should correct for the likelihood that some items were not reported as they were used, but only when new supplies arrived.

From the initial 26 sub-districts surveyed, sufficiently complete data on manpower were available from 22 sub-districts. Supply-use data were sufficiently complete from 14 of these 22 sub-districts.

Efficiency in the use of manpower

Using the data described above, we calculated the FTSE per sub-district for three important primary health-care functions: curative care, MCH/FP, and immunizations. With service output data from each sub-district we estimated the number of contacts per FTSE per working day, based on a 300-day year. These figures are shown in Table 13.1, which gives the average for the 22 sub-districts, followed by the figures for the highest and the lowest sub-district and the ratios between them.

The data in this table certainly reinforce the impression of a low overall productivity of personnel. Average client contacts per FTSE per working day for each function ranged from a high of about 10 for CC to a low of about 5 for MCH/FP. In other words, on average over the year, the equivalent of a full-time person doing curative care saw only 10 patients per day, with correspondingly lower figures for the other two functions. If one considers that a working day is officially about 7 hours long, these were low levels of output indeed. However, of equal or greater interest were the figures for the highest and lowest sub-districts; clearly there were areas of both much higher and much lower levels of manpower productivity. The differences varied by factors of 18 to 40, suggesting much scope for improving manpower productivity, even under existing conditions.

The 'FTSE' index combines all the different personnel into a single measure of manpower inputs. If larger amounts of lower-level and lower-cost manpower were being used to provide routine services, rather than scarcer more senior staff, this would appear to be less efficient in FTSE terms, even though it might be more efficient in cost terms. To correct for this possibility, Table 13.2 presents the average personnel cost per client contact for the sub-districts studied. Personnel cost included annual staff salaries and additional remuneration received by personnel. Costs for individual staff were allocated to functions proportionately to their reported time allocation. The totals for each function were then divided by the annual client contacts.

Table 13.2 first shows the average personnel cost per client

Table 13.1 *Variability in manpower productivity: contacts per full-time staff equivalent per day**

	Curative care	MCH/FP	IMM
Annual average (22 sub-districts)	9.9	4.9	5.6
Highest sub-district	53.8	42.8	33.2
Lowest sub-district	2.9	1.7	0.8
Ratio of highest to lowest	18.5	25.2	41.3

* 22 sub-districts based on 300 working days per year.

contact. As expected, the implication of low productivity was high cost – with average personnel costs alone ranging from $0.30 to $0.56 per contact in different functions. The official fee for outpatient care at the time of the study was $0.24, including drugs. Again the variation in efficiency – measured as personnel cost per contact – was high, although somewhat reduced from that shown in the previous table.

What factors were associated with this large variability in efficiency? We first explored differences in the pattern of allocation of manpower resources to sub-districts. The Indonesian rural

Table 13.2 *Variability in manpower costs per patient contact (US$)*

	Curative care	MCH/FP	IMM
Annual average (22 sub-districts)	0.30	0.56	0.56
Highest sub-district	1.38	1.98	2.71
Lowest sub-district	0.05	0.09	0.12
Ratio of highest to lowest	27.60	22.00	22.60

public-health system was organized at the sub-district level, with the rural health centre as the focal unit. If resources were distributed equally to sub-districts or per health centre, this might have accounted for difference in efficiency, as the size and population of each area were quite different, and there were differences in accessibility of services. However, the data showed quite large variations in manpower allocation by district, with differences ranging up to a factor of 8 from lowest to highest. When sub-district figures were corrected for population size the variability remained high.

With little evidence that personnel were assigned according to administrative area or population, we plotted FTSE indices for specific functions against the number of client contacts for those functions, to determine whether personnel assignments (to specific functions) were associated with utilization (of those functions). Manpower is generally considered to be a semi-variable resource, meaning that there should have been some association between the amount of manpower used (i.e. FTSE) and the resulting output (i.e. client contacts). If manpower was not allocated in response to utilization, but was in fact treated like a fixed resource, no association would appear. Figure 13.1 plots the FTSE for curative care against annual curative-care contacts. Clearly, there was no association. Nor did a similar plot for MCH/FP show an association for the sub-districts in the sample, though there was some suggestion of higher staff allocation for the few sub-districts reporting high levels of use.

These results suggested little systematic management of personnel resources so as to promote efficiency. While most of the personnel providing CC and MCH/FP services were multi-function staff, their work assignments did not appear responsive to differences in the demand for their services. Instead, personnel seemed to be managed more as a fixed resource: assigned to certain functions whatever the level of utilization. While this might be desirable at very low levels of use, in order to maintain a minimum level of service, the very low average levels of productivity showed that there was substantial excess capacity being wasted.

When inputs are fixed in a production process, the level of output becomes a powerful factor in determining efficiency. This is shown for personnel costs in the sub-district sample in Fig. 13.2 for both CC and MCH/FP. The sub-district observations showed a strongly declining average-cost curve. However, the decline was

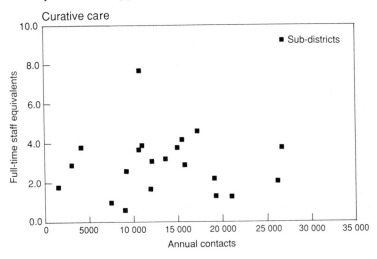

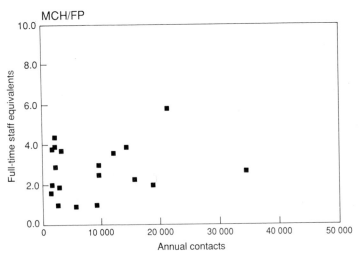

Fig. 13.1 Manpower allocations and outputs (curative care and MCH/FP).

not linear, suggesting some limited association with demand in the use of personnel.

These results suggested two possible strategies for improving efficiency. First, given the low overall level of manpower productivity, one could reduce the number of staff in low-utilization facilities. This was likely to be an unpopular process, and administratively difficult, if not impossible. Second, and more appropriate, we felt, was the better management of those staff. Health centres produced many types of services, and staff assigned to low-utilization functions should be reassigned to other activities, perhaps those involving outreach such as health education, supervision, and the support of community programmes. This would simultaneously increase the efficiency of personnel use in the 'low-utilization' functions, as well as raising the outputs of other activities.

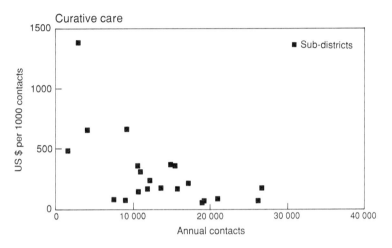

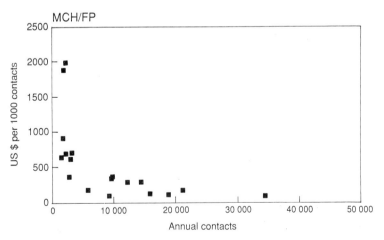

Fig. 13.2 Manpower unit costs and outputs (curative care and MCH/FP).

What were the potential financial incentives to government from improving personnel management? We calculated the manpower and cost saving that would have resulted from increasing the productivity of staff. If staff productivity in those sub-districts below the current average was raised to that average for CC and MCH/FP, this would have given the equivalent of an addition of 22 staff in the sample sub-districts. This was equal to a 17 per cent increase in personnel for those two functions, or the addition of one new staff member in each area. In cost terms, using the average salary for all professional staff, the improved productivity was the equivalent of a $20625 increase in the personnel budget, equal to 4.3 per cent of the total personnel budget for all sub-districts. This was certainly a minimum estimate of the benefits, which would be much greater if the average level of productivity could be increased substantially.

Efficiency in the use of expendable supplies

The second large component of the total costs of health services was expendable supplies. These consisted primarily of drugs, but also of items such as bandages and alcohol. Almost all the cost of these supplies could be attributed to the curative-care function of health services. A small proportion may have been related to MCH, but this was mainly low-cost items such as diet supplements (for example, ferrous sulphate and vitamin tablets).

In general, the quantity of supplies available at rural health facilities in Java was adequate at the time of this study. The central government made a substantial annual per capita cash allocation to local governments for purchasing drugs and other supplies for the health services. These funds were usually supplemented by direct local purchases as well. Our observations at the time of data collection suggested that almost all facilities had adequate supplies of drugs, although they might run out of specific items from time to time. In fourteen sub-districts for which we had complete data, the estimated average annual expenditure on supplies for 1982 was $9843. This gave an average of $0.27 per capita per annum.

Table 13.3 presents the supply cost per outpatient curative-care contact from the sample of sub-districts. This was estimated by dividing total supply costs by the number of CC contacts. The average for fourteen sub-districts was $0.83, varying by a factor of

6 from the lowest to the highest sub-district. This estimated average supply cost per contact was quite high, especially in relation to the fee per contact of $0.24. In addition – as we saw with manpower inputs – the variation in supply cost per contact was also high, indicating that some districts spent significantly less per contact than others.

As with the data on manpower, we plotted the average supply cost per CC contact against the number of contacts to identify any association of supply use with overall service use. This is shown in Fig. 13.3. Evidence of declining average cost suggested that prescribing practices responded to higher levels of utilization (i.e. by reducing the average supply cost per patient). Supplies did not appear to act as a true variable cost (in which case the points should have varied around a horizontal line), but rather were semi-variable. This may have accounted for some of the differences between sub-districts.

What do we mean by efficiency in the use of supplies? In principle, for every patient there should be a least-cost combination of supply inputs which is clinically adequate for his or her problem. Inefficiency occurs when providers deviate from this optimal input mix. Such inefficiences may be the result of various types of error in supply provision and use, such as providing excessive quantities of the correct drugs; providing unnecessary drugs; providing drugs that are unnecessarily costly compared to alternatives of equal clinical efficacy; and providing insufficient quantities of drugs. The first of these three errors would lead to increased costs, the last to lower costs but to lower effectiveness as well.

Available data provided only indirect evidence of inefficiency. The large variation in average supply cost per contact suggested a lack of discipline in the use of supplies. Poor management of drugs and poor prescribing has frequently been reported, and is likely to have been a main cause of inefficiency. For example, a previous

Table 13.3 *Variability in supply costs per curative-care contact (US$)*

Average for 14 sub-districts	0.83
Highest sub-district	1.91
Lowest sub-district	0.32
Ratio of highest to lowest	6.00

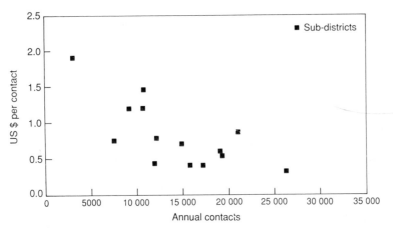

Fig. 13.3 Average supply costs per curative care contact.

review of more detailed information from two of the areas studied reported the lack of consistency in prescribing. Drugs were often given which had little relation to the stated diagnosis. Injectable vitamins were often used – a practice which often had dubious clinical justification. The usual prescribing pattern was to give a large number of different drugs – the average in that sample of patients was more than 4, but inadequate quantities of each one (Berman 1985). Public health facilities in Indonesia often lacked formal protocols for drug use. Supervisory review of prescribing practices was rare. The declining average cost with utilization shown in Fig. 13.3 suggests, however, that health workers did make decisions about drug use that had cost implications. With the data available, we were unable to assess how these decisions were made.

In compiling the drug-use and price lists, two factors related to the types of supplies provided stood out: syrups and inject-ables were much more costly than other forms of drugs; and local budgets for drugs were often used to purchase brand-name supplies which were more costly than the generic varieties also available. This latter factor was especially striking in the supplies available for use by insured civil servants. If providers are prof-ligate in the use of higher-cost supplies, this can significantly inflate costs.

Unfortunately, we were unable to control for differences in

case-mix, the proportion of insured patients, and patients' age-differences between sub-districts; these might have accounted for some of the variation in productivity and average costs without implying any difference in efficiency. In general, the vast majority of cases were of common diseases, such as respiratory and skin infections, diarrhoea, and malaria. Diagnoses in rural facilities were fairly unreliable, making even the reported case-mix data suspect. Perhaps more significant would be differences in the age-distribution of patients, since very young children often received medications in liquid syrup form, which were more expensive than capsules.

It should also be noted that these data represented the reported use of supplies, and not the amount provided to facilities, which would include unused stocks at health centres. The total cost of supplying these services was likely to be higher.

Thus, the data on supply costs were suggestive of significant inefficiencies. Previous research and our field observations did provide insights into their likely causes. But development of better indicators and more careful analysis of drug use was needed to formulate specific strategies for reducing waste in the use of supplies.

What was the 'excess' cost of high-supply-cost sub-districts? If the supply cost for those sub-districts above the overall average of $0.83 per contact were reduced to that average level, the total savings would have been $18165, which would exceed 13 per cent of the total supply expenditure from all fourteen areas. This amount would have been 'saved' from only five of the fourteen sub-districts. Clearly, this would be a significant quantity of resources, calculated only from those areas above the existing (high) cost of supplies per contact. If supply costs per contact were reduced in all areas, the savings could have been much greater.

Conclusion

Summary of results

These data presented here provided a number of useful insights into the productivity of rural health resources in Java. First, they suggested that for the two most important inputs to services – manpower and supplies – average productivity was low. This resulted in relatively high costs for routine services. The average personnel and supply cost for a curative care contact was over $1.10 – quite high for a rural health system spending on average $1 – $2 per person per year for all primary-care services.

Second, rough estimates of the potential financial gains from increasing productivity showed this to be a potentially important source of health-care financing at the margin. Increasing the efficiency of manpower and supply use in only those areas below the current low averages could have resulted in the equivalent of a 17 per cent increase in personnel available for CC and MCH/FP, and a 13 per cent increase in supply budgets. These were significant amounts of resources at a time when Indonesia had experienced sizeable absolute reductions in public-sector health expenditures.

Third, the data showed a large degree of variation across sub-districts in both manpower and supply use per contact. This variation suggested that there were some facilities achieving much higher levels of productivity than others within the existing administrative context. This evidence of 'positive deviance' was encouraging, as it implied that significant improvements in efficiency should be possible without waiting for major changes in health system administration.

Fourth, there were indications of several important causes of inefficiency in resource use which could be used to identify strategies for improving productivity. For example, the lack of association between personnel time allocated to CC and MCH/FP functions and the number of patient contacts suggested that improving task assignments and staff-time allocation in rural health facilities could bring large returns in productivity. Similarly, analyses of prescribing practices have shown sizeable wastage of drugs, which were a large component of total costs. This could be linked to the lack of standard treatment protocols and drug-use reviews, as well as to inefficient procurement practices.

Strategies for improving productivity

It is common these days to criticize public-sector services as being inefficient. In order to improve these systems, more analysis of the productivity of health-care resources is required. This analysis must be linked to administrative and management programmes which try to improve efficiency in existing services. The following are some suggestions on strategies to improve efficiency.

Assess current levels and variation in efficiency of different programmes and identify where large gains are possible. This requires practical studies of productivity using indicators of real resources (for example, staff time) and costs. These studies do not have to be expensive or excessively time-consuming. Efforts to improve efficiency should first address those programmes where large gains are possible or significant health benefits might be realized.

Develop facility-level indicators of productivity and use them to monitor and reward the performance of local managers. Some of the indicators used here, such as contacts per FTSE and supply cost per contact, have clear deficiencies. But they are feasible to calculate, and probably reflect the underlying resource efficiency of interest. There is a clear need for improving the efficiency of drug use, and indicators for monitoring the use of specific drugs relative to reported diagnoses could be added to health-facility supervision routines. With further development, health-system administrators could set parameters for such measures that would reduce waste. Such indicators should be made routine, and used in supervision of facility managers to encourage them to consider efficiency in their allocation of resources.

Encourage flexibility and resource reallocation within health facilities and programmes. In Indonesian health centres, it was not always easy to reassign personnel to other tasks, even if there was little demand for the services to which they were originally assigned: all programmes must be staffed. Administrative responsibilities multiplied through the addition of new vertical programmes. While there was much talk about management and efficiency in the health centre, it was unclear how much authority the health-centre manager had to allocate resources. Training health-centre physicians in management would not help if they did not have the authority to manage. Better management should be encouraged through decentralization of authority.

Reward higher productivity with additional services. As indicators of productivity are used for monitoring and supervision, allocation of new resources could also be channelled to those most able to use them.

Generate demand for under-utilized services. A major source of low productivity in Indonesia was under-utilization of services. One approach to raising efficiency when demand is lacking is reallocating resources as has just been suggested. However, for services of public health importance, demand-generation should is designed to ensure that money is spent on those things for which it was given and nothing else'. Accounts are generally aimed at ensuring financial control and accountability – there is more concern about *what* is purchased than *why* it is purchased (Waterston 1965). While not denying the importance – indeed the necessity – of financial audit and control, it is clearly necessary to consider other ways of presenting financial information if an attempt is to be made to use decision-making tools such as cost-effectiveness analysis (CEA) and cost-benefit analysis (CBA) to promote efficiency. CEA and CBA consider costs as they relate to the output achieved. Budgets must begin to make these connections between inputs and outputs if CEA/CBA-type thinking is to be used on anything like a routine basis.

Various ways exist to link budgets to the aims and objectives of plans. The ideal is *output budgeting*, which links costs to output data – i.e. to data on the impact of a programme. (For example, Programme A prevented Y number of deaths at a cost of x, whereas Programme B prevented more deaths at the same or a lower cost.) But such impact data are very rarely available, and, even when they are, the connection between cause and effect is often far from clear. Because output budgeting is in practice rarely possible, two less far-reaching approaches are often used. These are *programme budgeting* and *functional budgeting*.

Programme budgeting is defined here as the classification of expenditure according to programmes, which should relate to objectives, and may be defined according to client groups (for example, maternal and child health, antenatal care) or according to the type or level of service (for example, primary health care, public health). Examples of national programme budgets are shown in Tables 14.1 and 14.2.

Clearly, programme budgeting is conceptually inferior to output budgeting, as the effectiveness of expenditure is not considered. For example, it is impossible to tell from Table 14.1 whether or not the decline in the percentage of the budget allocated to rural facilities was a 'good' (i.e. efficient) trend. If, however, a decision were to be taken to increase the priority accorded to these rural health facilities (mostly health centres and nursing posts), this programme budget could be used to identify programmes which may be receiving a disproportionately large share of expenditure. Ex-post information could be used to compare budget shares over time, to monitor whether or not the intent to shift priorities was

be seen as an alternative strategy. This may be especially important for such programmes as MCH and immunization. Employment in social marketing, community meetings, and home visits might all be productive activities for otherwise idle clinic staff.

Concern with the efficient operation of public health services is not new. In general, previous efforts have focused on fine-tuning the micro-level operations of hospitals, clinics, and outreach programmes, often using operations-research methods. These approaches are important to provide the experimental data needed to estimate the potential efficiency of public services, since the discipline of profit or loss in the market-place is lacking. However, these efforts have not had the expected large-scale impact on public health systems. What we have proposed here is to give more explicit attention to cost measures as indicators of efficiency, combined with the development of incentives for facility managers and giving them the authority to reallocate resources. Rather than trying to develop rigid organizational protocols for peripheral facilities, managers should be encouraged to find their own methods for improving efficiency.

Some observers of the health systems of developing countries would like to write off the public sector as hopelessly inefficient. While the efficiency of existing public services is often distressingly low, there is no reason *a priori* that public health services must be inefficient. It is time that the health-system managers confronted the problems directly. To do that, they need more than just lamentations or dismissal. Practical analysis of the causes and costs of inefficiency and the benefits of increasing productivity can provide motivation. Experimentation and experience will show whether these systems, like other large public organizations, will respond to the new discipline required by the fiscal realities of the 1990s.

References

Berman, P. A. (1985). *Equity and cost in the organization of primary health care in Java, Indonesia*, Department of Agricultural Economics Publication AE 85–5. Cornell University, Ithaca, NY.

Berman, P. A. (1986). Cost analysis as a management tool for improving the efficiency of primary care: some examples from Java. *International Journal of Health Planning and Management*, **1**, 275–88.

Department of International Health (1976). *The functional analysis of health needs and services*. Asia Publishing House, New Delhi.

Mills, A. (1985). Economic evaluation of health programmes: application of the principles in developing countries. *World Health Statistics Quarterly*, **38**(4), 368–82.

Robertson, R. L. (1984). *Review of literature on costs of health services in developing countries*, PHN Technical Note 85–21. Population, Health, and Nutrition Department, The World Bank, Washington, DC.

Vogel, L. C., W'oigo, H. O., Swinkels, W. J. and Sjoerdsma, A. C. (1976). Cost analysis of out-patient services at Kiambu District Hospital, Kenya. *East African Medical Journal*, **53**(4), 236–43.

World Bank (1987). *Financing health services in developing countries: an agenda for reform*, A World Bank Policy Study. World Bank, Washington, DC.

Authors' note

The field research for this paper was supported by grants from the Ford Foundation and the US Department of Education. The Indonesian Institute of Sciences, the Indonesian Department of Health, and Gaja Mada University provided sponsorship and institutional support in-country. Data analysis was supported by a Biomedical Research Support Grant from the Johns Hopkins University.

14

Encouraging efficiency through programme and functional budg[...] lessons from experience in Ghar[...] the Gambia

Abdulai Issaka-Tinorgah and Catriona Waddingtor[...]

Input, programme, and functional budgeting

Encouraging health services to operate more efficiently lie[...] heart of health economics. Thus efficiency has been a re[...] theme in this volume. In the absence of competitive mark[...] health care – and hence in the absence of prices acting as [...] for efficient behaviour – institutional procedures determi[...] extent to which efficient resource-allocation occurs. If they [...] behave efficiently, decision-makers ideally need a reliable fl[...] information about the costs and benefits of health progran[...] Planners and managers should combine data on health need[...] the effectiveness of alternative interventions with the relevant [...] profiles. In reality, this link between benefits and costs – in e[...] between the objectives of plans and accounts information – is o[...] absent. All too often plans are pious statements of ambit[...] intentions, without being linked to the resources required to ens[...] their implementation.

This chapter looks at the potential for using budgets as an inf[...] mation tool relevant to the promotion of efficiency. It discus[...] case studies of attempted budgetary reform in Ghana and [...] functional budgeting in the Gambia. Finally, it draws conclusio[...] about the prerequisites for successful budgetary reform.

Traditionally, financial information is classified according t[...] input categories. Accounts are divided up into capital and curren[...] accounts, into categories such as wages and salaries and equipmen[...] and materials, and into administrative sectors such as Ministry o[...] Health expenditure and Ministry of Water Supplies expenditure. [...] As Culyer (1980) explains: 'administrative units demand cash [...] for spending on specific resources and traditional accounting [...]

Table 14.1 *Programme budgeting, Ministry of Health, Fiji (1984–1988)*

Programme	% of total annual expenditure				
	1984*	1985*	1986†	1987†	1988†
Urban hospitals/ health centres	54.9	70.0	65.7	63.0	63.0
Sub-divisional hospitals	14.4	10.7	10.0	15.1	10.9
Rural facilities	9.9	8.0	7.7	6.6	6.6
Public health	3.3	3.3	3.1	3.1	3.1
Drugs	6.7	7.7	7.6	6.9	6.9
Health education, training, administration and research	10.8	0.3	5.9	5.3	9.5
Total	100.0	100.0	100.0	100.0	100.0

* actual expenditure
† planned expenditure
Source: Ministry of Health and Social Welfare, Fiji (1986)

Table 14.2 *Programme budgeting, Ministry of Health, Ghana (1975–1976)*

Programme	% of total Ministry of Health Budget
Central and Divisional Headquarters	3
Medical care (hospital based)	79
[– Korle Bu Teaching Hospital	22]
[– Other hospitals	57]
Public health	12
Training	6
Total	100

Source: National Health Planning Unit. Ministry of Health, Ghana (1979).

reflected in a corresponding shift in resource-allocation. The advantage of programme budgeting is that it goes part of the way towards providing at least an output *orientation* to the presentation of financial information. It should encourage decision-makers to look at the alternative programmes on which money could be spent and to begin to question the relative expenditure of each programme. Moreover, when budgets are categorized according to programmes it is possible to monitor whether resources are being allocated according to stated priorities. The link between plans and budgets is thus established.

Functional budgeting is conceptually very similar to programme budgeting, but the term is normally applied to situations at a sub-national level, where each service unit has a separate budget. In a hospital there could be functional budgets for each ward and for the theatre, the laboratory, and the pharmacy. A public health office might have functional budgets for rubbish collection, inspection of buildings, and water supply and sanitation. Functional budgeting is in effect a local version of programme budgeting, and the terms are sometimes used interchangeably – neither classifies expenditure according to outputs. As in the case of programme budgeting, functional budgeting aims to encourage a questioning attitude to existing resource-allocation, and is not in itself an evaluation tool (Mooney 1984). Functional and programme budgeting can easily coexist with traditional input accounting. The audit requirement does not have to be threatened.

Because output, programme, and functional budgeting are designed to encourage efficiency, they are on theoretical grounds very attractive to economists. Unfortunately the history of the implementation of these types of budgeting has been far from successful. As was perhaps the case for cost-benefit analysis – extravagant claims were made that CBA might lead to the triumph of 'economically rational' decisions – the initial reaction to the inadequacies of traditional accounting systems was rather extreme. The dinosaurs of PPBS (Planning, Programming, and Budgeting System), ZBB (Zero-Based Budgeting), PESC (Public Expenditure Planning Cycle), and various other acronymic budgetary systems bear witness to this over-enthusiasm. At the heart of each of these reforms was an attempt to link budgetary allocations to the productivity of expenditures, and resource requirements to the achievement of various levels of objectives. Nationally, priorities were to be ranked, and expenditure was to be allocated so as to reflect these priorities (Caiden and Wildavsky 1974). Caiden and Wildavsky comment rather acridly on the fate of such ambitious interpretations of programme budgeting:

The experience with programme budgeting has been much the same in poor countries and rich; no one knows how to do it . . . No one understands how to put together the programme structures that relate the objectives to one another . . . Programme budgeting calls for a high degree of conceptual ability, a new accounting or information system, and political leadership ready and willing to use it. No one should be surprised, therefore, to find that programme budgeting runs into serious difficulties in poor countries.

The history of programme budgeting is indeed marred by unsuccessful attempts at reform. The US Federal Government has backed down on several attempts to change the budgetary system (Glennerster 1984). India, Argentina, and the Philippines have had similar unsuccessful experiences with programme budgeting. More recently, so too has the Ministry of Health in Ghana. The following section of this chapter presents a case study of this attempt to improve the budgetary system in the Ministry of Health in Ghana, and then discusses the lessons to be learnt from this experience.

Programme budgeting: the Ghanaian attempt

Before 1978 financial management in the Ministry of Health in Ghana followed the traditional incremental practice of setting expenditures by adding a certain percentage to the previous year's estimates, with regard to neither plans nor the availability of resources. Target (or objective) setting was conducted in isolation from financial considerations. Actual expenditure was often significantly different from the original financial estimates, yet no mechanism existed to question or remove such discrepancies. In short, the planning 'cycle' consisted of a series of virtually unconnected statements and events. Plans were rarely implemented.

Frustration with this system led to a proposal by the National Health Planning Unit of Ghana (NHPU) to improve the process of health planning and budgeting. The proposal was for a fairly sophisticated version of programme budgeting, which aimed to force managers to include financial considerations in the planning and management process.

The Ghanaian Ministry of Health proposed such radical changes to its planning and budgeting system because it wanted to realize the link between planning objectives and resource availability. Financial information was to be categorized according to both geographical areas (district and regions) and programmes (for example, Immunization, Manpower Training, and Mother and Child Health). Financial responsibility was to be decentralized, so that district programme officers would become budget-holders for the first time. Comparisons between areas and between programmes would then be possible to identify which budgets seemed to be disproportionately small. Ex-post data could be used to compare budget allocations over time to monitor whether or not intentions to shift priorities were fulfilled. The system would also encourage intra-programme consideration of priorities.

The basic idea of the new system was that financial estimates and implementation targets would be devised locally. The next tier up in the system would then consider the various statements about costs and benefits and decide how its budget was to be distributed amongst the competing interests. The estimation process began at sub-district level, and increasingly aggregated estimates were then to be considered at district, regional, and national levels. Costs and benefits were to be considered at all levels of the hierarchy, in order to improve efficiency both within and between programmes.

In order to implement this new system, an annual budgetary cycle was designed which stipulated dates by which consultations, meetings, workshops, guidelines, and draft estimates were to be completed. A standard 'programme worksheet' was used to estimate resource requirements. These requirements were specified using a standard cost list, which included the distinction between local and foreign currency expenditures. It was realized that Ghana's fluctuating economy meant that the list would require frequent up-dating. To complement the budgeting section, each worksheet also asked for a statement of objectives and targets, together with a time-scale. Objectives were required to be consistent with national health priorities.

This system demanded much more of sub-district, district, and regional staff than had the previous 'budgeting by default' system of incrementalism. To prepare staff for their new responsibilities, the NPHU prepared a comprehensive manual explaining the rationale for the new system and the mechanics of implementation.

Ten two-day workshops were organized by the NHPU throughout the country, and the worksheets, narrative statements of objectives, and standard costings were introduced and discussed. For many of the participants, these workshops were the first time that they had been encouraged to think explicitly in terms of priority needs and activities, as well as in terms of the availability of resources.

Though expectations of the NHPU's reforms were high, in practice few, if any, significant changes had been brought about by the late 1980s. Budgets in Ghana were still organized solely according to inputs. The current year's estimate was still the basis for the following year's budget, even if actual expenditure proved to be very different from the original estimate. Incrementalism had survived. The following reasons can be identified for the failure of the reforms.

Shortage of skilled staff. The new system required Ministry of Health staff to go through the process of formulating objectives, estimating targets, deciding on activities and services, and then computing the necessary resource requirements. To the district and sub-district staff who were to collect the data, the new process was radically different from their previous practice of unquestioning incrementalism. It was also probably too complex without more intensive training. To expect nation-wide implementation at once was therefore rather over-ambitious.

The complexity of the system meant that much of the proposal was doomed before it had begun – the budgetary exercise had to start with the peripheral staff before the regional and later national budgets could be compiled. Any system too complex to succeed at the peripheral level was doomed to failure. This problem of exaggerated expectations of the possibilities for data collection is not confined to Ghana. A manual for developing countries on financing the health sector (Mach and Abel-Smith 1983) describes a rational and comprehensive system of data collection. But the sophistication required to carry out such a proposal – to analyse budget by priority of health problem, by priority services, by geographical area, and disaggregated by source of finance, etc. – is more suited to one-off exercises by specialist teams than to routine use.

Lack of credibility. A system that aims to link forward planning to the likelihood of receiving resources will not work if promised resources do not materialize and if the plans are seen as unrealistic.

Many examples of problems in this area could be quoted, but two may suffice.

It was not officially recognized that the government-approved prices did not always represent the actual situation. Many items were available only at the black market rate, yet budgets had to be made in terms of the much lower government-approved rates. Inflation meant that these approved rates were often out of date. Spending officers developed ways of 'fictionalizing' the accounts in order to compensate for this discrepancy. This devalued the status of the budget document.

People had become used to the fact that the fluctuating economy of Ghana had led to frequent across-the-board cuts and restrictions in the use of even previously approved funds. There was thus a certain amount of justifiable suspicion about the validity of complex analysis and forward planning, when even approved budgets were not honoured.

Inadequate support from other Ministries. A prerequisite for the successful implementation of the new budgetary system was that the Ministry of Health could predict its next year's budget with at least a reasonable degree of certainty. In order to try to secure this, negotiations were conducted with the Ministries of Finance and Economic Planning. These negotiations were necessary because the Ministry of Health's proposals were out of line with the usual incremental-cum-muddling-through practices of spending ministries. In addition to the support required from these two Ministries, expenditure data were required from the Accountant-General's Department, which was responsible for monitoring annual expenditure and feeding the information back to the spending ministries. These data were not available, as the Department was working with information that was five years out of date.

Responsibility without power. The proposals envisaged that the plans would be devised and implemented at the district and/or sub-district levels. This relied on the release of the appropriate level of funds by the regions. In practice, however, funds were sometimes misappropriated for regional activities. This was clearly to the detriment of district activities and plans. There was thus little incentive for district-level officers to budget according to objectives, when their efforts were likely to be undermined by regional interference. Budgetary power must be linked to budgetary responsibility.

Absence of political will. The reforms assumed that the political system was able and willing to face the hard choices which the reforms were intended to highlight. But politicians are always eager to avoid forcing awkward political issues to a head. While successive Ghanaian governments have proclaimed their commitment to shifting resources into rural and preventive health services, when they have been faced with scarce resources, a fragile economy, and a vocal urban minority this change has not in fact been effected. A more sophisticated budgetary system would only have underlined this discrepancy between rhetoric and practice.

This section has dealt specifically with the Ghanaian experience. A similar scenario could, however, apply in many other developing countries. It is easy but ultimately unconstructive to analyse exhaustively the reasons for the failure of these reforms. Rather it is important to learn from such negative experiences. Thus the next section assumes that steps towards more 'rational' budgeting are desirable, but are unlikely to succeed unless certain criteria are fulfilled.

Possibilities for budgetary reform

It may be thought that a health economist's idea of bliss would be a Ministry of Health which followed the principles of a PPBS-type system whereby all expenditures were monitored on the basis of their contribution to the fulfilment of desired objectives, and unsatisfactory expenditures were curtailed. In reality, this is beyond the scope of most institutions, and attempts to introduce such a system merely result in counterproductive upheavals. If the desirable link between planning and budgeting is to be forged, however, the tradition of categorizing budgets solely according to input type must be changed. The following criteria represent a compromise between stultification and untenable complex reform. The message underlying all these criteria is 'don't try to change everything at once'.

Accept mixed scanning. 'Mixed scanning' means that a broad programme or functional budget is used to identify areas of particular concern or priority (Caiden and Wildavsky 1974). A closer, more output-oriented look can then be taken at these particular areas. Skilled staff concentrate on a particular topic. In Ghana, for example, Primary Health Care (PHC) was generally accepted as a priority area. In practice, implementation was rather unsuccessful. One of the main reasons for this was that plans bore no relationship to resource availability. Activities were started with enthusiasm, but they faltered and withered because of a belated realization that resources were inadequate for the scale of activities.

If skilled staff could focus their efforts on PHC issues, they could provide answers to the crucial questions of:

- How much can we realistically expect to achieve with our present resources? and
- How many more resources do we need to achieve our stated targets?

These answers would establish the basic link between resources and objectives. If the Ministry of Health focused on PHC in this way, and resource requirements were realistically estimated (instead of estimated through the practice of incrementalism), it would become clear that either the rate of implementation would need to be severely curtailed or else many more resources needed to be allocated to PHC.

Provide appropriate staff training. Changing and expanding a budgeting system has opportunity costs in terms of the use of skilled personnel. If planners, managers, and accountants are overwhelmed by the complexities of a system, they cease to work effectively. Moreover, many health workers acquire responsibility for budgets as their careers develop, without ever having had any training relevant to this duty. Economics is often described as a 'way of thinking', and programme and functional budgeting aim to provide information to encourage this thought process. But it is clearly unfair to expect personnel to produce and use budgets if they have not received any relevant training.

Ensure that budgetary power and responsibility are matched. Health managers will not have the incentive to link budgets to well-thought-out plans unless they feel that they have a reasonable chance of implementing those plans. If managers lack the necessary degree of managerial autonomy, budgets cannot mirror the economic function of prices, which is to encourage efficient behaviour. This is not to say that budgetary reform necessarily entails decentralization – as we have seen, national functional budgeting can be useful in itself. But what is certain is that people will not respond to budgetary incentives unless they have a reasonable degree of control over those budgets.

Acknowledge political realities. Rationality and politics are sometimes thought of as opposites. Indeed, as Charles Schultze pointed out in *'The politics and economics of public spending* (quoted in Caiden and Wildavsky 1974): 'The first rule of the successful political process is "don't force a specification of goals or ends".' A 'rational' budgeting system does not alter unwillingness to highlight the stark realities of resource constraints and choice, although the availability of relevant information may influence decisions. Writing about the relatively neglected 'Cinderella' services in the UK (community services; psychiatric and geriatric care; care of the mentally handicapped), Mooney (1984) stated:

. . . It would be foolhardy to suggest that without a considerable degree of political will any substantial movement in the direction of fostering these neglected services can be achieved. At the same time political will, without the appropriate information base to monitor, plan, set objectives, determine priorities, control resource use and evaluate service operations, is also unlikely to result in any great shift in priorities. Political statements on priorities need to be backed by an information structure which allows them to become a reality.

Accept throughput-oriented programme and functional budgeting. A recurring theme among reports of unsuccessful budgetary reforms is that of the difficulties inherent in output budgeting. Firstly, there is no universal acceptance in the health sector of how output should be measured. Secondly, such systems typically entail data collection and presentation requirements so excessive that they paralyse the system. In reality, it is often only possible to use throughput (i.e. intermediate or process) measures. Examples of such measures are numbers of fully immunized children, inpatient bed-days, and numbers of latrines built. It would thus seem wise to accept programme and functional budgeting, and to use their expenditure data in conjunction with throughput information. In the short term, however, even the introduction of programme budgeting can be a daunting task – indeed, a major problem with many budgetary reforms is that they have attempted to transform whole systems. The increased data needs and complex analysis required are beyond the capacity of most countries.

Functional budgeting offers a practical compromise between

traditional accounting and complicated reforms, as it is based on relatively simple amendments to existing accounting formats, yet can be used to assist in planning decisions. Small-scale functional analysis can also be used as a demonstration exercise, where wider changes are eventually intended. Because of the practical feasibility of small-scale functional budgeting and because it is potentially useful as a pilot analysis, we describe in detail in the next section an example of local functional analysis.

Functional analysis: a case-study from the Gambia

In 1985 a ward costing exercise was conducted in the Royal Victoria Hospital (RVH) in Banjul, the Gambia. The costing exercise was a one-off study, intended to provide planners with information relating to policy issues which were important at that time. Before this study, informed decision-making was well-nigh impossible, because information on costs was available only on traditional accounting lines, which classified expenditure according to the types of inputs (salaries, drugs and dressings, food, uniforms, etc.). Such information was of little use to planners, who were interested in comparing the different forms of throughput. It was impossible to tell from the hospital accounts how expensive an average paediatric case was compared with a patient on, say, the female surgical ward. It was also impossible to compare inpatient with outpatient costs.

The basic aim of this costing study was to reallocate the sums in the traditional accounting categories to the operational departments of the hospital – namely the surgical, medical, paediatric, obstetrics and gynaecology, ophthalmology, psychiatric, and private departments, and the sanatorium (all of which had both inpatient wards and outpatient clinics), plus the general, civil service, dental, and audiology outpatient clinics. These departments and clinics were called 'patient-service areas.'

There are essentially three levels of service in any hospital. These are listed below, with comments on how they can be related to patient activities.

Overhead support services. This category includes general administration (including nursing administration), transportation, the maintenance of hospital buildings, cleaning, and security. The costs of these services are difficult to allocate on a departmental basis, as they relate to the running of the hospital as a whole.

Overhead support services constituted approximately 18 per cent of total RVH expenditure. Within this category the largest input was the wages of orderlies (5.5 per cent of total expenditure). In theory these wages could have been allocated among departments if a 'time and motion'-type study of their work had been conducted. Whether or not such an exercise is worth while depends on the use to which it is intended to put the information.

Directly allocable support services. By far the largest component of this category is nursing salaries. Other services in this category are pathology, X-rays, physiotherapy, central sterile supplies, theatres, orthopaedics, uniforms, food, laundry, and the pharmacy.

Costs in this category had to be allocated to specific patient-service areas. This was done by one of two methods. The first was to use the information on actual allocations. This was possible for nurses' salaries, pathology, theatres, X-rays, uniforms, physiotherapy, the central sterile supplies unit, and orthopaedics. For example, for pathology records were used to determine the extent to which the various patient-service areas used the service. The duty rota for 1985 was used for the allocation of nurses' salaries after allowances had been added *pro rata* and amendments made for annual leave and unfilled posts. Most of the nurses worked directly in patient-service areas, but some were posted to the directly allocable support services, namely the pharmacy, central sterile supplies, and theatre services, and were allocated to patient-service areas along with the other costs of their department.

The second method was to allocate costs *pro rata*, in proportion to patient numbers. This method was used for the pharmacy, food, and laundry, because information was not available about the distribution of costs amongst the patient-service areas. The most difficult of the allocable support services to distribute amongst the various wards and clinics was the pharmacy. As drug usage had to be divided between outpatients and inpatients, it was 'guesstimated' (with admittedly more guess than estimate) that one inpatient was equivalent in terms of drug usage (and staff time) to two outpatient attendances. As drugs and dressings accounted for 18 per cent of the total RVH budget, it would be worth investigating further the ultimate destinations of drugs.

Patient-service areas. The hospital accounts included only medical staff in this category. The costs of medical time were added to the directly allocable costs to give total costs per patient-service area. The results are summarized in Table 14.3, and unit costs are calculated by relating information on expenditure to information on throughput. Before the functional analysis was conducted, only average hospital-wide unit costs were known. These were clearly misleading, since costs per inpatient day were found by this study to vary between departments by a factor of 4.5, and costs per outpatient consultation varied between clinics by a factor

Table 14.3 *Functional analysis and unit costs for the Royal Victoria Hospital, Banjul, The Gambia*

Patient–service areas	Expenditure*	No. of inpatient days	*Dalasi* per inpatient day
Wards			
Medical	292690	16351	17.9
Obstetrics and Gynaecology	368651	13620	27.1
Ophthalmology	69373	2835	24.5
Paediatrics	397998	21271	18.7
Private	57458	1191	48.2
Psychiatric	390070	15695	24.9
Sanatorium	154427	14600	10.6
Surgical	552410	25286	21.8
Total (wards)	2283077	110849	20.6

Clinics		No. of consultations	*Dalasi* per consultation
Audiology	32176	7376	4.4
Dental	120461	22974	5.2
General	345462	120952	2.9
Civil service	32207	10468	3.1
Medical	54573	11280	4.8
Obstetrics & Gynaecology	94044	14350	6.6
Ophthalmology	88598	20851	4.2
Paediatrics	130868	37603	3.5
Surgical	44348	8000	5.5
Total (clinics)	943737	253854	3.7

* Excludes overhead support services.

of 2.3. The discussion of a variety of policy issues was aided by the existence of a functional analysis for the RVH. For example, it had already been decided to expand the RVH. Current unit costs, disaggregated to the greatest extent possible, were required in order to estimate future operating costs. Since not all departments were to share equally in the expansion, isolation of the costs of units scheduled for expansion was thought likely to generate a more accurate cost prediction than use of a simple average cost for the whole hospital.

Another policy issue related to outpatient costs. A suggestion had been made to separate the general outpatient service from the RVH by locating it in a new urban polyclinic to be constructed on an adjacent site. This suggestion was made in the belief that outpatient costs at the RVH were much higher than for self-referred outpatients elsewhere in the country. The correctness or otherwise of this belief could not be established without a functional analysis.

Finally, the Ministry of Health was considering a policy of cost-recovery. No rational programme of cost-recovery could be devised in the absence of basic unit cost information. In particular, there was a desire to know the cost of providing private services, in order to see if private charges covered the full costs incurred.

Functional analysis of this type, and indeed functional budgeting, does not meet the ideal requirement of economics, to consider costs and alternatives in relation to effectiveness and overall benefits. It is, however, an improvement on the information in traditional accounts, and offers an implementable opportunity of making existing practices and budgeting and accounting documents a planning tool.

Conclusions

The commonest – and generally the only – financial analysis conducted in most ministries and organizations is the accounts. If scarce resources are to be used effectively, accounts must be transformed into planning tools. We have discussed the inadequacies of traditional accounting, and outlined the complex nature of most suggested reforms and the impossibility of their implementation. It is sobering to note that many of the conclusions about budgetary reform drawn from experience in Ghana are similar to those reached by Waterston, writing in 1965. Waterston attributed the failure of many budgetary reforms to the scarcity of skilled personnel, which led to the ineffective functioning of the public administration, the operating organizations, and the central budget office. He concluded that budgetary reform may even be counterproductive, because 'it may have been carried out at a high opportunity cost by absorbing the time of scarce technicians who may have been put to better use elsewhere. It may also have had the effect of obscuring inability or unwillingness to undertake needed reforms or other action elsewhere.'

Not much seems to have been learnt in the subsequent two decades. There is a need for action-oriented research to develop systems that are likely to be implementable in the difficult circumstances facing most Ministries of Health in the developing world.

References

Caiden, N. S. and Wildavsky, S. (1974). *Planning and budgeting in poor countries*. Transaction Books, New Brunswick and London.

Culyer, A. J. (1980). *The political economy of social policy*. Martin Robertson, Oxford.

Glennerster, H. (1984). Programme budgets and social planning. In *The fields and methods of social planning*. (ed. J. Midgley and D. Piachaud), pp. 107–28. Heinemann Educational Books, London.

Mach, E. P. and Abel-Smith, B. (1983). *Planning the finances of the health sector. A manual for developing countries*. WHO, Geneva.

Ministry of Health and Social Welfare, Fiji (1986). *Annual report for the year 1984*, Parliamentary Paper No. 1 of 1986. Parliament of Fiji, Suva.

Mooney, G. (1984). Programme budgeting: an aid to planning and priority setting in health care. *Effective Health Care*, 2(2), 65–8.

National Health Planning Unit, Ministry of Health, Ghana (1979). *Financial planning and budgeting for the delivery of health services*. The Ministry, Accra.

Waterston, A. (1965). *Development planning: lessons of experience*. Johns Hopkins University Press, Baltimore.

Authors' note

The authors wish to acknowledge the support of Mark Wheeler with the Gambia study.

Index

capital, malaria/malaria control and its
impact on supply of 20
capital stock, hospital, adjustment 254
catchment areas
in the Philippines, per hospital
95–6, 97
in Rwanda 143–52
see also distance
CCCD 141–2, 161–2
Cebu, Metropolitan, infant delivery
in 170–91
charges, *see* fees
charitable sources/sector
in Dominican Republic, for hospital
funding 126, 129
in the Philippines 87
chemotherapy, *see* pharmaceuticals
*and specific (types of)
pathogens/diseases/drugs*
childbirth, *see* delivery
children
diarrhoeal disease control, *see*
diarrhoeal disease
health services for mother and
(MCH), productivity of
manpower and supplies in, in
Java 314, 318, 319, 322, 323,
324, 325, 326, 327, 331
see also infant
Chitwan Valley, malaria control
and the 19
chloroquine-resistant malaria 57–8
cholera diarrhoeas
severity/seriousness and other
qualitative factors 240
vaccination in prevention of 217–19,
226–7, 232, 233
clinics (for outpatients)
costs, in the Gambia 348, 349
public and private, in the
Philippines 99, 100, 106
see also outpatients; primary
health care
Colombia, drug imports and prices 296
Combatting Childhood Communicable
Disease (CCCD), Programme
for 141–2, 161–2
community-based activities in
diarrhoeal disease control 239
community financing schemes for
drugs 307–8
compliance with drugs, patient
273–4, 304
consultation
in Côte d'Ivoire, numbers of 208–10

fees for
in Dominican Republic 126
in Rwanda 142, 162–3
co-operatives providing medical
services in Peru 70
corruption, pharmaceuticals and 298
cost(s)
of diarrhoeal disease control,
calculation 217–33
hospital
in Dominican Republic 114
in Ethiopia 11, 250–71
in the Gambia, exercise in
estimation of 346–9
models of 251–61
and prices (user fees), relating
136, 269
sharing, forms of 114
of hospital fee collection in
Dominican Republic 123
of infant delivery 269
output data linked to, *see* output
personnel, per client/patient
contacts, in Java 322, 323
of services in general (public and
private) in the Philippines
96–100
in Rwanda 144–50
supply, in public health services in
Java 321, 330
see also expenditure; fees;
financing
cost-benefit 336
cost-effectiveness
diarrhoeal disease control 11,
214–49
pharmaceuticals (in general) 292–4
schistosomiasis chemotherapy
11, 272–87
cost-minimization analysis 252–3
Côte d'Ivoire, demand for health care
in, quantity rationing and 10,
193–213
cotrimoxazole for urinary tract
infections, cost-effectiveness
293
credibility, programme budgeting and
lack of 341–2
credit(s)
accumulated by hospitals in
Dominican Republic 126
tied supplier, with drugs 309–10
crop production (farming/land
cultivation/agriculture) in Nepal
33, 36–42, 43–9 *passim*, 54, 57

Rapti Valley, malaria in 24
  control of 19
referral systems
  in the Philippines 87
  poorly functioning 5
rehydration therapy in diarrhoeal
  disease, oral 214–16, 238
resource(s)
  in Dominican Republic, of
    hospital/medical facilities
    124–131
  inputs, *see* inputs
  see also financing
resource-allocation
  macro 3–4, 332
    poor decisions on, factors
    compounding 4–6
  socially optimal 7
responsibility, budgetary
  with budgetary power, matching
    344–5
  without budgetary power 342
revenues
  health centre, in Rwanda 146
  hospital fee, in Dominican Republic
    125, 126, 127, 128, 130, 131–3,
    136, 137
  discretionary 133
  use/allocation 131–3
  see also income
rice (paddy) production in Nepal
  38, 40–1
rifampicin for tuberculosis, cost-
  effectiveness 293
risk factors for diarrhoeal disease,
  prevalence 234–5
road construction in Nepal 35
rotavirus diarrhoeas
  severity/seriousness and other
    qualitative factors 240
  vaccination in prevention of 226–7,
    232, 233, 241
Royal Victoria Hospital (Banjul,
  the Gambia), ward costing
  exercise 346–9
rural areas
  in Côte d'Ivoire, demand for health
    care 196–212
  in Java (Indonesia), public health
    services 313–34
    manpower and expendable
    supplies in, efficiency of 314–34
    organization 318–19
  in the Philippines, urban compared
    with 98–100

infant delivery in 171–91 *passim*
rural health units (RHUs) in the
  Philippines 83, 106, 108
Rwanda, financing of health care
  at government health centres
  10, 140–64
Rwankuba health centre in Rwanda
  144–66 *passim*

scale of intervention in diarrhoeal
  disease control 236–7
schistosomiasis 11, 272–87
  chemotherapy 11, 272–87
    cost-effectiveness 11, 272–87
    mass group 275, 277–8, 279–86
    passim
    mass population 274, 275–6,
    279–86 *passim*
    screened group 275, 278,
    279–86 *passim*
    screened population 274–5, 277,
    279–86 *passim*
  prevalence rate 285–6
  screening test 285–6
school children
  diarrhoeal disease control aimed at
    education of 239
  as diarrhoeal disease source 225
screening tests for schistosomiasis
  285–6
  population receiving, chemotherapy
    274–5, 277, 279–86 *passim*
  selected groups receiving,
    chemotherapy 275, 278,
    279–86 *passim*
season in the Philippines, infant
  delivery related to 174, 184
Secretariat for Public Health and
  Social Welfare (Dominican
  Republic) 117
self-medication 303
services, health care, *see* health
  care services
settlement in Nepal 33, 34, 46,
  50–1, 57
Singapore, health system comparisons
  with other ASEAN countries
  and Japan and USA 82–3, 84
soap, diarrhoeal disease control and
  availability of 225–6
socially optimal resource-allocation 7
spending, *see* expenditure
spouses, infant delivery in the
  Philippines and 178